The Open University Press, Celtic Court, 22 Ballmore, Buckingham, MK18 1XW.

First published as *Caring for Health: Dilemmas and Prospects,* 1985. This completely revised edition first published 1993.

A catalogue record of the book is available from the British Library.

Library of Congress Cataloging-in-Publication Data

Dilemmas in health care/edited by Basiro Davey and Jennie Popay.—
    Rev. ed.
    p. cm. — (Health and disease series; book 7)
    Rev. and updated ed. of: Caring for health, 1985.
    Includes bibliographical references and index.
    ISBN 0–335–19119–3
1. Medical care—Great Britain. 2. Medical policy—Great Britain.
I. Davey, Basiro. II. Popay, Jennie. III. Caring for health. IV. Series.
RA395.G6D55 1993
362. 1′0941—dc20   92–44760
CIP

Edited, designed and typeset by the Open University.

Printed in the United Kingdom by Page Bros, Norwich.

ISBN 0 335 19119 3

This text forms part of an Open University Second Level Course. If you would like a copy of *Studying with the Open University,* please write to the Central Enquiry Service, PO Box 200, The Open University, Walton Hall, Milton Keynes, MK7 2YZ.

2.1

6384C/u205b7i2.1

Acknowledgements

Grateful acknowledgement is made to the following sources for permission to reproduce material in this book:

Figures

Figure 2.1 Haywood, S. (1979) Team management in the NHS: what is it all about? *Health and Social Service Journal*, 5 October 1979, Macmillan Magazines; *Figure 3.4* DHSS (1988) *Review of the Resource Allocation Working Party Formula: Final Report by the NHS Management Board*, reproduced with the permission of the Controller of Her Majesty's Stationery Office; *Figure 5.1* Clinical Accountability, Service Planning and Evaluation (1988) *CASPE patient satisfaction questionnaire*, King's Fund Centre, by permission of CASPE; *Figure 5.2* Green, J. (1988) On the receiving end, *Health Service Journal*, 4 August 1988, Macmillan Magazines; *Figure 7.1* Courtesy of Pharmaceutical Proteins; *Figure 7.2* Department of Health (1991) *Research for Health: A Research and Development Strategy for the NHS*, reproduced with the permission of the Controller of Her Majesty's Stationery Office; *Figure 7.6* Camera Press; *Figures 7.7, 7.8* Siemens plc; *Figure 8.1* Audit Commission (1986) *Making A Reality of Community Care*, reproduced with the permission of the Controller of Her Majesty's Stationery Office; *Figures 9.1, 9.2* Royal College of Physicians (1991), *A Report of a Working Party of the Royal College of Physicians*; *Figure 9.3* Cancer Research Campaign (1992) *Lung Cancer and Smoking, Factsheet 11.1*, CRC; *Figures 9.4, 9.5* Cancer Research Campaign (1991) *Breast Cancer, Factsheet 6.2*, CRC; *Figure 9.6* adapted from British Medical Association (1990) *The BMA Guide To Living With Risk*, Penguin Books Ltd; *Figure 10.3* Davey Smith, G. and Marmot, M. (1991) (Suppl) Trends in Mortality in Britain, *Annals of Nutrition and Metabolism*; *Figure 10.6* Chaitman, B. R. (1981) Effect of coronary bypass surgery on survival patterns, *American Journal of Cardiology*, **48**, Cahners Publication Company; *Figure 10.8* Doll, R. and Peto, R. (1976) Mortality in relation to smoking: 20 years' observation on male British doctors, *British Medical Journal*, **2**, British Medical Association; *Figure 10.9* Ball, K. P. (1979) *The Heart Patient 1, Epidemiology*, Update Publications; *Figure 10.10* MRC Working Party (1992) Medical Research Council trial of treatment of hypertension in older adults, *British Medical Journal*, **304**, British Medical Association; *Figure 10.12* Brisson, G. (1982) *Lipids In Human Nutrition*, MTP Press, Toronto; *Figures 10.13, 10.14* Isles, C. G. *et al.* (1992) Relation between coronary risk and coronary mortality in women of the Renfrew and Paisley survey, compared with men, *The Lancet*, **339**, The Lancet Ltd; *Figure 11.1* Marsh, C. (1988) *Exploring Data*, Polity Press; *Figure 11.2* Luxembourg Income Study, Working Paper 26, World Bank, World Tables, 1990; *Figure 11.3* Blaxter, M. (1990) *Health and Lifestyle*, Routledge.

Tables

Table 2.1 Leathard, A. (1990) Health Care Provision: Past, Present and Future, Chapman and Hall; *Table 4.1* Adler, W. *et al.* (1978) Randomised controlled trial of early discharge for inguinal hernia and varicose veins, *Journal of Epidemiology and Community Health*, **32**, BMJ Specialist Journals; *Table 4.2* Kane, R. L. *et al.* (1984) A randomised controlled trial of hospice care, *The Lancet*, **(i)**, The Lancet Ltd; *Table 4.3* Reprinted from, by permission of the publisher, *Canadian Medical Association Journal*, **115** (1976); *Table 4.4* Reprinted from *Social Science and Medicine*, **14a**(6), Pendleton, D. and Bochner, S. The communication of medical information, p. 671, copyright 1980, with kind permission from Pergamon Press Ltd, Headington Hill Hall, Oxford OX3 0BW, UK; *Table 4.5* Buck, N., Devlin, B. and Lunn, J. N. (1987) *Report of a Confidential Enquiry into Peri-Operative Deaths*, Nuffield Provincial Hospitals Trust; *Table 4.6* Department of Health (1990) *Health Service Indicators Package 1989–90*, reproduced with the permission of the Controller of Her Majesty's Stationery Office; *Table 5.1* Department of Health (1991) *Return of Written Complaints By Or On Behalf Of Patients: England 1990/91*, reproduced with the permission of the Controller of Her Majesty's Stationery Office; *Table 6.2* Department of Health (1991) *Health and Personal Social Services Statistics for England*, reproduced with the permission of the Controller of Her Majesty's Stationery Office; *Table 7.1* Kirchberger, S. (1991) *The Diffusion of Two Technologies for Renal Stone Treatment Across Europe*, King's Fund Centre; *Table 7.2* adapted from OECD (1990) *Health Care Systems in Transition: The Search for Efficiency*, OECD Social Policy Studies No 7, OECD; *Table 7.3* adapted from Burstall, M. L. (1990) *1992 and the Regulation of the Pharmaceutical Industry, IEA Health Series No. 9*, Institute of Economic Affairs; *Table 7.4* Royal Commission on the NHS (1978) *Patients' Attitudes To The Hospital Service, Research Paper No. 5*, reproduced with the permission of the Controller of Her Majesty's Stationery Office; *Table 9.1* Royal College of Physicians (1991) *Preventive Medicine: A Report of a Working Party of the Royal College of Physicians*; *Table 9.2* Cohen, D. and Henderson, J. (1983) A minister for prevention: an initiative in health policy, *HERU Discussion Paper 2/83*, University of Aberdeen; *Table 9.4* adapted from Daly, E. *et al.* (1993) Hormone replacement therapy in a risk-benefit perspective, paper delivered at the 7th International Congress on the Menopause, Stockholm, June 1993; *Table 10.1* Davey Smith, G. and Pekkannen, J. (1992) Should there be a moratorium on the use of cholesterol lowering drugs?, *British Medical Journal*, **304**, British Medical Association; *Table 10.2* Phillips, A. N. *et al.* (1988) Parental death from heart disease and the risk of heart attack, *European Heart Journal*, **9**, The European Society of Cardiology, Academic Press Ltd; *Table 10.4* Blane, D., Davey-Smith, G. and Bartley, M. (1990) Social class differences in years of potential life lost, size, trends and principal causes, *British Medical Journal*, **301**, British Medical Association; *Table 11.2* Oppenheim, C. (1990) *Poverty: The Facts*, Child Poverty Action Group.

Text/boxes

p. 6 Hall, C. (1992), Clot-busting drugs 'cut heart deaths', *The Independent*, 3 September 1992; *Box 2.1* Drucker, P. F. (1979) *Management*, Butterworth-Heinemann Limited; *Box 2.2* Butler, P. (1992) Academics urge trust managers to take on doctors over performance, *Health Service Journal*, 26 June 1992, Macmillan Magazines; *Box 4.1* Johns, C. (1992) Developing clinical standards, in Vaughan, B. and Robinson, K. (eds) *Knowledge for Nursing Practice*, Butterworth-Heinemann; *Box 4.2* Mahoney, F. I. and Barthel, D. W. (1965) Functional Evaluation: The Barthel Index, *Maryland State Medical Journal*; **14**(2), pp. 61–5; *Box 4.3* Hunt, S., McEwan, J. and McKenna, S. (1980) *The Nottingham Health Profile*, © the authors; *Box 4.4* Reprinted from *Social Science and Medicine*, **14a**(6), Pendleton, D. and Bochner, S., The communication of medical information, p. 670, copyright 1980, with kind permisson from Pergamon Press Ltd, Headington Hill Hall, Oxford OX3 0BW, UK; *Boxes 4.5, 4.6* adapted from Boulton, M., Tuckett, D., Olson, C. and Williams, S. A. (1986), Social class and the general practice consultation, *Sociology of Health and Illness*, **8**, Basil Blackwell Ltd; *Box 5.1* Department of Health (1991), *The Patient's Charter*, reproduced with the permission of the Controller of Her Majesty's Stationery Office; *Box 7.1* McKinley, J. B. (1981) 'Promising report' to 'standard procedure': seven stages in the career of a medical innovation, *Milbank Memorial Fund Quarterly/Health and Society*, **59**, Daniel M. Fox, Milbank Memorial Fund; *Box 8.1* Green, H. (1988) *Informal Carers, OPCS Social Survey Division, Series GH5, No. 15, Supplement A*, reproduced with the permission of the Controller of Her Majesty's Stationery Office; *Box 8.2* Audit Commission (1986) *Making A Reality of Community Care*, reproduced with the permission of the Controller of Her Majesty's Stationery Office; *Box 8.3* Hunter, D. J., Judge, K. and Price, S. (1988) Community Care: Reacting to Griffiths, *King's Fund Institute Briefing No. 1*, King's Fund Institute; *Box 8.4* Wistow, G. and Hardy, B. (1991) Joint management in community care, *Journal of Management in Medicine*, **5**(4), MCB University Press Ltd; *Box 11.1* Mack, J. and Lansley, S. (1991) *Breadline Britain 1990s*, HarperCollins.

Un-numbered photographs/illustrations

p. 7 Yorkshire Post Newspapers Ltd; *p. 9* King's College Hospital, London; *p. 67* The Spastics Society; *p. 75* John Smith/Profile; *p. 76* Leon Grech, The Open University; *p. 77* Leon Morris; *p. 82* BMA News Review; *p. 85* Gina Glover/Photo Co-Op; *p. 111* CORDA, the Heart Charity; *p. 124, p. 135(b)* Gina Glover/Photofusion; *p. 139* Gwynedd Mental Health Services; *p. 146* Health Education Council; *p. 149* Health Education Council and *British Medical Journal*; *p. 159(a), p. 161(a)* Advertising Archives; *p. 159(b)* Health Education Authority; *p. 161(b)* Health Education Authority, 1992, *Tobacco and the BBC*, photo 15, p. 11; *p. 167* Department of Pathology, Edinburgh University; *p. 187* Mike Abrahams/Network; *p. 189, p. 194, p. 198* Glaswegians Photo Archive/Cranhill; *p. 191* Crispin Hughes/Photo Co-op.

Contents

About this book   2

1 Universalising the best: an impossible dream?   5
Basiro Davey

2 Managing health care: balancing interests and influence   12
Stephen Harrison and Gerald Wistow

3 Rationing and choice   27
Alastair Gray

4 The evaluation of health care   43
Clive Seale

5 The consumer voice   64
Clive Seale

6 Health work: divisions in health-care labour   81
Gillian Pascall and Kate Robinson

7 Innovations in health care   103
Nicholas Mays

8 Care in the community: rhetoric or reality?   121
David Hunter

9 Disease prevention and health promotion   143
Helen Lambert and Klim McPherson

10 Coronary heart disease: a cautionary tale   165
Richard Holmes

11 Poverty, economic inequality and health   184
Chris Pond and Jennie Popay

Appendix: Table of abbreviations used in this book   200

References and further reading   201

Answers to self-assessment questions   209

Index   217

About this book

A note for the general reader

Dilemmas in Health Care considers a range of major and enduring dilemmas arising from the organisation and delivery of health care in the United Kingdom in the 1990s. The book analyses 'health care' in its widest possible sense, encompassing conventional health services, social and community services, disease prevention and health promotion initiatives and, finally, economic and fiscal policies that could have an impact on health. Throughout the book, we acknowledge the nation's reliance on lay carers as the principal mediators of health care in this (as in other) countries.

The book contains eleven chapters, written by specialist authors whose academic affiliations are given in the study comment box at the start of each chapter.

Although the topics chosen for inclusion in the book are highly varied, each author has identified the principal dilemmas facing those involved in formulating policy, or delivering or receiving health care, and has analysed the reasons underlying the difficult and incompatible choices that may have to be made. In particular, the authors address the extent to which effective health care can be reconciled with efficiency in a cost-limited health-care system, while keeping in view the aim of distributing services equitably and delivering them humanely.

Chapter 1 serves as a general introduction to the main themes of the book, and defines some essential terms and concepts. Chapters 2 to 4 focus primarily on health-care policy and the influences that are shaping the organisation of the National Health Service (NHS); these include relationships between managers and doctors and the need for rationing and evaluation. In Chapters 5 to 7 the focus shifts to the concerns of health-service users and the health-care workforce, particularly in relation to 'consumerism', professionalisation and new medical technologies. Chapters 8 to 11 move beyond the boundaries of the health service, to discuss community care, disease prevention and health promotion, coronary heart disease, and strategies to improve health by alleviating economic inequality.

Dilemmas in Health Care is the seventh in a series of eight books on the subject of health and disease. The book is designed so that it can be read on its own, like any other textbook, or studied as part of U205 Health and Disease, a second level course for Open University students. General readers do not need to make use of the study comments, learning objectives and other material inserted for OU students, although they may find these helpful. The book also contains references to a collection of articles and extracts[1] prepared in association with the OU course: it is quite possible to follow the text without reading the articles referred to, although doing so will enhance your understanding of this book's contents. The book is fully indexed and referenced and contains an annotated guide to further reading and an appendix of abbreviations.

A guide for OU students

Dilemmas in Health Care continues the analysis of the British health-care system, which began with the historical and comparative background to the present health service in *Caring for Health: History and Diversity.*[2] It also builds on skills and concepts taught in other books in the Health and Disease series.

Study comments are given in a box at the start of each chapter. These primarily direct you to other books in the course series where connections should be made, or to other course components. Major learning objectives are listed at the end of each chapter, along with self-assessment questions (SAQs) that will enable you to check that you are able to achieve those objectives. The text and the index show key terms printed in bold type, indicating the page on which a definition or explanation of that term can be found. There is also a further reading list for those who wish to pursue certain aspects of study beyond the limits of this book.

The time allowed for studying *Dilemmas in Health Care* is four weeks, or about 40–48 hours. The following table gives a more detailed breakdown to help you to pace your study. You need not follow it slavishly, but try not to let yourself fall behind. If you find a section of the work difficult, do what you can at this stage, and then return to the material when you reach the end of the book. There is a tutor-marked assignment (TMA) associated with this book; about three hours have been allowed for completing it, *in addition to* the time spent studying the material that it assesses.

[1]*Health and Disease: A Reader* (Open University Press, 1984; revised edition 1994).

[2]*Caring for Health: History and Diversity* (Open University Press, revised edition 1993).

Study guide for Book 7 (total 40–48 hours, including time for the TMA, spread over 4 weeks). Chapter 1 is the shortest in the book, and Chapters 2 to 11 are approximately the same length, but notice that there is an unusually large number of Reader articles associated with this book and you should pace your study accordingly.

A television programme 'Who calls the shots?' relates to Chapters 1 to 8 of this book and can be watched at any point during your study of those chapters.

1st week

Chapter 1	**Universalising the best: an impossible dream?**, including extracts from an Audit Commission Report (1990) in the *Reader*
Chapter 2	**Managing health care: balancing interests and influence**, including audiotape 'Dilemmas in hospital management'
Chapter 3	**Rationing and choice**, including *Reader* article by Williams (1993)

2nd week

Chapter 4	**The evaluation of health care**, including *Reader* articles by Cochrane (1971) and extracts from a correspondence entitled 'Ethical dilemmas in evaluation' (1980–2)
Chapter 5	**The consumer voice**, including *Reader* article by Winkler (1993)
Chapter 6	**Health work: divisions in health-care labour**, including *Reader* articles by Paterson (1981) and extracts from the House of Commons Health Committee Report (the 'Winterton Report') (1991–2)

3rd week

Chapter 7	**Innovations in health care**, including revision of extracts from a report by the Audit Commission (1990) in the *Reader*
Chapter 8	**Community care: rhetoric or reality?**
Chapter 9	**Disease prevention and health promotion**, including *Reader* articles by Breslow (1990) and La Vecchia *et al.* (1991)

4th week

Chapter 10	**Coronary heart disease: a cautionary tale**
Chapter 11	**Poverty, economic inequality and health**
TMA completion	

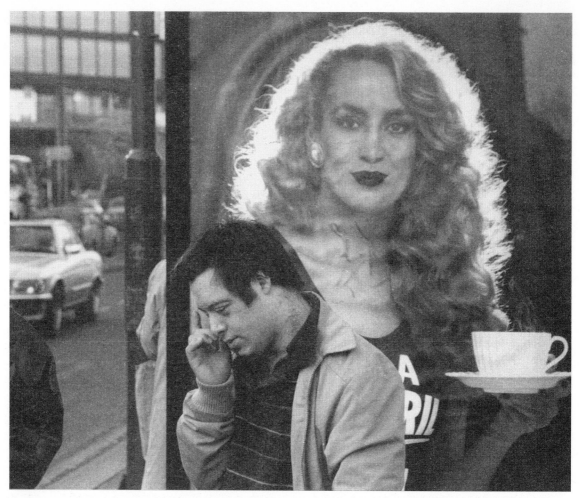

Dilemmas abound in the British health-care system in the 1990s. Prominent among them is the pursuit of appropriate strategies to meet the complex health needs of the population against a backdrop of resource constraints. How are humane priorities to be decided? What is the desirable balance between basic research, community care and support, high technology medicine and policies to reduce poverty and economic inequality? And how much of the nation's wealth should be spent on health?

Frontispiece: *a young man, described as 'mentally handicapped' in offical jargon, waits for a bus in a city street (Photo: Mike Levers). Cover background: an electron micrograph of influenza virus particles (Photo: Heather Davies). Cover middleground: elderly people pass the time in local-authority residential care (Photo: Mike Levers). Cover foreground: an anaesthetist using advanced medical technology in the operating theatre at Northampton General Hospital. (Photo: Mike Levers).*

1 Universalising the best: an impossible dream?

This book has been written with two assumptions about the essential background knowledge that readers bring with them: first, we assume a general understanding of how the structure and funding of the National Health Service (NHS) in the United Kingdom evolved from the patchwork provision of health services that it replaced in July 1948; second, we assume a general knowledge of the main policy changes in the organisation of the NHS from 1989 to 1992, which began with the Government White Paper 'Working for Patients'. This information may be found most readily in Caring for Health: History and Diversity, particularly Chapters 6, 7 and 9.[1] A television programme ,'Who calls the shots?', is relevant to almost every chapter in this book and may be watched at any convenient time.

During your study of Chapter 1, you will be asked to read an article in the Reader,[2] entitled A Short Cut to Better Services: Day Surgery in England and Wales, published by the Audit Commission (1990).

This chapter was written by Basiro Davey, Lecturer in Health Studies in the Biology Department of The Open University.

[1]Caring for Health: History and Diversity (Open University Press, revised edition 1993).

[2]Health and Disease: A Reader (Open University Press, revised edition 1994).

Introduction

This book is about dilemmas in health care in the United Kingdom in the 1990s. It is concerned particularly—but not exclusively—with dilemmas that are wrapped up in the organisation and delivery of formal health care by the NHS. Private health care is barely mentioned. We also consider dilemmas associated with the prevention of disease and the promotion of health, which extend well beyond the remit of formal health services.

A number of common threads run through the book and it is essential that you start out with a map of the territory, before plunging into a detailed analysis of the dilemmas in contemporary British health care that we have chosen to include. The purpose of this opening chapter is to give you a framework into which each of the following chapters will fit and, in the process, introduce some key terms that will occur many times in the book. At the end of this chapter, we very briefly describe the contents of Chapters 2 to 12.

The title of this chapter reflects the primary aims of the book: to examine the seemingly irreconcilable constraints on achieving Aneurin Bevan's vision of the NHS as 'universalising the best', and to consider whether this is an impossible dream *even* if we use a wider definition of formal health care to include social services and government policies that affect the nation's health. We begin by considering what 'universalising the best' would entail.

Effectiveness, humanity, equity and efficiency

How can 'the best' be evaluated? Four criteria are commonly identified as the most useful yardsticks against which health care can be measured.

If health care is to be the best available, then it must demonstrate its **effectiveness** at curing, or alleviating, or preventing illness and disability. This implies some means of *evaluating* the outcome of health care which takes into account quality as well as the quantity of life thereafter. An intervention might be judged effective in scientific tests of outcome, yet still fall short of the best in the judgement of the person who receives it, for example because treatment was too painful or prolonged, involved unacceptable surgery or removal from familiar surroundings. In other words, the health care was lacking in **humanity**; it failed to take account of personal needs and preferences. The 'best' health-care system should also offer humane working conditions to the people it employs (around a million worked in the NHS in the early 1990s).

'Universalising' effective and humane health care requires delivery of services according to the principle of **equity**; that is to say health care must be delivered according to each person's *need* for it, without discrimination on grounds of the means to pay or the age, sex, social class, place of residence, ethnic status or any other socio-demographic characteristic of the recipient.

    ☐ Suppose that true equity in the delivery of health care was somehow achieved. What effect would you expect this to have on the distribution of illness and disability in the population?

    ■ The health experience of individuals from different socio-demographic groups should become more similar, reducing the gradients of inequality in health that persist today. The gradients could not be expected to be abolished altogether because health care is not always effective and *alone* is not enough to ensure health.

Note that equity is not the same as *equality,* which implies equal *share* of health care to all *regardless* of need, and which therefore may produce *unequal* health outcomes. True equity seems an impossible dream; it could only be achieved in a health-care system that has the human and financial resources to meet all needs. And, even in this ideal world, some might argue that devoting these resources to health care regardless of *cost* would be wasteful since the resources might be better spent on some other human activity—the arts perhaps, or defence, or education. This raises the question of **efficiency** in health-care delivery, which means obtaining the maximum output for any given level of resources—often referred to as the most *cost-effective* use of resources. The more that resources are limited, the greater becomes the need to evaluate their efficient use.

These four goals of health-care systems—effectiveness, humanity, equity and efficiency—are the pillars on which this book rests. The tensions between them form the basis for several of the key dilemmas we analyse in later chapters.

Dilemmas in health care

Reconciling competing demands

We deliberately used the term **dilemma** in the title of this book, rather than problem or issue, because it means 'being forced to choose between less than ideal, even unpleasant, alternatives'. If you reflect for a moment on the laudable aim of universalising the best health care, you will see that dilemmas are an inevitable consequence of trying to resolve the often competing demands of effectiveness, humanity, equity and efficiency. Consider the following news report of a drug intervention trial in Scotland:

> Deaths from heart attacks could be halved in rural areas if family doctors carried 'clot-busting' drugs and gave them to patients at home immediately they had made the diagnosis... Professor John Rawles, of the University of Aberdeen told the [14th Congress of the European Society of Cardiology in Barcelona] that rural GPs should carry the drugs in any area that was more than 30 minutes from the nearest hospital. He also warned that in some urban areas lives could be saved even though patients lived closer to hospitals. 'In central inner cities having got to hospital patients can sit in the accident and emergency department for an hour before being seen,' he said. Professor Douglas Chamberlain, president of the British Cardiac Society, said 'These are very significant results and highlight the value of giving clot-busting drugs quickly. It is a very exciting study.' But he warned GPs about the pitfalls of the drugs, which can cause brain haemorrhages in one in 200 patients. (Hall, 1992, *Independent,* 3 September, p. 5)

    ☐ Suggest ways in which this news report reveals dilemmas in reconciling the competing demands of effectiveness, humanity, equity and efficiency in health-care provision.

    ■ Rapid use of the drugs is judged to be *effective* in reducing mortality after a heart attack, and you might argue that this is a *humane* intervention since most patients would wish to live longer. But this might not be true for *all* patients and the benefits would be offset for a minority of patients by the danger of a brain haemorrhage. There is thus a dilemma in reconciling effectiveness with humanity each time the GP is called out. If GPs carried these drugs routinely, *equity* of treatment would improve for patients in rural areas, and for those waiting in busy casualty departments in towns, but we cannot evaluate from the report whether supplying these drugs to all GPs would be an *efficient* use of resources. Some other intervention might be better 'value for money'. The goals of improving equity and efficiency may pull against one another and the dilemma is in deciding which should be given priority.

Notice that the dilemmas inherent in this situation were *created* by an innovation in *medical technology* (new clot-busting drugs) confirmed by scientific evaluation of the outcome of drug treatment, compared with the therapy available previously. If adopted for routine use, the drug will also create innovations in *medical practice* (doctors will do things differently), and because mortality is reduced there are also *resource implications* in terms of provision of hospital beds and staffing for patients who would otherwise have died. Unless additional beds are created to meet this demand, other users of those beds may have to wait longer. This example should alert you to the need for caution when reading triumphal reports of 'breakthroughs' in medical science—what is good news for one group of health-service users or workers is frequently bad news for someone else. Remember it is in the nature of a dilemma that even the best compromise available between conflicting alternatives leaves someone worse off than before.[3]

Who decides who gets what?

Situations such as the one reported above are commonplace in health care and may be characterised as dilemmas about 'Who gets what?' This leads to other questions addressed in this book: Who *decides* who gets what? Are their decisions *rational*, in the sense of being informed by systematic evaluation of the pros and cons of conflicting alternatives? Are the decision-makers able to decide the merits of each case *dispassionately*, or are they influenced by ideological or political imperatives, pressure from service-users, the media and the workforce, innovations in health-care technology, and advancing biomedical knowledge?

At the top of the hierarchy of decision-making, the ultimate dilemma is faced by government Ministers. They must decide how much of the nation's wealth should be allocated to the NHS, how much to social services, or

[3]This is amply illustrated in a television programme for Open University students entitled 'Who calls the shots?', in which the radical reorganisation of services for acutely sick children in part of Buckinghamshire is examined.

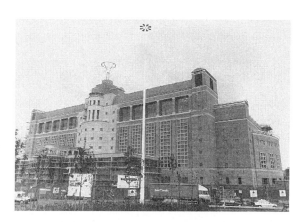

Quarry House, the new headquarters of the NHS Management Executive in Leeds (known locally as 'Gotham City'), which were opened in 1993. (Source: Yorkshire Post Newspapers Ltd*)*

income support, and how much to other sectors. They can also influence the scope of private health care, for example by giving financial incentives such as tax concessions. The Secretary of State for Health and the Ministers and officials in the Department of Health (DH) bear the responsibility for directing national policies affecting the nation's health and allocating resources to different areas of the health sector.

Next come the managers in the NHS Management Executive, under direction from the DH, who decide how the resources available to the NHS should be divided up between (say) acute hospital medicine, or community care, or health education programmes. Closer to the users of health services come managers in the health authorities and health boards of the United Kingdom, who take policy decisions about the nature and extent of the health services required by their resident populations, and—since the reforms of the early 1990s—decide which provider units to purchase those services from (the so-called *purchaser–provider split* in the internal market in health care).

Together, the Department of Health, the NHS Management Executive and the new purchasing authorities form the **strategic level** of health-care management; that is, the level at which decisions are taken about the overall national and regional strategy for resource allocation and the organisation and delivery of health services.

☐ Can you suggest examples from the early 1990s of a major strategic policy decision affecting resource allocation to, or organisation and management of, health services, in addition to the creation of the internal market?[4]

■ You may have thought of the following:

1   The decision to allow opting-out of health-authority control of a range of provider units such as hospitals, community and mental health services, to become self-governing NHS Trusts, able to negotiate contracts to provide specific services for the residents of *any* purchasing authority, set their own staffing levels and determine spending priorities within the Trust.

2   The decision to allow GPs to manage their own budgets received directly from the Regional Health Authority (RHA) to provide health care for their patients and purchase specialist care on their behalf from hospitals and other providers such as community and mental health services.

3   The decision by the DH to allocate responsibility for community care to local authorities from 1993 and to provide a certain level of funding in support of those services.

Lower down the hierarchy of decision-making in health care is the **operational level** of management, seen at work in individual provider units—for example, a day-care centre for adults with mental health problems, or a health centre housing a group of GPs, or a long-stay geriatric hospital. Unit managers face daily dilemmas about how best to keep their unit operating efficiently to meet the needs of service-users and the workforce as effectively, humanely and equitably as possible.

At the 'coalface', in wards and consulting rooms and in people's own homes, the **clinical level** of health-care management is exercised primarily by doctors, but increasingly by nurses and other health-care professionals, who decide what interventions are appropriate for their clients, within constraints imposed upon them from higher up the line of management. As you will see later in this book, the clinical freedom of doctors to treat as they see fit often conflicts with the increasing pressure from strategic and operational levels to contain health-care costs.

[4]See *Caring for Health : History and Diversity* (revised edition 1993), Chapter 7, and the article 'Britain's health-care experiment' by Patricia Day and Rudolf Klein in *Health and Disease: A Reader* (revised edition 1994).

The case study that follows serves to illustrate many of the dilemmas that arise as a result of the need to reconcile competing demands between and within the strategic, operational and clinical levels of decision-making.

Day surgery—a case study

This case study is based on a substantial extract from a report published by the Audit Commission in 1990, entitled *A Short Cut to Better Services: Day Surgery in England and Wales*.[5] Before reading it, briefly consider the purpose of the Audit Commission. It was originally set up as an independent body by the Local Government Finance Act 1982 to promote the efficient use of resources allocated to the public services, while helping them to maintain effective standards. Its role was extended to the NHS by the NHS and Community Care Act 1990 and among other activities it took over responsibility for the external audit of health authorities and family practitioner services.

The Audit Commission is staffed by experts in the public services, including the health service, who work in small teams over very short time-scales to produce up-to-date and highly influential reports, each focused on a particular aspect of service organisation and delivery which has resource implications. The primary concern in these reports is with economy, efficiency and effectiveness in the use of resources (*economy* is taken to mean using the least volume of resources). After publication, the reports are used to implement 'good practice audits' by the Commission's local auditors.

The extract you are about to read is taken from the first Audit Commission report published on the NHS (two more reports on community care are discussed in Chapter 8). Read it now and then answer the following questions. Several of the later chapters in this book will also refer to this report.

☐ Identify recommendations in the report that would lead to changes in (a) the strategic, (b) the operational, and (c) the clinical levels of management.

■ You may have thought of the following:

(a)   The primary concern of the Audit Commission's study is 'the scope for more day surgery' in the NHS. Expanding both the volume of day surgery and the types of surgical procedures that are routinely conducted as 'day cases' is a *strategic* change in health-care management.

[5]See *Health and Disease: A Reader* (revised edition 1994).

(b) In order to effect this change in strategy, various *operational* changes are recommended. For example, managers are encouraged to estimate the potential for more day surgery in their units and provide adequate facilities with appropriately trained staff. This will entail dedicating a theatre and a recovery ward to day surgery, and developing operational policies to cover such things as admissions procedures and allocation of 'beds' to consultants.

(c) *Clinical* management of patients would also have to change if the volume of day surgery is to increase. The report notes that a significant proportion of surgeons are resistant to performing certain surgical procedures as day cases.

When this report was written, a substantial volume of **elective surgery** (i.e. non-emergency procedures, including minor operations suitable for day-case admission) was being performed outside the NHS, in the private health-care sector. To some degree this resulted from the long waiting times faced by patients in some parts of the country for scarce in-patient beds for elective surgery. An increase in NHS day surgery could be expected to reduce the volume of minor surgery performed privately, as the report points out, and this has implications for the equity of health-care provision.

☐ The report summarises a considerable number of benefits of day surgery. Can you list some of them? As you do so, ask yourself '*who* benefits?' in each case.

■ Benefits identified by the authors fall into three groups:

1 Benefits to patients, e.g. quicker treatment, less likelihood of cancellation, less time spent away from home, and better care in a specialist setting.

2 Benefits in terms of reduced health-service costs, principally by savings in the 'hotel' costs of keeping patients in hospital overnight. (Indirectly this should benefit patients and staff as savings are reallocated to other parts of the hospital service.)

3 Benefits in terms of nurse recruitment and retention; the authors presume that the regular hours, no weekend duties and less stressful conditions in a day surgery unit would be attractive to nurses.

☐ Three groups with rather differing interests in health care can be identified: the managers, the doctors and other health-care workers, and the service-users. Which of these groups do you consider this report most strongly attempts to influence, and which group is least considered?

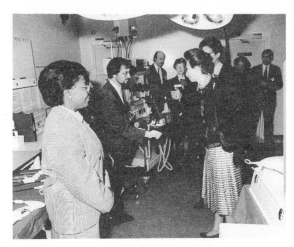

The shift towards day surgery in the NHS has been actively promoted in the 1990s. Considerable publicity surrounded the official opening by the Princess Royal of the largest day surgery unit in Europe in October 1992, at King's College Hospital in London. It cost £8 million and can cope with 40 operations per day. (Source: King's College Hospital, London)

■ The report is aimed primarily at managers; doctors and nurses are discussed mainly in terms of the operational problems that managers have to overcome, by changing surgeons' attitudes and helping to recruit more nurses; patients are the least considered—even though the benefits of day surgery to patients are clearly *invoked* (see above) and patients are *assumed* to prefer this form of treatment, they were not actually asked as part of this study. (Research into patient satisfaction and attitudes to day surgery was being carried out on behalf of the Commission, but was not completed when the report was published in 1990.)

This example illustrates a more general situation: service-users generally have the smallest voices in resolving dilemmas about 'who gets what' and where priorities should lie when effectiveness, humanity, equity and efficiency are in conflict. Historically, the health-service agenda has been set principally by *doctors* at the clinical level of management. Their decisions have tended to determine local operational policy. The Audit Commission reports are part of a wide-ranging strategy by central government to enhance the power of health-service *managers* at the operational level and enable them to increase the efficiency of provider units, even if this opposes the traditional clinical freedom of doctors. The balance of power in health-service decision-making is a recurring theme in the remaining chapters in this book.

Introduction to Chapters 2 to 11

Each of Chapters 2 to 11 of this book takes a particular topic of interest in British health care in the 1990s, and examines it from the viewpoint of the dilemmas it raises for those involved in getting the best compromise between effectiveness, humanity, equity and efficiency. We have had to leave out a great many important issues for lack of space, but those that we tackle illustrate *enduring* dilemmas that we predict will remain unresolved into the next century. Many of them have been with us for much longer than the lifetime of the present NHS and are also relevant to health-care systems elsewhere. Others have been generated by recent developments, or take us beyond the ability of health care to affect health.

The book begins with dilemmas inherent in the shape and direction of health-care policy, particularly in institutional settings dedicated to health care such as hospitals and general practices (Chapters 2–4). Then the focus switches from policies generated at the top of the health-service hierarchy, to the policy dilemmas generated to some degree by those at the bottom—the service-users and the health-care workers (Chapters 5–7). The rest of the book moves beyond the boundaries of the health service into the wider community, and examines the dilemmas raised by strategies to prevent disease and promote health (Chapters 8–11). In the following brief overview of each chapter, connections with the Audit Commission report that you have just read can sometimes be made.

We begin in Chapter 2 with 'Managing health care: balancing interests and influence', which considers how the changing balance of power between the three main groups involved in health-care decision-making—managers, doctors, and service-users or their representatives such as Community Health Councils and pressure groups—has altered the dilemmas they each face. The ability of doctors to commit resources that managers have subsequently to supply creates major dilemmas for both parties in what sometimes resembles a battle between clinical freedom and cost containment.

Financial constraints on health care are the source of many intractable dilemmas, a subject to which we turn in Chapter 3, 'Rationing and choice'. Limits on health-care spending are common to all nations, but on what should we spend the money we have available and who decides the priorities? The Audit Commission report advocates day surgery as a cost-effective use of resources, but it also stresses the need to evaluate the success of policy changes. In Chapter 4, 'The evaluation of health care', we consider systematic methods of determining whether health care is an effective means of increasing health.

You might consider that the choice of *evaluation method* is straightforward, but we show that compromises must be made between the most desirable and the most practical methods, and this in turn influences the choice of *subject* for evaluation. What should we evaluate when choices are limited?

Chapter 5, 'The consumer voice', considers dilemmas created by conflicts between local preferences concerning health care and national planning priorities. Can the individual influence the health service, even in the internal market where 'consumers' have replaced patients and providers are supposed to compete for contracts to secure their custom? The focus on the individual continues in Chapter 6, 'Health work: divisions in health-care labour'. Here we examine the dilemma facing health workers of how best to maintain or achieve humane working conditions, adequate pay and status, together with effective care for patients, within a service that is strictly cash-limited and riven by boundary disputes between different occupations. In particular, we focus on the strategies adopted by nurses to break free of their traditional role as doctors' 'handmaidens' and emerge as a high-status independent profession.

Chapter 7, 'Innovations in health care', discusses the influence of business interests, research-funding bodies, service-users and the workforce on the acquisition of new medical technology, new drugs and new working practices in the health service. The profitability of innovations in health-care practice ensures that a steady stream of options are generated by suppliers (for example, the clot-busting drugs mentioned earlier), and these have to be costed and priorities decided by health-service managers under pressure from doctors and potential beneficiaries of the change. In addition, costs must be held down and savings from changes in working practices (e.g. more day surgery) must be considered.

In Chapters 8 and 9 we move out of the clinical setting and into the wider community. Chapter 8, 'Care in the community: rhetoric or reality?', considers the dilemmas inherent in the accelerating policy of community care in the 1990s. Can community care be made a more humane and effective service than the institutional care it is intended to replace, or is it a cost-cutting exercise concealed in rhetoric? Will community care in reality use resources more efficiently? Prevention of illness and disability is another option for reducing health-service costs but, as Chapter 9, 'Disease prevention and health promotion', shows, the switching of resources to further this apparently uncontentious aim creates its own set of dilemmas. The evaluation of prevention or promotion strategies is extremely difficult, so should health-care resources be committed to unproven interventions?

How much are we prepared to pay to save a life—for example by screening for cancer? Are we justified in trying to constrain individual behaviour in the interests of producing a healthier society?

Chapter 10, 'Coronary heart disease: a cautionary tale', draws together many of the dilemmas raised in previous chapters through the medium of a single case study. Coronary heart disease illustrates dilemmas arising from the uncertainty surrounding the causes of the disease, which generate heated debates about prevention versus treatment, the value of innovations in surgery and drugs, and the extent to which individual 'lifestyles' or social circumstances hold the key to reducing mortality rates.

Finally, Chapter 11, 'Poverty, economic inequality and health', brings the book to a close by raising the question of whether formal health care *alone* can tackle the health problems faced in the United Kingdom in the 1990s. Against the background of sharp inequalities in health experience between different sections of the population, should we give greater priority to measures aimed at alleviating poverty, or reducing economic inequality, in the expectation that an indirect consequence of either will be an improvement in health and a reduction in disease? Are attitudes to poverty in the United Kingdom supportive of change in the tax and benefit systems to 'make the poor less poor'? And would attempts to improve health by redistributing income and wealth result in damage to productivity and business confidence? The book ends in speculation about the future.

A note about the authors

In this book, we have been careful not to take sides when competing options are being discussed; our aim has been to reveal the *nature* of the dilemmas—not to offer solutions. The chapters that follow have been written by specialists in certain areas of health policy or health-care research, mostly from educational or research institutions outside the Open University. The editors of this book have not attempted to disguise the somewhat different 'voices' expressed in each chapter, but we would like you to be aware of who the authors are and where their interests and priorities may therefore lie. This information is given at the start of each chapter, in the box containing study comments for Open University students.

OBJECTIVES FOR CHAPTER 1

When you have studied this chapter, you should be able to:

1.1 Use examples to illustrate the meaning of effectiveness, humanity, equity and efficiency in health care.

1.2 Distinguish between strategic, operational and clinical levels of management in health care.

1.3 Suggest ways in which achieving simultaneous improvements in effectiveness, humanity, equity and efficiency may create dilemmas for health-service managers, health-care workers and service-users.

QUESTIONS FOR CHAPTER 1

Question 1   (*Objective 1.1*)

Identify options in the Audit Commission report on day surgery that (according to the authors) would result in greater effectiveness, humanity, equity and efficiency in health care.

Question 2   (*Objective 1.2*)

Suggest some possible consequences for the strategic, operational and clinical management of heart disease arising from the research into the use of clot-busting drugs reported in Chapter 1.

Question 3   (*Objective 1.3*)

What dilemmas might face each of the three groups involved in health-care decision-making (managers, health-care workers and service-users) if the recommendations in the Audit Commission report were adopted?

2 Managing health care: balancing interests and influence

During your study of this chapter you will be referred to an article in the Reader[1] by Patricia Day and Rudolf Klein, entitled 'Britain's health-care experiment', which was set reading for the previous book in this series, Caring for Health: History and Diversity.[2] Chapter 7 of that book describes the successive reorganisations of the NHS in the 1970s, 1980s and 1990s, and we assume you are familiar with those events and the debates generated by them. Early in your study of this chapter you will also be asked to listen to an audiotape band entitled 'Dilemmas in hospital management' and to consult the notes that accompany that band. A television programme, 'Who calls the shots?', is highly relevant to this chapter; it deals with the management of health services for chronically sick children from both the 'purchaser' and 'provider' viewpoints.

This chapter was written by Stephen Harrison, Senior Lecturer in Policy Studies, and Gerald Wistow, Professor of Health and Social Care, both at The Nuffield Institute for Health (formerly Health Services Studies), University of Leeds. The Institute was set up in 1958 and has established an international reputation for teaching in the areas of health policy and health and social care management.

If Florence Nightingale were carrying her lamp through the corridors of the NHS today, she would almost certainly be looking for the people in charge. (Griffiths, R., 1983, p. 12)

[1] Health and Disease: A Reader (revised edition 1994).

[2] Caring for Health: History and Diversity (revised edition 1993).

Management: why the concern?

Who manages and influences the health service is rarely an immediate concern for those who use it. Contacts with the NHS generally centre on encounters with individual health-care professionals such as doctors and nurses. What counts is their capacity for listening, understanding, diagnosis and treatment. In such encounters, managers and the management process are largely hidden influences. There has, moreover, been a tendency to equate management with a wasteful and unnecessary bureaucracy which diverts resources from patient care. The former Prime Minister (1979–91), Margaret Thatcher, was well-known for her statement that 'the NHS is safe in our hands'. It is much less well-known, however, that this statement was originally expressed in the following terms at the 1982 Conservative Party Conference.

> The NHS is safe only with us because the government will see that it is prudently managed and financed, that care is concentrated on the patient rather than the bureaucrat. (Thatcher, M. quoted in Small, 1989, p. 104)

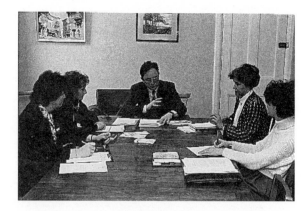

For patients, health-service management is generally an invisible process compared with their direct contact with doctors and nurses. (Photo: Mike Levers)

At the same time, however, Margaret Thatcher's governments gave more attention to issues concerning the management of the NHS than had any of her predecessors. As the quotation at the start of this chapter indicates, questions about who should manage and influence the NHS have become increasingly important. They are important both to the staff employed within the service and also those who use it. Staff have to work with the different styles of organisation and work priorities that managerial changes bring with them. Most fundamentally, who manages the health service, and in whose interests it is managed, determines 'who gets what' from the substantial sums of public resources spent on the NHS each year.

Understanding something about the nature of the debate about management and the relationships between the three principal interest groups within the health service will help you to understand some of the main factors influencing the dilemmas that face the NHS. Questions of who is in charge and who should be allowed to influence the health service form a backdrop for many of the issues explored in subsequent chapters in this book.

Traditionally, the *medical profession* has been the interest group with the primary role in shaping the NHS:[3] managers, in the form of hospital administrators, had limited influence. Then in the 1980s, a new breed of *general manager* was appointed by central government to solve a perceived leadership and accountability vacuum in response to the 'Griffiths Report' (from which the first quotation in this chapter was taken). Both groups would claim to be serving the best interests of a third interest group, the *members of the public* who pay for and use the service and their *representatives* (for example, members of Community Health Councils, CHCs). This chapter explores the relationship between doctors, managers and those appointed to reflect the interests of patients and the general public in the management of the service. These three interest groups are defined in more detail in a moment. The purpose of our analysis is to address two specific questions:

1   How has the balance between these interest groups been changing in the 1980s and what are the prospects for further change in the 1990s?

2   What is the *desirable* balance of influence between these interest groups and what are the arguments that inform this judgement?

The first question is a largely *empirical* one, which we shall address by drawing upon evidence collected in a wide range of research studies. Of course the assessment of probable further change is a matter of judgement at the time of writing in 1992, so we shall be asking you to be alert for further evidence as it emerges.

The second question is more directly *normative*; that is, it involves a value judgement. We shall, therefore, at the end of the chapter undertake a critical analysis for each of our three interest groups of claims that they might make for greater influence within the NHS. Since, as you will see, none has a wholly convincing case for overwhelming influence, there exists an important dilemma concerning the desirable balance of influence.

These two questions are important, for beneath them lurk a number of dilemmas about what is meant by 'universalising the best' and how to achieve it. It may not be possible to achieve both efficiency and equity, or efficiency and humanity. And if the different interest groups who provide the focus for this chapter have different views about (say) efficiency, whose view should prevail? And as in any other large organisation, there may be conflicts between long-term strategy and the shorter-term considerations of operational and clinical management.

Between these broad but fundamental questions about the balance of influence over the management of health services, the middle of the chapter—together with the accompanying audiocassette band[4]—seeks to bring alive what it is that managers do when they go to work. In an organisation the size of the NHS—and it has been said to be the second largest in Europe after the former Red Army—some degree of selectivity is necessary. Consequently, we focus on aspects of purchasing and providing, the two principal management functions at local level. In so doing, we illustrate some of the key issues around which the interplay between different interests takes place, and expose some of the dilemmas that managers face in their day-to-day activities.

The nature of management

Before addressing any of these issues, however, it is important to define what is meant by '**management**'. There is a voluminous literature on the nature and purpose of management in general and in the NHS more specifically, as well as on the similarities and differences between management in the private and public sectors.

[3] See *Caring for Health: History and Diversity* (revised edition 1993) Chapters 5–7.

[4] Open University students will listen to an audiocassette band entitled 'Dilemmas in hospital management' later in the chapter.

For example, Peter Drucker, a long-established management theorist, has argued that there are certain basic 'disciplines' of management which apply irrespective of the nature of organisations and the context in which they work. These disciplines are listed in Box 2.1.

Box 2.1 Basic disciplines of management

1 The need to define function and mission

2 The need to derive clear objectives and goals

3 The need to determine priorities and set targets

4 The need to set standards of performance

5 The need to make individuals accountable for results

6 The need to build self-control from results

7 The need to audit objectives and results

Source: based on material in Drucker, P. F. (1979) Management, *Heinemann, London, Chapter 1.*

Equally, there is much empirical evidence to suggest that managers do not actually work in such a systematic and goal-directed fashion. (Some of the evidence relating to the NHS is discussed below.) However, recent changes in the management of the health service have been based on a view that the management process *ought* to be consistent with the kinds of principles reflected in Drucker's disciplines. Thus, the established prescriptions about management in the NHS are that it should attempt to fulfil the following processes:

1 Determination of objectives, priorities and standards

2 Commitment of resources (finance, workforce, buildings and equipment) to secure those objectives

3 Review of performance against objectives

4 Review of objectives

As noted in Chapter 1, these management processes can be found at a number of different levels of organisation in the health service. Thus, taking process 1 in the list—*determination of objectives, priorities and standards*—as an example: *strategic* management by purchasing managers such as those in a District Health Authority (DHA) will include decisions about which are the most important health services for local residents to have access to;

operational managers in a provider unit such as a hospital will have to make decisions about (say) the most important new technology to obtain (an issue that features in Chapter 7) or the areas most in need of extra staff; *clinical* management by doctors will include decisions about which types of patients to treat with what degree of urgency. In each case, the management process involves setting objectives, priorities and standards. You might suggest examples of management decisions at the strategic, operational and clinical levels for processes 2–4 in the list above—perhaps drawing on the Audit Commission report on day surgery which you read during study of Chapter 1.

Three interest groups

It is also necessary to define in more detail the three interest groups upon which we shall be focusing in this chapter. By *doctors* we mean those medically qualified individuals whose main work is to diagnose and treat patients. For the sake of clarity we shall confine ourselves to hospital consultants and general practitioners (GPs), omitting consideration of junior doctors in training. By *managers* we mean all of those who hold formal managerial roles in the NHS; a few of these are medically qualified, and many more qualified in other health professions, especially nursing, but all are here regarded as managers. In practice, our concern is with more *senior* managers rather than, say, first-line supervisors. Table 2.1 gives a flavour of the professional backgrounds of such people in the period immediately after the Griffiths reforms.

☐ What does Table 2.1 show about the background of senior NHS managers?

■ The majority of general manager posts went to former NHS administrators and treasurers. Among all other categories of NHS staff, more doctors than nurses were appointed to senior posts. Very few posts were taken by managers from outside the NHS.

The third interest group—*citizen representatives*—is taken to mean the members of CHCs, and the non-executive members of health authorities (RHAs and DHAs in England and Wales; Health Boards in Scotland, and Health and Social Services Boards in Northern Ireland), Family Health Services Authorities (FHSAs) and non-executive directors of NHS Trusts.[5] None of these persons are 'representative' in the sense of being directly elected;

---

[5]The composition, main responsibilities of, and relationships between these organisations are described in *Caring for Health: History and Diversity* (revised edition 1993), Chapter 7.

Table 2.1 The background of NHS general managers in 1987

Former occupation	Regional general manager/number	District general manager/number	Unit general manager/number	Per cent of all
NHS administration and finance	9	132	355	61
NHS medicine	1	16	110	16
NHS nursing	1	5	71	9
NHS other	–	–	14	2
outside NHS	3	36	57	12
vacancies	–	2	4	1
Total	**14**	**191**	**611**	*

*Percentages do not sum to 100 due to rounding. (Data from: Leathard, A. 1990, *Health Care Provision: Past, Present and Future,* Chapman and Hall, London, p. 89)

indeed, the various non-executives referred to above are formally appointed (for example, by local authorities) for the individual contribution that they are expected to make and in legal terms are part of management. At the same time, however, it is common for them to be regarded as representative of local citizens in an indirect way:

> Of the non-executive directors (of NHS Trusts) at least two will be drawn from the local community, for example from hospital leagues of friends and similar organisations. (Department of Health, 1989a, *Working for Patients,* Cmnd. 555, p. 23)

Moreover, the members of health authorities have been specifically urged by the Department of Health to become 'champions of the people'. You should note however, that citizen representatives are only one of the vehicles by which the views, preferences and interests of the public can be expressed. Moreover, the interests of different 'publics', including patients, their families and the wider citizenry may not coincide (as discussed in Chapter 5). Here we are purposely restricting our focus to those individuals whose role is in some sense formally representative of the public as a whole.

However, it is important to recognise that the three groups discussed here are not the only significant interest groups to be found in the NHS, either as employees or service-users. Chapter 5 looks in much more detail at how citizens or consumers of health care have been perceived and involved in influencing the services that they use. In Chapter 6, attention is given to other important professional groups within the NHS workforce where, once again, issues of influence and significance loom

large, especially in relation to nursing, which forms the largest single group of workers in the service.

Who dominates?

In choosing the three interest groups on which this chapter focuses, we have followed the approach employed in Robert Alford's influential study of health care in New York in the 1970s, *Health Care Politics: Ideological and Interest Group Barriers to Reform.* An 'interest group' in this sense does not indicate a tightly organised association (doctors and managers are loosely organised, citizen representatives hardly at all): nor does it presume that there are no conflicts of interest within such groups. Rather, the interest groups are 'structural'; that is, they are differentiated according to how they are

> ...served or not served by the way they 'fit' into the basic logic and principles by which the institutions of society operate...*dominant* structural interests are those served by the structure of social, economic and political institutions as they exist at any given time.... *Challenging* structural interests are those being created by the changing structure of the society. *Repressed* structural interests are the opposite of dominant ones.... (Alford, 1975, p. 14)

Later in the chapter, when we have discussed the three interest groups in more detail, we shall be asking you to consider how they correspond to Alford's three categories of structural interests (dominant, challenging and repressed), and whether there are likely to be any changes in the balance of power in the foreseeable future.

In the next section of this chapter, we look back at the historical balance of influence between the three interest groups, and in particular we focus on the pivotal changes that surrounded the Griffiths Report of 1983.

The introduction of general management

Following the Griffiths Report of 1983, the government introduced a series of measures, usually summarised as **general management**, which were intended to strengthen the role of senior NHS managers.[6] The essential character of the new general managers is well summarised in the report's advocacy of

> ...a driving force seeking and accepting direct and personal responsibility for developing management plans, securing their implementation and monitoring their achievement. (Griffiths, 1983, p. 12)

The report also emphasised that doctors should be more closely involved in management. The impact of these changes upon the relative influence of our three interest groups can be considered under three broad headings: medical influence, managerial objectives and evaluating services.[7]

Medical influence

An examination of the research literature shows that, before Griffiths, senior managers were not the most influential 'actors' in the NHS; rather, doctors were. It is important not to misunderstand this, for it was neither a conspiracy by doctors, nor a matter of a few highly influential doctors of the mould of Sir Lancelot Spratt (found in Richard Gordon's books, such as *Doctor in the House*). Rather, it was rooted in both the concept of professional autonomy and the implicit bargain negotiated between the profession and the government when the NHS was created in 1948.[8] In the specific case of doctors, the notion that they should be free to exercise their professional judgement independent of lay or managerial control is known as **clinical autonomy** or **clinical freedom**. We can summarise this concept as the extent to which a (fully trained) doctor is, or should be, free to employ his or her own judgement in the selection, diagnosis, and treatment of patients.[9] As Patricia Day and Rudolf Klein point out in their article 'Britain's health-care experiment' (1991),[10]

> The NHS has always been based on an implicit, unspoken concordat between state and profession. The former set the budgets within which doctors operated. The latter, however, had complete autonomy to decide whom to treat, and how, within the limits of those budgets. (Day and Klein, 1991, p. 44)

Consequently, and despite managerial influence over such matters as new buildings and major equipment purchases, it was hospital doctors who made decisions about which were appropriate patients to accept, how to diagnose and treat them, and, thereby, how much to spend on them. In a sense, therefore, the aggregate of all these individual clinical decisions about laboratory tests, X-rays, treatments, and whether (and for how long) to hospitalise patients became the pattern of service offered by the NHS. Clinical management determined operational management and strongly influenced strategic policy-making. Moreover, this clinical freedom also provided doctors with a good deal of obstructive ability to resist changes of which they disapproved. You will not be surprised to learn that, in such circumstances, health authority members and CHC members had little discernible influence.

General management did not immediately bring about a situation in which either citizen representatives or top managers were more influential than doctors; the latter retained their obstructive ability and clinical freedom to decide how to treat which cases. There were, however, three immediate differences.

---

[6] These measures are described more fully in another book in this series, *Caring for Health: History and Diversity* (revised edition 1993), Chapter 7.

[7] See the review of 25 pre-Griffiths research studies of NHS management by Harrison (1988) and a review of 25 post-Griffiths studies by Harrison *et al.* (1992), in the Further Reading list at the end of this book.

[8] See *Caring for Health: History and Diversity* (revised edition 1993), Chapter 6.

[9] Clinical freedom and its impact on doctor–patient relationships is discussed in another book in this series, *Medical Knowledge: Doubt and Certainty* (Open University Press, revised edition 1994); the history of clinical autonomy is a theme in *Caring for Health: History and Diversity* (revised edition 1993). Also see Johnson (1972), and Schulz and Harrison (1986) in the Further Reading list.

[10] Included in *Health and Disease: A Reader* (revised edition 1994). This article is set reading for *Caring for Health: History and Diversity* (revised edition 1993).

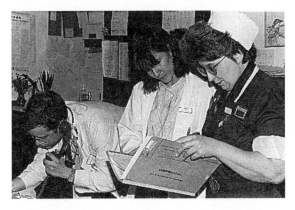

NHS resources are committed by the day-to-day clinical decisions of professional staff, principally doctors and nurses. (Photo: Mike Levers)

First, the medical profession was seen to suffer two major defeats at the hands of government over, respectively, the introduction of restrictions on prescribing, and the introduction of general management itself, to which the British Medical Association (BMA) had objected. Second, managers, under government pressure to 'balance the books' were able to enforce such changes as bed closures, which might previously have been obstructed by doctors. Third, there was the introduction, on a progressive basis, of management techniques such as *performance indicators* (see Chapter 4) and *activity-related budgets* (budgets based on actual workload). The effect of such techniques, which record, and in some cases cost, the work of doctors is beginning to make medicine more transparent to managers, and therefore potentially more controllable by them.

The following remark from Richard Banyard's study of unit general managers (UGMs) summarises the modest increase in management influence over doctors in the period immediately following the implementation of the Griffiths Report.

> Only limited progress has been made towards ensuring that UGMs exercise greater control in the setting of clinical targets and monitoring of clinical activities, while progress towards establishing closer links between UGMs and medical advisory systems has been patchy. The perceived impact of general management at 'front line' level has apparently been slight, and general managers are not infrequently regarded as somewhat remote figures. (Banyard, 1988, p. 916)

Managerial objectives: the agenda changes

The standard management prescriptions, referred to above, decree that top managers (at least) should be *proactive*, in seeking to achieve previously established objectives. By contrast, before the introduction of general management, research has shown that top managers' work was largely driven by problems, that is, it was largely *reactive*. A great deal of this work could be considered as 'organisational maintenance': smoothing out conflicts and helping doctors and other health-care workers to obtain the resources necessary for their work. This was neatly illustrated in Stuart Haywood's 1979 study of decision-making by pre-Griffiths management teams. Figure 2.1 summarises the findings of this study.

☐ According to Haywood's study, what kinds of items took up most of the agenda in NHS management team meetings prior to the Griffiths reforms?

■ 90 per cent of team agenda items consisted of information exchange, deciding to whom issues should be referred (process items) or routine decision-making.

Haywood concluded by describing senior managers as 'directors of process...reactors rather than initiators' (Haywood, 1979, p. 59). Further examination of the pre-Griffiths research suggests that managers' agendas were also *producer-oriented*; that is, that the problems to which top managers gave most attention were those coming from *inside* their organisation: problems raised by

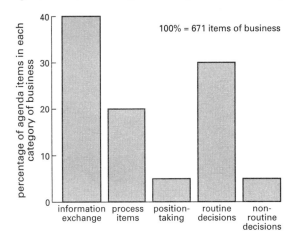

Figure 2.1 *A sample of NHS management team agenda items. 'Process items' are decisions about to whom an issue should be referred. (Source: Haywood, S., 1979, Team management in the NHS: What is it all about?, Health and Social Service Journal, 5 October, p. B.54, Table 1)*

doctors, other professionals, and trades unions, rather than problems raised by patients, their relatives, or by citizen representatives on health authorities or CHCs.

Research since the Griffiths reforms shows a marked change in all this. Management is as reactive a process as ever, but many of the problems which concern it now come from *outside* the organisation: not from consumers or local citizen representatives, but from central government, as the NHS has become increasingly politicised. Thus, for example, the government's initiative to reduce hospital waiting lists has occupied a good deal of management capacity, as has the need to cope with balancing the books in the face of expenditure restrictions. This shift is summarised by Philip Strong and Jane Robinson in their study of reactions to management changes in the NHS:

> Griffiths, then, for all its radicalism, was only a partial break with the past. There was now a chain of command which reached from the top to the bottom of the organization. There was also a new headquarters staff with a potential flexibility to match the exigencies of local need and form. But the service was still trapped, for general managers at least, within a national straitjacket. Local initiative was frustrated by ministers, by civil servants, by supervisory management tiers, and by powerful professional bodies. Doctors still gave orders, nanny still knew best. (Strong and Robinson, 1990, p. 164)

At the same time, however, doctors came to accept the existence of general management. Any opposition from the BMA soon faded and the legitimacy of the new management arrangements gradually ceased to be challenged.

Evaluating the service

In general, research on the period before the Griffiths reforms concludes that very little evaluation took place in the NHS, since everyone involved tended to regard the services provided as basically good. Individual complaints might certainly arise and be dealt with, but the basic 'goodness' of the service meant that it was not felt necessary to engage in any form of systematic audit or evaluation. On the contrary, a good deal of time was spent by all three of our interest groups in deciding how to spend the additional resources which were available each year. A large number of initiatives ostensibly aimed at making services more 'consumer responsive' or improving their 'quality' (in a somewhat undefined sense), followed on from Griffiths, but the research findings have tended to reveal these as broadly cosmetic in character (see Chapter 5). This point was made neatly, if

not very kindly, by one of the respondents to the Strong and Robinson study mentioned above:

> …some of the nurses in quality [control] terrify me!…. I've been really shocked by some of the ones I've met. They hadn't a clue. They thought it was all about dealing with patients' complaints…some of the ones I've met think the idea is to get quality printed on T-shirts! (quoted in Strong and Robinson, 1990, p. 182)

Moreover, since by the 1980s growth money was less readily available, managers might have taken the opportunity to link evaluation of services with continued funding. In practice, they were unable to do so. In the following quotation, Rob Flynn is summarising the view expressed by a health-service manager who was a respondent in his research study:

> …there *was* something special about managing cutbacks. It means asking fundamental questions—'Do we really need an Accident and Emergency Unit here? If not, then close it.' But there were limits to this approach, first the consultants and second the 'very real commitment' of staff to health care. (Flynn, 1991, p. 228)

□ Drawing on the previous discussion, how would you relate the three interest groups (managers, citizen representatives and doctors) to Alford's categories of dominant, challenging and repressed interests referred to earlier in this chapter?

■ Clinical autonomy was literally rooted in the political and financial structure of the NHS, so that doctors were the *dominant* influence on the allocation of resources and the kinds of services available to patients. However, the introduction of general management was designed, in part, to *challenge* that position, especially by subjecting clinical practice to more scrutiny. Better information about the activities of doctors, and the costs and effectiveness of their work would make it more transparent and less mysterious. By contrast, however, the Griffiths changes appear to have done little to enhance the role of citizen representatives, who remain a *repressed* interest within the NHS.

Future prospects for general management

Since the research cited in the above account was carried out, there have been important further changes to the organisation of the NHS, arising largely from the 1989

White Paper, *Working for Patients*.[11] In considering the probable impact of these changes on the relative influence between our three interest groups, we can draw upon earlier research findings, informal evidence (for instance, from reports in the news media), together with a large slice of the authors' own judgement (see for example Harrison and Wistow, 1992).

The doctor–manager relationship

We begin by examining the doctor–manager relationship and, for the first time in this chapter, consider hospital consultants and GPs separately.

At least three sets of factors seem likely to continue the shift, begun by the Griffiths changes, of relative influence from consultants towards managers. First, there is now more information available to managers concerning the activities of doctors. Methods of obtaining information and evaluating activity are described in detail in Chapter 4, and include measures of the efficiency with which beds and other facilities are utilised (performance indicators); the relationship of clinical workload to budgeted expenditure (resource management); and the aggregated results of reviews of clinical decisions conducted by medical colleagues (medical audit). This information will make medical activity more transparent to managers.

Second, the system that followed *Working for Patients* has introduced management involvement in the appointment of consultants (sometimes on short-term contracts), their merit pay, and in the job descriptions of those appointed. This is a significant shift away from a system in which such matters were decided entirely within the medical profession. Indeed, job descriptions were largely left to incumbents of the posts to devise for themselves.

Third, the 'purchaser–provider split' created by the *Working for Patients* reforms is showing early signs both of providing a degree of managerial leverage over hospital consultants, and of changing the balance of influence *within* the medical profession, from consultants to GPs. For example, a study conducted by the authors of this chapter found GPs and DHA purchasing managers identifying a number of areas in which the performance of provider units was considered to be deficient (Harrison and Wistow, 1992). These included waiting times for

ophthalmic (eye) treatment, attitudes of consultant obstetricians to patients, outcomes of orthopaedic (bone and joint) surgery, and direct access by GPs to physiotherapy services. The DHA purchasing managers said they would consider threatening to move contracts elsewhere, but they were careful not to issue direct threats because they feared a destructive spiral of deteriorating relationships. However, hospital (provider) managers made clear to consultants the possibility of losing their contracts under the new arrangements and it was anticipated that this would lead to peer group pressure being applied to improve the quality of services where this was necessary.

The potential shift in the balance of influence from consultants towards purchasing authority managers and fund-holding GPs has been more generally appreciated by provider unit managers, who see the external threat to remove contracts as a source of additional leverage over the consultants in their units. The introduction of the 'contract culture' certainly seems, therefore, to be beginning to shift the balance of influence away from hospital doctors and towards managers, though it should not be forgotten that treatment decisions, and consequent expenditure, are still primarily controlled by doctors. Indeed, 'clinical directorates' headed by consultants are an increasingly common tier of management at the level of the medical specialty (e.g. geriatrics, obstetrics, etc.).

Impact on citizen representation

The new management arrangements in the 1990s, however, have not led to significant changes in the influence of citizen representatives. CHCs have been weakened: their members lost the right to attend the meetings of DHAs. Moreover, the *Working for Patients* reforms included changes in the membership of RHAs, DHAs, and Family Health Services Authorities (FHSAs, formerly Family Practitioner Committees, FPCs).[12] We confine ourselves here to the membership of DHAs, where the changes included;

- Reduction in overall size

- Addition of several senior NHS managers (executive members)

- Removal of local government appointees and trade union nominees (non-executive members)

- Removal of automatic medical and nursing membership

[11]The reorganisation of the NHS in the early 1990s, commencing with reforms set out in *Working for Patients,* is described and discussed in *Caring for Health: History and Diversity* (revised edition 1993), Chapter 7.

[12]See *Caring for Health: History and Diversity* (revised edition 1993), Chapter 7.

The self-governing NHS Trusts are new creations following *Working for Patients;* each Trust's management team must include two 'community' non-executive directors, though these may be unrepresentative of the population at large. For example, a report by Tony Sheldon in 1991 showed that non-executive members of NHS Trusts tended to be white, male and from business backgrounds. In summary, then, the early signs are that the influence of citizen representatives, never strong to start with, has been marginally weakened by the NHS organisational changes of the 1990s.

Local management in practice

We turn now to the second task identified in the introduction to the chapter: to give you an insight into the substance of management agendas and tasks. The level of analysis needs to shift, therefore, to a much more specific concern with the kinds of issues and dilemmas with which managers grapple on a day-to-day basis. In what follows, our focus is on *local* management rather than management at either regional or national levels (except in so far as the last two impinge upon the first).

Three tasks lie at the heart of local management in the health service:

1   Deciding what health services and treatments to purchase on behalf of local residents, and what to provide in local NHS units

2   Ensuring the delivery of services and treatments within available resources

3   Assessing the performance of services and treatments, for example in terms of their effectiveness, efficiency, equity and humanity.

Following the *Working for Patients* reforms, different aspects of each of these tasks are shared by two different kinds of organisations at local level: purchasers and providers.

☐   Which organisations are included in each of these categories?

■   Purchasers include DHAs (in England and Wales)[13] and fund-holding GPs. Providers consist of

primary health-care services together with self-governing Trusts and other NHS units providing hospital, community and mental health services. (You will find that the Reader article by Day and Klein provides a useful summary description of these arrangements.)[14]

It follows from our earlier analysis that the performance of local management tasks and their outcomes is heavily influenced by relationships between the three interest groups you have been studying. It was also at least implicit in our earlier observation that the nature and results of local management processes are also substantially influenced by external factors. Two such factors were shown to be of increasing importance: *resource constraint* and the decisions of *central government.* These two factors are linked since the overriding concern of successive governments has been to strengthen budgetary controls and secure greater value for money.

The research on which we drew earlier in the chapter demonstrated that management agendas had become increasingly dominated by financial pressures in the period following the implementation of the Griffiths Report in 1983, and also that managers had become increasingly 'cost conscious'. These developments point up the relative powerlessness of managers over the way in which resources are spent within the health service. Thus a central dilemma for local management is how to reconcile its responsibility for managing limited resources with its limited control over the doctors and other health-care workers who commit resources.

The audiocassette band which accompanies this chapter provides examples of actual situations in which managers are seeking to reconcile such forces. It also provides examples in which the influence of government and parliament is felt upon local management agendas. However, in listening to the audiotape, you should note that the scenes depicted are based in a large *provider* unit—a district general hospital—and that this is not typical of all settings in which the NHS is managed. You should now listen to the audiotape entitled 'Dilemmas in hospital management'.[15]

[14]Day, P. and Klein, R. 'Britain's health-care experiment' in *Health and Disease: A Reader* (revised edition 1994).

[15]The audiocassette band 'Dilemmas in hospital management' has been recorded for Open University students; please read the Audiocassette Notes which accompany it before listening to the audiotape.

[13]Health Boards in Scotland; Health and Social Services Boards in Northern Ireland.

As we noted in the commentary on the audiotape, much of the concern of the managers involved in operational decisions is with making the best use of scarce resources such as staff and hospital beds.

☐ Consider the conversations between the hospital Chief Executive and the manager of the Intensive Therapy Unit (ITU). Summarise the dilemma they faced over trying to reconcile equity with efficiency in the delivery of ITU services.

■ Equity in the health service means that everyone receives health care appropriate to their needs. The hospital has resources, such as ITU beds, which have been provided to meet some expected level of need, but if actual need exceeds this (as was the case when this audiotape was recorded) then some patients will not get appropriate treatment. However, if more ITU beds were provided so that all needs could be met, or if elective (pre-booked) patients were not accepted to keep beds free for emergencies, then beds would often be empty and hence the unit would be using resources less efficiently.

This section of the audiotape also raised the conflict between efficiency and humanity, both in the treatment of patients who may have to be relocated to an ITU bed in a distant unit or moved onto a general ward when ideally they should stay in the ITU, and in the working lives of overstretched staff in a particularly stressful area of health care. Later chapters in this book will refer back to other sections of this audiotape.

The audiotape was recorded in a provider unit, and thus did not cover examples of the role of managers in carrying out the *purchasing* function.[16] Purchasing managers do not have direct responsibility for the 'hands-on' operational management of particular services; their task is to address the same questions about who gets care, how, and with what results but from a more strategic perspective. Indeed, their responsibility is to address such issues from the perspective of the local population as a whole. Thus, the purchasing manager's role may be defined as consisting of the identification of health-care needs, priorities and standards within a defined population and the direction of resources to ensure those needs are met.

[16]The day-to-day dilemmas facing purchasing managers are illustrated in a television programme for Open University students, 'Who calls the shots?'.

A desirable balance of influence?

We conclude this chapter by moving away from what has actually been happening in the NHS, and addressing instead the more speculative question of the *desirability* of possible shifts in the balance of influence between our three interest groups. We begin by considering doctors.

Should clinical freedom predominate?

Arguments concerning the relative influence of doctors focus very much on the concept of *clinical autonomy*, which—as we noted earlier—is the extent to which a doctor is, or should be, free to employ his or her own judgement in the selection, diagnosis, and treatment of patients. Clearly, the greater a doctor's autonomy, the less he or she is influenced by others.

An important argument in favour of extensive clinical autonomy for doctors is that it is necessary in order to safeguard the patient's interests. One strand to the argument relates to technical expertise; no one else is technically capable of doing a doctor's work, and he or she should not therefore be overruled by a non-doctor. But this argument on its own is not sufficient to justify clinical freedom, since it could be satisfied by saying that doctors could be given management instructions by other doctors. Hence, there is a second strand to the argument, which says that it is the doctor's ethical duty to do everything medically possible for someone whom he or she has accepted as a patient, and that this ethic needs to be protected from interference by any other party, including managers. The end point of this justification is that it is in *patients'* best interests for individual doctors to be clinically free, and that the profession as a whole should be largely *self-regulating*.

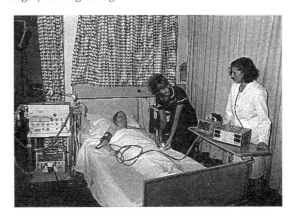

Doctors have extensive clinical autonomy about who receives health services and how they should be treated, but increasingly they are asked to consider the financial costs. (Photo: Mike Levers)

☐ Make a list of any arguments you can think of *against* doctors having extensive clinical freedom. (Some of these points were raised in the audiotape you listened to earlier.)

■ Your arguments probably fell into one or more of the following three categories:

(a) Why should doctors not be subject to managerial control? It is possible to see clinical autonomy as something which is propagated by the medical profession for its *own* interests; thus, it could be used to avoid doctors' clinical work being managed by 'outsiders', or to protect the incompetent. Clinical autonomy can also be 'stretched' to include freedom to decide how much of what kind of (interesting?) clinical work to do, and the organisation of the working week, etc.

(b) Are users of health-care services (and their citizen representatives) really so unqualified to make decisions about treatment and services? Clearly, they are unlikely to develop the level of technical understanding of a skilled medical professional, but this does not mean that they cannot and should not be given greater opportunity to influence treatments and services.

(c) Health services raise many ethical, political and financial issues that fall outside the spheres of doctors' technical competence. For example, health care involves legitimate issues of public accountability for taxpayers' resources which cannot be ignored by either citizen representatives or managers. The argument for substantial clinical autonomy fails to deal with the problem of finite resources—clinical decisions are also decisions to commit public money.

More power to the managers?

As we indicated above, over the last decade government has given increasing priority to strengthening management processes and thus the influence of managers. We also suggested at the beginning of the chapter that the public's contact with, and awareness of, NHS management was limited compared with its direct contact with doctors and other staff involved in 'hands-on' care of patients. At the same time, however, the ways in which health services are organised and managed do have direct consequences for patients, their relatives and friends. Government policy in the 1990s has given some priority to certain aspects of the management task which impact directly on users of the service, through initiatives concerned with, for example, waiting lists and the need

for different categories of health-care workers to collaborate in providing 'seamless care'. You may also have seen a copy of the *Patient's Charter*, published by the government in 1992, which sets certain targets for the health service in meeting patients' needs (a document we examine in detail in Chapter 5).

☐ Drawing on your experiences of the NHS and the audiotape on hospital management (and, if you wish, the news media), list some ways in which the NHS could be 'better managed' from the patient's point of view.

■ We cannot expect to anticipate all the items that you might have listed, but here are some common examples:

(a) Quicker allocation of appointments and admissions, and shorter waiting times when attending an appointment (the difficulties in finding beds for emergency admissions were well-illustrated on the audiotape).

(b) Better information for service users about their condition, the treatment, and its likely outcome (the hospital Chief Executive on the audiotape had decided to provide in-patients with information booklets).

(c) Better integration of the different parts of health (and social) services, so that those involved in diagnosis, treatment and support, work together to provide the right care at the right time and place.

(d) Greater emphasis on ensuring the effectiveness of services and treatments offered by the NHS (Chapter 4 examines this topic in greater detail).

It is clearly possible to make the case that managers would be able to tackle these (and other) problems if they were more influential in relation to doctors and other health-care professionals. Earlier in this chapter, we stressed the potential impact of new forms of information about doctors' activities upon this relationship, but some commentators have gone further in arguing that doctors should be increasingly subject to managerially-devised *incentive* systems. Box 2.2 presents a discussion of this issue from a journal whose main audience is NHS managers; the article uses an academic report (Centre for Health Economics, 1992) as its provocative starting point, and adds comments on the report by medical and management representatives. You should study it now.

One obvious counter-argument to the above is the danger that a more managerially oriented NHS will be *less* responsive to the differing needs of individual

Box 2.2 Academics urge trust managers to take on doctors over performance

Trusts should use their freedoms to take the lead in reforming the 'inefficient' and 'indefensible' system of hospital doctors' pay, a report recommends. The existing system is anachronistic and contains no incentives to reward efficiency, despite the NHS reforms, according to a York Centre for Health Economics paper published this week.

> 'The consequence of this payment system is that hospital doctors are neither penalised for poor performance nor rewarded for good work, and it is difficult to encourage specialisation in areas of short supply.'

The report, which calls for the introduction of short-term contracts and performance-related pay, is likely to be greeted sceptically by consultants' leaders, who are opposed to the replacement of nationally agreed terms and conditions. John Chawner, chair of the BMA consultant committee, said last week that paying doctors at different rates could lead to a two-tier system and may provoke doctors to leave the NHS.

The report suggests trusts—with their ability to appoint their own consultants and set local pay rates—could use short-term contracts to increase performance incentives. Short-term contracts would also make doctors more accountable to managers, which, says the report, would go some way to 'redressing the highly uneven balance of power' in hospitals. Performance-related pay could encourage greater activity and efficiency, the report suggests. But it warns that performance measures should be appropriate, and should try to take into account medical outcomes.

> 'Measures should try to take account of the work input of doctors and the value of outcomes from this, rather than just encouraging doctors to meet political targets.'

It calls for consideration of a system based on the US Medicare doctor remuneration method, which links fees to time input and intensity of activity of doctors' work. Despite some reservations, including the difficulty of adapting the system to the NHS, the system could provide the basis for an 'open and systematic' method of reimbursement.

Several trusts have implemented or are considering introducing short-term contracts, including St James' Trust in Leeds, where doctors are offered the choice of five-year rolling contracts or existing NHS terms and conditions. Andy Black, chief executive of the Central Middlesex Trust, said changes to hospital doctors' pay were inevitable:

> 'People all over the health service are facing up to the fact that employment details are changing.'

Source: Butler, P. (1992) Academics urge trust managers to take on doctors over performance, Health Service Journal, 26 June, p. 6.

patients. For example, the use of information systems about the costs and outcomes of care (including performance indicators, resource management, and medical audit) could result in crude labelling of individuals simply as members of a particular diagnostic (or whatever) category. On the other hand, the new style of NHS management also places considerable emphasis on being more responsive to consumers (e.g. by achieving the targets set in the *Patient's Charter*). If this proves to be anything more than mere rhetoric, it could form a counter-weight to any tendency towards a remote and insensitive form of managerialism.

A second argument against managers having more power springs from asking a question which we asked earlier about doctors: why should we trust them? More precisely, why should we expect managers to display any less self-interest than doctors? Managers may be too dependent on political approval for their present position and promotion prospects to represent the public interest fully. On this argument, giving greater influence to managers will not necessarily improve matters for users or the population in general. To take one frequently cited example, managers might use their new powers to award themselves large pay increases. Looking back at his own work after almost eight years, Sir Roy Griffiths commented in a speech to the Audit Commission in 1991 (and published a year later) that:

> One or two things I did not intend. Whilst my name at the time was primarily connected with general management, I personally took this as a shorthand for the introduction of an effective management process. I did not intend that the result should be yet another profession... (Griffiths, 1992, p. 67)

Greater influence for citizen representatives?

There seem to be three main arguments to support the view that citizen representatives should be given greater relative influence in the NHS than is currently the case.

The first is that since the NHS is publicly funded, citizens should have an influence over its activities. Since it is known that substantial *local* variations in service exist, it follows that the citizen voice should be a local one, and that accountability to the national government is insufficiently democratic for this purpose. According to this argument, the limited professional/technical knowledge of citizens is not a crucial factor; if the public wants (say) neonatal intensive care to be provided for very tiny newborn babies, even if they have little chance of survival, then that is the choice of those who are, indirectly, paying. (For a formal statement of this line of reasoning, see Goodin and Wilenski, 1984.) It should be noted that, at the time of writing in 1992, this is a somewhat radical argument, opposed to the economists' view that only *effective* health care should be provided by the NHS (for a careful exposition of this argument, see Culyer, 1992).

A second argument in favour of greater influence for citizen representatives is that some of them (primarily CHC members) are far more accustomed to close contact with the users of health services than are NHS managers and so are better placed to know what 'consumers' want. Indeed, a large proportion of CHC members are involved with voluntary organisations which either act as pressure groups for users and/or actually provide services which fill the gaps in NHS provision.

Third, there is a more general argument that citizen representatives of all kinds bring an outside perspective to the NHS. They may be able to challenge long-standing 'insider' assumptions about the kind of services that ought to be provided, and about the standards that should be aimed for. Of course, there is little point in the ritual airing of these alternative perspectives if their proponents lack the influence to have them taken seriously.

There are, however, a number of arguments *against* the allocation of greater influence to citizen representatives in the NHS. The first essentially says that having citizen representatives is not the only, nor necessarily the most effective, method for taking into account public views about health services in the decision-making process. Managers could solicit the views of people who are current or recent service-users by means of opinion surveys, and in fact many hospitals and health authorities routinely employ such devices, which are further discussed in Chapter 5. Moreover, it is possible for the managers in a purchasing authority to consult its resident citizens on topics such as relative health-care priorities, though methods for doing this are not yet well-developed.

The study by the authors of this chapter mentioned earlier found DHAs in England and Wales beginning to approach this task in a number of ways (Harrison and Wistow, 1992). For example, one DHA had circulated 2 500 copies of its draft health plan, together with a supporting questionnaire, to community and business organisations within its area. Preliminary results were seen to be threatening to the main provider unit (a hospital) because they suggested that community rather than hospital-based care for elderly people was emerging as a priority. A market research firm had also been commissioned to carry out a postal questionnaire of GPs, with follow-up interviews, and also to conduct interviews with over a thousand local people. Moreover the DHA was planning to stimulate public debate by the publication of an adversarial dialogue between proponents and opponents of the funding of a procedure to treat infertility.

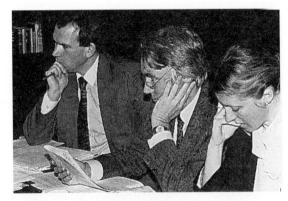

Non-executive members of DHAs bring an external perspective to NHS management. (Photo: Mike Levers)

However, another DHA was more cautious about consulting the public and appeared to be restricting itself to the provision of more information to local people rather than obtaining information from them. One of the respondents in this health authority suggested that public surveys ran the risk of creating unrealistic public expectations and that 'the public are not well enough educated to make choices about health care'. Accepting that non-executive members of the DHA did not represent the public, the respondent envisaged using GPs as proxies for public opinion.

A second category of argument against giving more influence to citizen representatives centres upon the notion that in the NHS they are not, in fact, representative of citizens, either in the sense of being elected by citizens, or in the socio-demographic sense: women, ethnic minorities and manual workers are usually under-represented. The *present* citizen representatives can therefore be said to lack legitimacy. This could also be used to argue that an equitable health service can only be achieved through national rather than local action.

The corollary to this argument is that any attempt to allocate greater influence to citizen representatives should be preceded by measures to improve their representativeness. Thus, some commentators have argued for the transfer of the NHS to the control of elected local government authorities, or alternatively for the direct election of health authority members. In their 'Essay in the government of health', published in 1982, D. E. Regan and John Stewart argued that:

> Either solution would give the legitimacy required for independent action. Either solution would give a basis for local accountability. The members of the governing body would have the authority that comes with the fact of election. Either solution would provide an independent authority justified, within the framework set nationally, in independent action. Each would provide a basis on which the authority could legitimately meet local needs. Each would provide a basis for local experiment and the learning that goes with it. Each would meet the requirements for an authoritative basis for independent decision-making at the local level. Each would increase the capacity for difference within the government of health. (Regan and Stewart, 1982, p. 40)

In their conclusion, Regan and Stewart preferred the local government option, largely on the grounds that it would assist the integration of health services with other relevant services (such as social services).[17] For a more recent version of this argument, evaluated in the new context of the purchaser–provider split in health care, see Harrison *et al.* (1991). Other commentators, however, have considered that the retention of separate, though elected, health authorities might be a positive advantage; in his essay *The Governance of Health Services*, published in 1985, the health-service analyst Chris Ham noted that it might

> ...be argued that separately elected authorities offer an advantage in that they would help to stimulate a local debate about health service issues, a debate which would not occur so readily if health services were included with other services under a broad local government umbrella. (Ham, 1985, p. 16)

Both of these approaches are open to the common objection that an increase in *local* decision-making could lead to greater variations in standards, priorities and services between different parts of the country—in other words, present a threat to equity in health care. You should recognise that there is an inherent dilemma involved in strengthening *local* decision-making by citizen representatives on the one hand, and securing *national* standards of provision and access to care on the other.

Future prospects?

It should by now be clear that it is difficult to make the argument that one or other of the three interest groups with whom this chapter is concerned should simply have overwhelming influence. The arguments for and against increasing the influence of each group, whether or not you agree with all of them, seem to suggest that it is the *balance* that is important, though there is clearly room for considerable variation in opinion about what that balance should be at any particular point in time.

[17]Similar (unsuccessful) arguments were put forward in favour of local government control of a national health service when the structure of the NHS was being developed in the 1940s; see *Caring for Health: History and Diversity* (revised edition 1993), Chapters 5 and 6.

We noted earlier that in the 1980s and early 1990s the balance of influence seemed to be moving away from doctors and (to a lesser extent) citizen representatives, and towards managers. But of course, managers did not achieve this on their own—rather, they had behind them an 'interest group' which we have mentioned only in passing in this chapter—central government. Central government could choose to back other interest groups in the future, for example by promoting the rapid expansion of the GP fund-holding scheme. All other things being equal, the effect of this would be to shift back a degree of relative influence to the medical profession, though in this case to GPs rather than to the hospital consultants who were dominant in the past.

Similarly, you should recall that giving more influence to citizen representatives is only one way in which the 'consumer' interest might be better expressed; we have noted a range of ways in which purchasing authority managers are seeking out local views. In addition, the *Working for Patients* changes include some emphasis on patient choice and greater responsiveness to their needs. The *Patient's Charter* is part of that approach. You may wish to reserve final judgement on the future prospects for influence by citizens until you have studied Chapter 5.

A central and persistent dilemma for managers is how to reconcile their responsibility for seeking out need with their responsibility for operating within cash-limited budgets. Strategic issues about equity and the relevant weights to be placed on different categories of need must also be addressed in more explicit ways than in the past. Thus it is not only clinical practice which is becoming more transparent and fully described: separating-out purchasing from providing functions also encourages more clearly-expressed decisions about which needs will be met, how, and to what extent (rationing is discussed in Chapter 3).

We began this chapter by remarking on the largely hidden nature of management in the NHS so far as present and future service-users are concerned. You should now reflect on the extent to which the changes in the NHS in the 1990s are leading to decision-making processes—and their consequences—which are more explicit at the level of individual professional practice as well as the local management of the service as a whole. It is a paradox that the future management of the NHS will be more than ever subject to public scrutiny because of the explicit nature of its decision-making processes, yet these same processes fail to give the consumer any significant degree of formal involvement.

OBJECTIVES FOR CHAPTER 2

When you have studied this chapter you should be able to:

2.1   Summarise the historic balance of influence within the NHS between doctors, managers and citizen representatives, and the effects of the Griffiths Report on this balance.

2.2   Comment on the probable impact upon this balance of the *Working for Patients* reforms.

2.3   Summarise and comment on a range of arguments which have been proposed as the justification for changes in the balance of influence.

2.4   Summarise the main operational responsibilities of NHS managers in provider units, and show how this differs from the more strategic role of NHS managers in purchasing health care.

QUESTIONS FOR CHAPTER 2

Question 1 (*Objective 2.1*)

The basic disciplines of management set out in Box 2.1 imply that managers are the most influential group within an organisation. How far has this been the case in the NHS from its inception to the present day?

Question 2 (*Objective 2.2*)

Which aspects of the reforms contained in *Working for Patients* are likely to strengthen the position of managers?

Question 3 (*Objective 2.3*)

What arguments have been put forward in this chapter about increasing the influence of (a) doctors, (b) managers, and (c) citizen representatives?

Question 4 (*Objective 2.4*)

Summarise the main difference in the role of a health-service *purchasing* manager, and a manager in a health-care *provider* unit.

3 Rationing and choice

This chapter begins by looking back to the Beveridge Report of 1942 and the foundation of the NHS in 1948, which were discussed in Chapters 5 and 6 of Caring for Health: History and Diversity.[1] Chapter 9 of that book introduced the concept of 'supplier–induced demand' for health care, which is discussed further here. During study of the present chapter you will be asked to read an article in the Reader,[2] 'Priority setting in the NHS' by Alan Williams.

This chapter was written by health economist Alastair Gray, Research Associate at the Centre for Legal Studies, Wolfson College, Oxford University, and a member of the Open University team which wrote the first edition of the 'Health and Disease' series.

Economics and health care

> We never will have all we need. Expectation will always exceed capacity. This service must always be changing, growing and improving, it must always appear inadequate. (Aneurin Bevan in 1948, cited in Foot, 1975, pp. 209 and 210)

In this comment, made to some of its future staff just before the NHS came into existence in 1948, Nye Bevan pin-pointed one of the basic dilemmas the NHS faces. With, on the one hand, an intention to provide comprehensive health services and, on the other hand, limited resources at its disposal, the NHS (like any health-care system) has to perform a continual balancing act: reconciling the demands placed upon it with a supply of resources that is not limitless. Inevitably, the result is some form of health-care *rationing*.

This predicament of scarce resources in a world of apparently boundless desires, of the interplay of supply and demand, is the very stuff of economics. Indeed, on some accounts the identification of economics with the concepts of demand and supply is well-nigh total:

> Some of us, when visiting hospitals, have discovered that by putting on a white coat and talking rudely to nurses it is easy to pass as a physician. To be mistaken for an economist is often even simpler. All one need do is nod gravely and say 'demand and supply'. (Fuchs, 1972, p. 39)

The relationship between these two quantities lies at the heart of providing health care, and it is not surprising, therefore, that economists have become increasingly involved in the health sector. So this chapter begins by examining the ways in which the demand for and supply of health care are formed in the United Kingdom. It then looks at the ways in which rationing of health care takes place in the United Kingdom, and how this compares with rationing in the USA. Next, the chapter considers the extent to which the NHS has succeeded in achieving *equity* in terms of equality of health-care provision. It then examines the various methods that have been proposed to make rationing more explicit and rational, and concludes by considering whether proposed ways of resolving some of these dilemmas have any chance of success. Notice that our focus is primarily on the *strategic* level of policy and decision-making about 'who gets what from the NHS, and why?'

The demand for health care

'Demand' is a word with many meanings. In economics it is conventionally linked to price. Thus, if health care were bought and sold like tomatoes in a market-place, then the demand for health care would normally be defined as the amount of health care that people are prepared to purchase at any particular price. In the NHS, however, although charges are made for a range of items such as prescriptions or spectacles, for courses of dental treatment, and for services such as single rooms, people

[1] *Caring for Health: History and Diversity* (revised edition 1993).

[2] *Health and Disease: A Reader* (revised edition 1994).

generally do not pay at the time they use the health service (it is *zero-priced*). Indeed, removing financial barriers to access and providing a service free at the time of use was one of the founding objectives of the NHS.

If the amount of health care provided by the NHS was not going to be rationed by having price barriers, just how much demand would there be for its services? How much formal health care would people want, if they no longer had to pay for it? In 1948 when the NHS began, nobody was entirely clear about this. The view expressed in the Beveridge Report of 1942 (which formed the basis for the NHS) was that there was an untreated 'pool of sickness' in society because financial barriers had deterred many people from obtaining medical treatment. By offering a free and comprehensive range of treatments, the NHS would initially have to deal with a backlog of demands but, once that had been accomplished, the NHS would be catering for a healthier population and the number of cases it had to treat would fall and then stabilise at a lower level. Consequently, overall expenditure was projected to remain broadly constant for at least twenty years into the future.

□ Which two basic assumptions are embedded in this view?

■ The first is that the demand for the health service is finite; the second is that the health service will cure people and reduce illness, and therefore expenditure will be self-limiting.

In one or two areas of the service there was indeed some evidence of a backlog of demand. For example, in the three years up to 1951 the average number of spectacles supplied free by the NHS was almost 7 million per annum. In the three years after 1951, however, this fell to around 3.5 million per annum. One explanation for this was that direct charges to patients were introduced in 1951 to cut the cost of the ophthalmic services, but there seems little doubt that there had been a backlog of demand caused by an inability to afford spectacles in the past, and that this backlog was being cleared in the first few years of the service. The same pattern occurred with dentures, and again the argument that there was a backlog seems much more plausible than the lurid tales in popular newspapers at the time that people were frantically amassing dozens of free dentures in their cupboards.

These limited exceptions apart, however, the assumptions of the Beveridge Report were rapidly exposed by events as mistaken (as Aneurin Bevan believed they would be). Far from quickly reaching some finite limit and then declining, the number of people turning up at out-patient clinics, accident and emergency departments, and at dentists' or GPs' surgeries, steadily increased from year to year. In fact, according to almost any measure of the amount of services being used—often referred to as **activity data**—the demands on the NHS have increased fairly constantly throughout its existence.

Influences on the level of demand

There are a number of explanations for this turn of events. Most importantly, the demand for services from the NHS has not turned out to be self-limiting, because the *need* for health care is not absolute but relative. If somebody is ill and potentially something can be done to improve her or his condition or prevent it from becoming worse, then she or he is likely to be described as 'in need'. Thus one reason for removing the price barrier to health care derived from the idea that people had needs for health care which were not being met because they did not have the money to express their needs as demands. This was not entirely wrong-headed: as you have seen, it is probable that many people needed spectacles but had not been able to express that need as a demand backed by money.

What *was* wrong was the idea that the need was absolute or fixed: wrong, because the range of things that medical care can do is not fixed, and thus any innovation or development creates a new set of needs (a subject discussed further in Chapter 7); and wrong, because the decision as to whether an individual has a need for health care—and if so, how much of what sort of care—is often made not by that individual alone (referred to as a person's **felt need**), but with the involvement of health professionals. Indeed the concept of the **clinical iceberg**—that is, the notion that the population contains a submerged mass of treatable but untreated conditions—takes us even further away from the idea that need is absolute. For in this case need can be detected not by individuals themselves, but only by clinical examination (**professionally defined need**). The conclusion to be drawn from some estimates of the 'clinical iceberg'—that almost the entire population is in need of medical care, and those who appear not to be have simply been insufficiently examined—demonstrates forcefully just how relative the concept of need can be. It is, at least in part, in the eye of the beholder.

This involvement of others—experts, administrators, researchers, or 'society' as a whole—in judgements about the need for health care is crucial to understanding how demands on the NHS are generated. By and large, patients initiate contact with the NHS themselves, for example, by calling or visiting a GP. But having done so, they are largely in the hands of the doctor, and it is therefore the doctor who makes decisions about what forms of treatment they need and hence (as the previous chapter described) what further demands are placed on the resources of the NHS. It is the GP who decides whether to refer someone to a consultant, the consultant who decides whether hospital in-patient care is required, what pathology tests to order, what drugs to use, and how long to keep the patient in hospital. The doctor, whose role is to supply care, is also cast in the role of demanding care on the patient's behalf. But the doctor may supply more health care than the patient would have chosen had the patient been fully informed (hence the expression *supplier-induced demand*),[3] and so the demand for health care is constantly pressed against the limits of what is supplied.

There are, of course, other factors influencing the demand for health care in the United Kingdom, which are to some extent independent of changing definitions of need, or the existence of supplier-induced demand. Trends in tobacco and alcohol consumption, or in factory and road safety, may all result in a change in the demand for health care, as may long-term changes in overall patterns of disease.

Changes in the demographic structure of the population have also had an effect: the demand for health care is not spread evenly throughout the population and therefore if the proportion of the population in high-demand groups increases, the overall level of demand will rise. For example, in England in 1991 the NHS spent on average just over £500 for every person in the population. However, whereas it spent only around £250 per person aged between 5 and 64 years, it spent around £900 on every person aged 65 to 74 and £2 200 on every person aged 75 or over. So as the proportion of the population who are old or very old rises, so too do the demands placed on the NHS. Similarly, people who are widowed or divorced generally use more health care than those who are married (even after taking account of differences in their ages), so if an increasing proportion of the population were widowed or divorced, all else remaining constant, the demand for health services would increase.

However, let us return for a moment to the idea of shifting definitions of need. Figure 3.1 shows the percentage change between 1979 and 1985 in discharge rates from hospital (that is, the annual number of people discharged from hospitals relative to the size of the local population) by age-group.

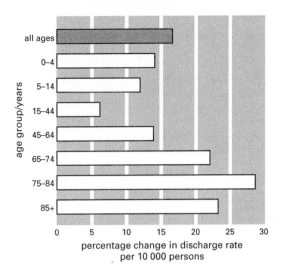

Figure 3.1 *Changes in the discharge rate from non-psychiatric hospitals in England, 1979–85, by age-group. (Source: Bosanquet, N. and Gray, A. (1989)* Will You Still Love Me? *National Association of Health Authorities, Birmingham, Table 7, p. 15)*

□ What pattern does Figure 3.1 reveal?

■ It shows that discharge rates rose in all age-groups, but especially among those aged over 65.

In other words, the demand for hospital services by elderly people has increased not only because the age-structure has altered, but also because the demands made by elderly people have increased. These demands have risen because, for example, technological changes such as new anaesthetics have made it much safer to operate on elderly people. So new needs have been created, increasing the level of demand placed on the NHS.[4]

In fact, these new demands have been a much more significant cause of rising demand for health care than alterations in the demographic structure *per se,*[5] and prompt the question: if demands for health care are constantly increasing, partly induced by the health professions themselves and partly by scientific and technological innovations, then what is to stop the entire economy from gradually becoming an extraordinarily elaborate health-care system? The answer, of course, is

---

[3]See *Caring for Health: History and Diversity* (revised edition 1993), Chapter 9.

[4]Technological changes such as these are discussed in Chapter 7.

[5]Evidence on this is presented in *Caring for Health: History and Diversity* (revised edition 1993), Chapter 9.

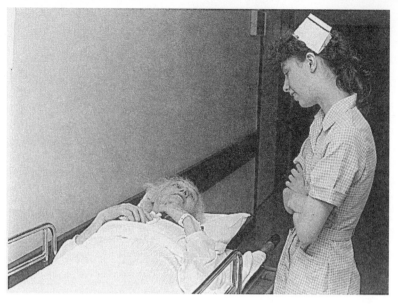

An elderly woman waits in a hospital corridor for treatment. More elderly people receiving a growing range and amount of care means that the NHS devotes a far higher proportion of its resources to elderly people than it did in the 1950s and 1960s. (Photo: Mike Levers)

that central government and the Health Departments (the DH in England, and its parallels in Scotland, Wales and Northern Ireland) are also involved in making strategic decisions about just how many demands are to be met: they have to decide what level of resources to supply to the health service. So before looking at the way in which managers, doctors, nurses and other health workers come to terms with having to operate within these limits we need to look at how these limits are set.

The supply of health care

Every day, many people involved in the strategic, operational and clinical management of the NHS make decisions about the supply of health care, whether this be the size of food portions served by catering staff, or the decision by a consultant to implant a pace-maker in someone with a heart condition. Since 1948, however, the overall supply of health care in the NHS has been limited by the amount of money available in any year. The responsibility for setting this annual limit, and limits on many other expenditure programmes, rests with central government.

Limits on health-care expenditure

All governments have some general policy towards what total public expenditure should be, quite apart from the policies towards programmes within the total, and have

sought either to increase or reduce it for various reasons. From 1941 to the 1970s, for example, successive governments manipulated the total level of public expenditure in an attempt to regulate the economy as a whole. In consequence, individual programmes were affected by wider national economic policies and events. In 1976, for example, an economic crisis resulted in the International Monetary Fund requiring the government to reduce spending across the board; the NHS, like other programmes, experienced a squeeze.[6] In contrast, during the 1980s, this regulatory view of public expenditure was supplanted by a view that public expenditure was inherently harmful to the economy and should be reduced wherever possible.

In general terms, therefore, the decision about how much money to make available to the NHS is part of the government's wider economic strategy and reflects its attitude towards what the level of total public expenditure should be.

In 1948 there was no definite view as to how much the NHS would cost to run. For some services, for example, the family practitioner services, it was decided that expenditure would simply have to be 'demand-led', and the bill picked up afterwards. But for the bulk of services,

[6]See *Caring for Health: History and Diversity* (revised edition 1993), Chapters 7 and 9.

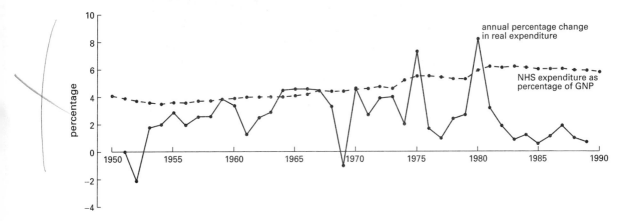

Figure 3.2 *Spending on the NHS as a percentage of Gross National Product, and annual changes in real expenditure on the NHS, 1949–90. (Source:* Annual Abstract of Statistics, HMSO, various years)

the initial level of expenditure was determined largely by the past: enough to continue to run the buildings and pay the staff that the NHS had inherited.

Even so, in the first few years of the NHS there was a great deal of confusion over precisely how much it was costing and whether the amount was changing.

□ Why might it be difficult to compare the cost of running the NHS over different years?

■ The main difficulty is inflation (a sustained rise in the general level of prices) which makes it necessary to distinguish expenditure in current money prices from expenditure adjusted to take account of changing money prices (usually known as expenditure in constant prices or real expenditure).

When the cost of the NHS was fully investigated in the early 1950s, it was found that it had increased very much less than generally thought, not just because general inflation had been ignored, but because the rate of inflation experienced by the NHS was higher than the general rate. The general rate of inflation is normally measured by the **Retail Price Index (RPI)**, which measures the changes in price from year to year of a 'basket' of goods and services (e.g. food, drink, tobacco, clothes, energy, transport, housing) bought by an average consumer. But some items change in price more rapidly than others, so anybody buying a 'basket' of goods and services that isn't average may experience a higher or lower rate of inflation than that measured by the RPI. The 'basket' bought by senior citizens has tended to have a higher than average rate of inflation, and so too has the 'basket' bought by the NHS, mainly because it is so labour-intensive.

In the 1950s, after post-war austerity gave way to a long phase of fairly continuous economic growth in the United Kingdom and the world economies, real expenditure on the NHS began to rise. So too did the share of the United Kingdom's Gross National Product (GNP)[7] devoted to it, as Figure 3.2 shows.

□ What does Figure 3.2 reveal about NHS expenditure in the early 1950s?

■ During this period it was actually declining as a percentage of GNP.

□ What happened during the later 1950s and 1960s?

■ NHS expenditure as a percentage of GNP grew fairly continuously over this period.

Throughout the 1960s and into the early 1970s the strategy underlying central government decisions about what to allocate to the NHS was geared towards growth and was relatively informal: government ministers collected the views of regional hospital boards about requirements and future developments, and then discussed with the Cabinet and the Treasury the amount of money likely to be available, all within a tacit understanding that the economy was growing and some real increase in NHS funding would be forthcoming. Because there was growth in the economic system as a whole, there was no

---

[7]Gross National Product (GNP) is the money value of all the goods and services available to the nation, including income from abroad, e.g. from foreign investment.

necessity to make painful decisions about the relative priority of one area of government expenditure compared with another; and within the NHS, there was little inducement to think about the relative priorities of different parts of the service.

In the 1970s, however, the growth of the economy slowed down, government control over expenditure began to tighten, and the whole relationship between central government and the NHS began to change. This continued into the 1980s. One important feature of this tightened control was the introduction of **cash limits**. Until 1974–5, the annual sum allocated for the NHS included an allowance for the predicted level of inflation. But if prices subsequently rose by more than predicted, extra money was voted through Parliament to cover the increases. This process is known as **volume planning**, because it allows the volume or quantity of services to be maintained despite any changes in prices.

But in the mid-1970s, as the rate of inflation increased and became more unpredictable, this procedure changed, and in 1976–7 a fully-fledged system of cash limits was introduced: if inflation turned out to be higher than allowed for, no extra cash was automatically forthcoming, and the volume of services might have to be reduced. By 1985, cash limits were being applied to all NHS spending except the family practitioner services, which remained 'demand-led'.

☐ Look back at Figure 3.2. What happened to NHS expenditure during the 1980s?

■ As a percentage of GNP it peaked around 1982 and then began to decline.

Establishing the amount of total national wealth being devoted to the NHS is relatively straightforward, but it is no easy matter to establish how NHS expenditure has changed from year to year in real or volume terms—that is, after allowing for inflation in the NHS. However, Figure 3.2 also shows an estimate of the annual percentage change in real spending on the NHS. As the figure reveals, this has varied substantially from year to year, but there have been very few years indeed when real spending actually fell.

Charging patients for services

Apart from this grip on the purse-strings of the NHS, the government also has at its disposal a more direct control over the level of demand for the NHS—by setting charges for services. The government raises the money to fund the NHS from three main sources. The great bulk is drawn from general funds raised through taxation, duties, excises and so on (known as the Consolidated Fund). Eighty-three per cent of NHS funds came from this source in 1990. Another source is the National Insurance contributions deducted from wages and salaries, a portion of which is set aside for the NHS. In 1990 around 15 per cent of NHS funds came from this source. The third source is from direct charges to patients for services.

Conservative and Labour governments have different attitudes to health-service charges, as Figure 3.3 shows. Although these charges have never raised more than five per cent of the total cost of the NHS, they are not evenly spread across its services: the dental service (excluding hospital dentistry), for example, raised around 25 per cent of its costs through charges in 1990. The main

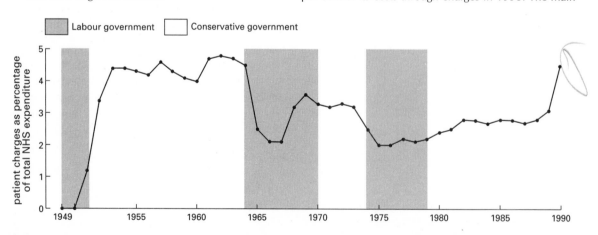

Figure 3.3 *Proportion of the total cost of the NHS raised by direct charges to patients, 1950–90. (Source: Department of Health:* Health and Personal Social Service Statistics for England, *various years)*

argument for charges is that they may reduce the 'trivial' use of services, although responsibility for this must lie mainly with the health professionals who prescribe treatment. The main argument levelled against direct charges is that they re-introduce financial barriers which may discourage people from seeking health care, even though many patients are, in principle, exempt. Research has generally concluded that they do have disincentive effects on patients: typically, a 10 per cent increase in the charge for a service reduces demand for that service by approximately 2 per cent. Moreover, some evidence from the very large-scale Rand health insurance experiment in the USA has indicated that reduced use because of increased charges may have adverse effects on the health status of the population (e.g. Bailit *et al.*, 1985; Brook *et al.*, 1983).

Controls on private health care

Although this chapter is primarily concerned with the NHS, it should be noted that the government can exercise some strategic control over the supply of health care by the *private* sector. For many years there were few deliberate attempts to expand the private sector and a number of controls to restrain it. Despite this, in the years after 1948 the number of people holding private health insurance policies rose steadily, from 120 000 persons insured in 1950 to one million in 1960 and two million by 1970. However, from the late 1970s onwards the private sector expanded rapidly: the number of people covered by the main insurance companies jumped from 2.2 million in 1977 to 4.1 million in 1981, and reached over 5 million by 1990—or around 9 per cent of the United Kingdom population. Most of this increase during the 1980s occurred in company or employee schemes, encouraged by government policy through tax breaks which made it cheaper for companies to offer private health insurance as a fringe benefit.

Finally, a spectacular example of the government relaxing the expenditure controls was provided during the 1980s by the growth of private nursing and residential homes. These are not normally considered to be part of the health-care system as such, but increasingly have taken in people who otherwise might have been in long-term hospital accommodation. In 1979 the government was paying around £10 million each year towards the support of people requiring such accommodation, but by 1988 this had grown to £1 *billion,* paid via the Department of Social Security (DSS) rather than the various Health Departments.

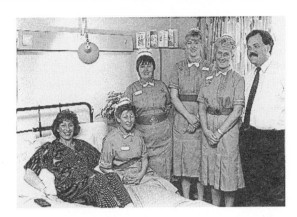

Scene in a private hospital. The private sector expanded rapidly in the 1980s, especially in the area of elective surgery for adults of working age. (Photo: Mike Levers)

Rationing of health care

You have now seen that on the one hand, the overall amount of health care supplied through the NHS is limited, in the last resort, by central government, and on the other hand that there appears to be no limit to the potential demands for NHS services. Rationing is the inevitable result. How in practice does this occur?

Waiting lists

One highly visible way in which health care is rationed in the NHS is by means of queues or *waiting lists* for treatments. In 1991, 830 000 people were on hospital in-patient waiting lists in the United Kingdom, and although the average wait to admission was less than five weeks, around one in five people had to wait for at least six months, and for some of these the wait could be much longer. Surveys have found that up to 20 per cent of in-patients are caused some inconvenience or distress by waiting for admission, and that those waiting for out-patient appointments are frequently distressed, in physical pain or discomfort, or anxious. It is perhaps not surprising, therefore, that the areas in which waiting lists are greatest—for elective (non-emergency) surgery—are precisely the areas in which the private sector has experienced the biggest growth. The Audit Commission Report recommending the expansion of NHS day surgery (which you read during Chapter 1) is one response to the problem of waiting lists.

Of course, waiting lists have a number of other causes besides being rationing devices: for example, to try to ensure that people have some advance notice of admission, or to obtain a stable mix of patients, so that theatre sessions are not comprised of a large number of minor operations one day and complicated operations the next. They may also reflect professional preferences: the medical conditions most commonly found on long waiting lists tend to be poorly researched and 'unfashionable' with the medical profession. And waiting lists are not always what they seem to be: they can be artificially inflated by consultants or hospital or purchasing authorities trying to obtain extra funds for their area. There is also widespread evidence that waiting lists can be inefficiently kept, and may include names of people who have recovered, moved to another area or had treatment elsewhere. So they are not an infallible guide to 'shortages' in the NHS or the extent to which services are rationed.

Influences on rationing decisions: a comparison of Britain and the USA

To get beyond the waiting lists, let us look at a study published in 1984, entitled *The Painful Prescription: Rationing Hospital Care*, in which two Americans, Henry Aaron, an economist, and William Schwarz, a physician, examined the differences in the provision of a range of services between the NHS (excluding Northern Ireland) and American health care. Their starting-point was the observation that the per capita expenditure on hospital in-patient care in Britain in 1981 was barely a half (53 per cent) of that in the USA. Their objective was to explore the way in which rationing occurred in these circumstances, by selecting ten different forms of hospital treatment and comparing the rates of use in the two countries.

In three of their ten case studies—treatment of haemophilia (failure of the blood to clot), mega voltage radiotherapy for cancer patients, and bone-marrow transplants—approximately the same level of treatment was provided in Britain as in the USA. In another instance—chemotherapy for cancer patients—it was not clear how levels of treatment compared in the two countries. But in the remaining six examples they studied, the levels of provision in Britain in 1981 were markedly lower than in the USA. These included X-ray examinations, carried out half as often in Britain; the treatment of chronic renal (kidney) failure, where the rate of dialysis adjusted for population size was one-third that in the USA, but the transplantation rate was similar; and coronary artery surgery, performed in Britain at one-tenth the rate of that in the USA. Similarly, the CT scanning[8] capability of Britain was found to be one-sixth that of the USA, and the

number of intensive-care beds relative to population in Britain was only 10 to 20 per cent of the number in the USA.

To increase the provision of just these six forms of treatment in Britain to the same rate as in the USA would involve increasing the total hospital budget of the NHS by 18 per cent. Moreover, in the instances where rationing in the NHS seems most clearly marked, as in dialysis treatment for kidney failure, resource limits are not necessarily mentioned by GPs or others when explaining their rationing decisions to a patient (or to her or his family):

> I would say that mother's or aunt's kidneys have failed or are failing and there is very little that anybody can do about it because of her age and general physical state, and that it would be my suggestion or my advice that we spare her any further investigation, any further painful procedure and we would just make her as comfortable as we can for what remains of her life. (Cited in Aaron and Schwarz, 1984, p. 37)

Age, diabetes, physical disability, mental illness, hepatitis and lack of facilities for home dialysis are all incorporated to some degree into the decision whether or not to provide treatment. Moreover, GPs become attuned to the likelihood of patients being accepted or rejected if they are referred to a renal specialist, and therefore adjust their referral patterns accordingly. Rationing thus becomes part of accepted standards of clinical practice: doctors not only commit resources, they may also withhold them.

It should also be noted that the difference between the NHS and the USA is not uniform: the provision of some treatments is much lower in the NHS, but others are provided at almost comparable rates. Aaron and Schwarz deduced from these observed variations a set of seven factors that appeared to result in a greater likelihood of obtaining services:

1   Age: likelihood of treatment increased for children compared with adults (particularly elderly people).

2   'Dread' disease: likelihood of treatment increased for diseases inspiring fear, especially cancers.

3   Visibility of illness: likelihood of treatment increased if suffering is severe and obvious.

4   Advocacy: likelihood of treatment increased if organised pressure groups exist.

5   Aggregate cost: likelihood of treatment increased if the total cost of a programme seems negligible.

6   Need for capital funds: likelihood of treatment increased if capital outlays are fairly low.

---

[8]'CT' stands for 'computer-aided tomography', a method of scanning the soft tissues of the body. It is described further in Chapter 7 of this book, and in another book in this series, *Studying Health and Disease* (Open University Press, 1985; revised edition 1994).

7   Cost of alternatives: likelihood of treatment increased if the costs of not treating exceed the costs of active intervention (for example, providing hip replacements may be much cheaper than caring for people with osteoarthrosis of the joint).

Given the systematically higher levels of provision in the USA, it is tempting to conclude that health care is not rationed in the USA. However, if the NHS were compared with health-care services for the majority of the population in, say, Bangladesh, then the temptation would be to see the NHS, not as a heavily rationed system, but as a model of the *absence* of rationing. You might then draw a range of conclusions about the way accepted standards of clinical practice in Bangladesh have been altered to accommodate the lack of resources. The whole point of this comparison is to emphasise that rationing is only useful as a concept which summarises a *relationship* between supply and demand. The existence of a higher level of supply of health care in the USA must therefore be placed in the context of the level of demand in the USA.

When this is done, two facts emerge. First, there has been a long-standing concern in the USA that some treatments are over-supplied relative to their demonstrated effectiveness, or to the level of need for them; this is partly because the economic structure of American health care provides powerful incentives for supplier-induced demands.

    ☐ Can you suggest why?

    ■ Many American doctors' incomes increase the more operations they perform or the more drugs they prescribe.

Second, in some respects the American health-care system also rations, but in different ways from that of the United Kingdom. In particular, the absence of universal health insurance in the USA results in rationing of health care by means of price barriers; in practice, around 18 million people, or 8.6 per cent of the population, are permanently uninsured, and a further 16 million people, or 7.5 per cent of the population, are temporarily uninsured for part of any year, while many others are insufficiently insured to cope with serious illness.

The point is not, therefore, that health care in the USA is *un*rationed, but that rationing takes a different form from that in the NHS, occurring on the basis of financial means or employment status, for example. This is also incorporated into accepted standards of clinical practice in the USA, as the following two cases reported in *The Lancet* in 1984 demonstrate:

A 86-year-old Cuban refugee was taken to a private hospital emergency room in California after being beaten. He lapsed into a coma as two neurosurgeons refused to respond to the emergency physician's calls for assistance because the patient lacked health insurance. After transfer to a public hospital, a skull fracture and irreversible brain damage due to intracranial bleeding was discovered.

A woman of 21 was hit by a truck and taken to the nearest (private) emergency facility. Despite multiple leg, ankle, pelvic, and rib fractures, and a rapidly falling haematocrit (evidence of severe bleeding), she was transferred 30 miles to a public hospital because she was uninsured. A ruptured aorta was diagnosed, and she was transferred to another private hospital for surgical repair because the thoracic surgery programme at the public hospital had been closed several years earlier. (Himmelstein and Woolhandler, 1984, p. 392)

Thus, whatever the level of overall resources, and whatever the system of health care, the services provided inevitably finish up being rationed, but in very different ways and according to widely differing criteria.

In search of equity

Health care may be rationed, therefore, but is it rationed in a way that might be regarded as fair? The 1944 White Paper on the NHS stated that one objective of the NHS would be to ensure that everyone 'shall have equal opportunity to benefit' from the services available. To what extent has this been achieved? Let us start by noting some different interpretations of the phrase. *Equal* might refer to an equal share of health care between individuals, or between different social groups: social classes, sexes, age groups, disease groups, or groups in different regions of the country. *Opportunity to benefit* might refer to the availability of health services, having access to health services, making use of health services, or trying to get everyone onto the same level of health—in other words, some approach towards *equity,* i.e. a share appropriate to the person's need for health care.

    ☐ Suppose 'opportunity to benefit' from the NHS was interpreted as the achievement of equality of levels of health between different social classes. What implications might this have for other interpretations of 'opportunity to benefit' described above?

■ In trying to attain equal levels of health, it might be necessary to create deliberately unequal access or use of health services, so that those in poorest health received most health care.

□ What other assumptions are contained in this particular objective?

■ It assumes that health care can have significant effects on health, and that health inequalities between social classes can be tackled through the health service. It also implicitly excludes inequalities other than those of social class: for example the gender inequalities in health that exist within each social class.[9]

Each different interpretation of this objective of equality contains a different set of implications for the NHS. For example, if equality of *use* of services is sought, should the NHS actively seek out people who might benefit from health care, rather than waiting for them to turn up? Expanding such 'outreach' services has its advocates, but how far should it go before it becomes an authoritarian intrusion rather than a service? Perhaps because there are so many difficulties associated with different ways of defining 'equality', the strategic management of the NHS has tended to devote most attention to just one particular aspect: the *availability* of services in different regions of the country. To a lesser extent, it has also sought to reduce differences in the standard of care offered to different patient groups. How much has it achieved?

Regional differences in service provision

In 1948, one of the most glaring aspects of the uneven distribution of health services between regions was the availability of GPs:

> ...the number of residents per GP was twice as great in Kensington as in Hampstead, thrice as great in Harrow; four times as great in Bradford, five times in Wakefield, six times in West Bromwich, and seven times in South Shields. (PEP, 1944)

By means of agencies called Medical Practices Committees, the distribution of GPs was significantly altered after the NHS was established. Different areas of the country were classified as relatively over- or under-doctored, and GPs wishing to set up practice had to apply to the committees for permission. Those applying to practise in over-doctored ('restricted') areas were almost certain to be refused, while those applying to practise in under-doctored ('designated') areas were automatically permitted.

The main advantage of the system was that it used powers of refusal and was therefore less coercive than a system compelling doctors to relocate. The disadvantage was that the system could have only a gradual effect, as each year only a small proportion of GPs entered practice and had to apply for permission. However, the proportion of the population in areas classified as under-doctored did fall very sharply; in England and Wales, for example, from around 50 per cent in 1952 to barely 2 per cent in 1982. In important ways, therefore, the scheme was successful, though *within* the areas classified by the Medical Practices Committees the distribution of GPs could still be highly uneven. In particular, access to primary health care was very poor in London and some other inner-city areas, as the Acheson Committee on primary health care in inner London reported in 1981 (London Health Planning Consortium, 1981). By 1992, an evaluation of progress since the Acheson Report noted considerable improvements, but the provision of primary care in the capital remained relatively poor (Jarman and Bosanquet, 1992).

Plans to reduce inequalities in the resources distributed to different regional hospital boards took longer to appear: the more hospital facilities a region had, the more funding it received, and vice versa. But in 1970 a formula aimed at ironing out the regional differences in expenditure on the hospital services in England was introduced, and in 1976 this was refined by the *Resource Allocation Working Party* (RAWP), and therefore became known as the **RAWP formula**.

The RAWP formula, like its predecessor, only covered the Regional Health Authorities (RHAs) of England, not the United Kingdom as a whole. The relative needs of each region were calculated on the basis of two main factors: the size of the population served, taking into account its age and sex composition; and the standardised mortality ratio of the region, which was taken as a measure of underlying morbidity. Various adjustments were then made to take account of flows of patients across regional boundaries, the existence of teaching hospitals, and so on. The resulting revenue requirement or target was then compared with the actual resources each region received. If they were below requirement, they would get extra resources each year until they reached the target; if they were above requirement, their allocation of resources would be held back. There would not be any actual cutback, rather some regions'

[9]The unequal distribution of health and disease in different groups in the contemporary population of the United Kingdom is described in another book in this series, *World Health and Disease* (Open University Press, 1993), Chapter 9.

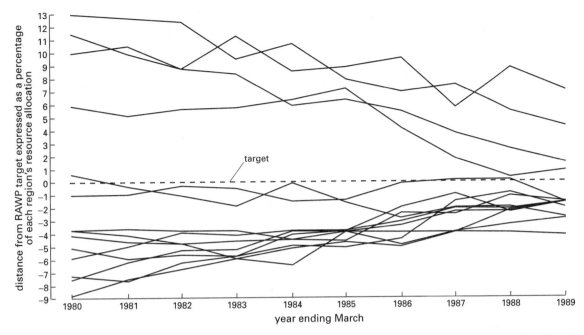

Figure 3.4 *Distances from the RAWP revenue target of the 14 RHAs in England, 1979–89. (Source: Department of Health and Social Security (1988)* Review of the Resource Allocation Working Party Formula: Final Report by the NHS Management Board. *DHSS, London, Figure 1.1)*

allocations would grow less rapidly than others; neither was it to be too sudden, instead the adjustments were to take place over a ten-year period.

Figure 3.4 illustrates the progress of the 14 English RHAs towards the RAWP target between 1979 and 1989.

☐ How would you describe the pattern in Figure 3.4?

■ Generally, the distances from the target allocations were reduced, but very few regions had reached the target by 1989.

The application of the RAWP formula raised many complex issues: it only altered the *funds* given to regions, not the services themselves; it did not acknowledge that some regions might be more efficient than others in the way they used their resources; and it did not address the many important inequalities in provision *within* regions, although some RHAs did devise similar formulae to distribute resources to their District Health Authorities (DHAs). But despite these limitations, it did begin seriously to alter the status quo for the first time since the NHS had begun.

The RAWP formula was devised on the assumption that no region would actually lose anything: the idea was

that continued growth in the total NHS budget would make redistribution painless, through a gradual *levelling up* of resources. During the 1980s, however, this assumption was severely strained by tight restrictions on total NHS spending, so that increasingly it seemed that regional inequalities could only be reduced by *levelling down* of the better-off RHAs, a very much more painful exercise than being held constant. The NHS reforms begun in 1989 with *Working for Patients* and the creation of an 'internal market' in health care, encouraged the idea that money should follow patients to wherever treatment was on offer,[10] and led to the RAWP formula being adapted in favour of a simpler mechanism. However, it was not clear at the time of writing (1992) what the implications of this might be for equitable resource allocation in the NHS.

The RAWP formula also exposed a much older issue. It only covered resource allocations between regions within England, not between England and other parts of the United Kingdom. Scotland, Wales and Northern

[10]See *Caring for Health: History and Diversity* (revised edition 1993), Chapter 7 and 'Britain's health-care experiment' by Patricia Day and Rudolf Klein, in *Health and Disease: A Reader* (revised edition 1994).

Ireland have all produced their own formulae for distributing resources in their own areas, but there is no explicit formula for deciding how to distribute resources to the component parts of the United Kingdom, although wide disparities exist in the level of health funding between the four parts of the United Kingdom.

Priority groups

Another dimension of inequality in health-care provision can be found between patient or disease groups. Not every patient in the NHS receives equal priority in treatment or attention. For example two-thirds of the psychiatric hospitals the NHS inherited in 1948 had been built in the nineteenth century. In 1954, when Parliament debated the subject of mental health for the first time in twenty-four years, it was pointed out that although mentally ill and mentally handicapped patients occupied 42 per cent of the NHS's beds, they had attracted only 16 per cent of all NHS capital investment, and a miserly 1 per cent of research funds.

During the late 1960s, a fresh wave of criticism of the low priority being given to patients in psychiatric, geriatric and psychogeriatric hospitals was set in motion by the publication of a book in 1967 entitled *Sans Everything—a Case to Answer*, by Barbara Robb.[11] The ensuing official inquiries did not fix the blame solely on lack of money. Local hospital problems were also cited, as were management difficulties. However, it was clear that the problems could not be solved without additional money. In 1976, the Department of Health and Social Security (DHSS) published its first *priorities document*—a general review of existing patterns of expenditure on different patient groups, and how it wished to see these patterns of expenditure alter in the future. In particular, it identified a list of priority groups which became known as the **Cinderella services** because of their traditionally low level of funding:

> ...the central proposal in this document is that much of the available 'growth money' should be concentrated on services used mainly by the elderly and the physically handicapped, the mentally ill and handicapped, and children. (DHSS, 1976, p. 27)

[11]*Sans* is the French word for 'without'; the title of the book refers to Shakespeare's description of the seventh age of mankind as 'Sans teeth, sans eyes, sans taste, sans everything', (*As You Like It,* II. vii, written *c.* 1599). Criticism of mental health services in the 1960s is discussed more fully in *Caring for Health: History and Diversity* (revised edition 1993), Chapter 6.

Table 3.1 shows the priority ('Cinderella') and non-priority services in the NHS, and the change in expenditure on them between 1976–7 and 1986–7.

Table 3.1 Hospital and community current expenditure on priority and non-priority services in England, 1976–7 and 1986–7

Service area	Expenditure (£million) in 1986–7 prices in:		Percentage growth in expenditure between 1976–7 and 1986–7
	1976–7	1986–7	
Priority Services			
mental handicap in-patient	479.3	495.6	3.4
mental handicap out-patient	0.6	1	66.7
mental illness in-patient	942.4	998.2	5.9
mental illness out-patient	44.3	71.4	61.2
geriatric in-patient	776.6	902.4	16.2
geriatric out-patient	4.7	8.1	72.3
sub-total	**2 247.9**	**2 476.7**	**10.2**
Non-Priority Services			
acute in-patient	3 456.4	3 519.2	1.8
acute out-patient	915.3	1 134.5	23.9
obstetric in-patient	438.5	431.9	–1.5
obstetric out-patient	57.7	81.3	40.9
sub-total:	**4 867.9**	**5 166.9**	**6.1**

Data from Social Services Committee (1988) *Public Expenditure on the NHS: A Memorandum Received from the DHSS*, House of Commons session 1987–88, Table 3.1.

☐ In Table 3.1, look first of all at the size of the budgets of the different services. Which part of the service dominates the overall expenditure?

■ Acute in-patient care is by far the largest single area of expenditure.

☐ How much evidence does Table 3.1 give for a shift towards priority services?

■ Between 1976–7 and 1986–7 the priority services as a whole grew more rapidly, but around £230 million of the additional moneys went to the priority services, compared with £300 million extra for non-priority services (although priority groups such as elderly people are in fact heavy users of non-priority services such as acute hospital care).

The generally slow progress towards changing priorities in the NHS has raised a number of questions. In the first place, the priorities documents have only been advisory, with no mechanism for forcing health authorities to follow them. Some health authorities have made more progress than others, but it is not clear that any sanctions can be imposed on those that are not following the advice. There are other problems. Altering priorities is an exercise affecting many groups of health-service staff, whose own priorities seem in some instances to be contrary to those of the various Health Departments. For example, there exist long-standing difficulties in getting nursing staff to work in 'Cinderella services', and this, coupled with a lack of resources, is reflected in the low nurse-staffing levels in such hospitals.

Between two and three times as much is spent per in-patient day in the hospitals providing non-priority services as in the hospitals providing priority services, and this order of difference is reflected in the amounts spent on nursing care. It is also reflected in many other aspects of hospital care: for example, in long-stay hospitals standards of catering generally remain lower than in short-stay hospitals, and the status attached to medical careers in the priority areas is also generally lower than in the non-priority areas. So the officially designated priority areas in the health service are not by and large the priority areas for some health-care occupations.

A further problem is that the policy guide-lines contained in the priorities documents do not affect only the NHS. In particular, the emphasis on increasing care to dependent groups 'in the community', rather than in hospital or other residential accommodation, requires the close participation both of local authorities and lay carers. This will be examined in more detail in Chapter 8.

Finally, to what extent is it possible for the NHS to set priorities independently of the attitudes of people *outside* the health service? A number of surveys of public attitudes to health-care priorities have suggested that highest priority seems to be given to the officially low-priority acute hospital services, while officially high-priority services tend to be well down the list. (Such discrepancies between public and government preferences were also noted in Chapter 2, over the provision of care that was not

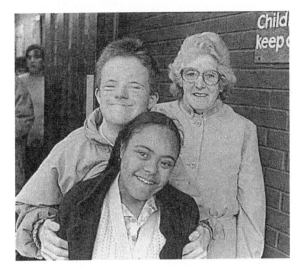

Although a 'priority service', spending on care of mentally handicapped people grew more slowly than on the 'non-priority services' between 1977 and 1987. (Latterly the term 'learning disabled' has been preferred.) (Photo: Mike Levers)

demonstrably effective, e.g. for extremely low-weight babies.) Of course it is possible that most people are generally unaware of the poor standards of care for some of the official priority groups, and would modify their priorities if they had more information. However, as the Aaron and Schwartz research discussed earlier in this chapter suggested, factors such as public 'dread' of particular diseases, or the public visibility of particular illnesses, do seem to be reflected in current patterns of rationing, and it is not clear that this could or indeed should be ignored.

The pursuit of efficiency

As you have seen, some form of rationing permeates all health-care systems, posing many dilemmas for all concerned, whether patients, health professionals, politicians or tax-payers. Although these dilemmas are often profound, a number of methods have been proposed to make them more tractable, and one of these is cost-effectiveness analysis.

Cost-effectiveness analysis

Suppose, to begin, there are two methods of treating a particular disease: for example, treatment of a duodenal ulcer using a drug or by means of surgical removal. If the evidence suggests that these are equally *effective* treatments, so that the same proportion of people are freed of all symptoms in the same period of time, then it would seem to make sense to compare the costs and use the method that costs least: in other words, the treatment that costs least would be more **cost-effective**.

This example illustrates the basic procedure of a **cost-effectiveness analysis** in health care, which is the basis of many *evaluations* of health services, as you will see in Chapter 4. Put simply, the costs of a health-care treatment or programme are compared with the benefits obtained. The result would normally be expressed in terms of a cost/effectiveness ratio: for example, £200 per person cured of a duodenal ulcer by drug therapy, compared to £300 per person cured of a duodenal ulcer by means of surgery.

Going on one step, it may often be desirable that comparisons are not just restricted to different ways of treating the same condition—drugs or surgery for a duodenal ulcer—but are made between different conditions: for example, is it more cost-effective to spend limited health-care resources on hip replacement operations than on heart transplants? However, it will not be possible to make such a comparison if the effectiveness of the treatments is measured in different units: *avoidance of death* from heart transplantation, but *reduction in disability* from hip replacement.

What is required is some common measurement of effectiveness, such as lives saved, or years of life (life-years) gained. If a measure of effectiveness such as life-years saved can be used in different appraisals, it becomes possible to compare the relative cost-effectiveness of different treatments or programmes by comparing the costs per life-year saved.

Taking another step, life-years saved are not an adequate measure of outcome if a health-care programme makes an important impact on morbidity or disability, or allows someone to live longer but at less than full health. In such instances, it would be desirable to find some measure of effectiveness that incorporates changes both in the quantity and in the *quality* of life.

QALYs

A possible candidate for such a measure is the **quality-adjusted life year**, or **QALY**. For example, if a treatment programme delays death by six months but leaves the patient in pain or bedridden, then that 0.5 of an additional life year can be 'weighted', so that in units of QALYs it amounts to *less* than six months. Similarly, if a treatment improves physical status or reduces the duration of pain or disability, the change in weights will result in an *increased* number of QALYs.

Cost-effectiveness analyses[12] that make use of QALYs as the measure of benefit/effect are increasingly referred

to as **cost-utility studies**. They may be a suitable method of evaluation if:

1 Quality of life is one of the outcomes, or is the important outcome;

2 The programme being investigated affects morbidity and mortality, and the investigators wish to combine these into a single outcome measure;

3 The investigators wish to compare a programme to others that have already been evaluated using cost-utility analysis.

(Torrance, 1986, p. 5)

Some of these issues are explored in an article by health economist Alan Williams entitled 'Priority setting in the NHS', which is in the Reader.[13] You should read it now.

☐ According to Williams, what is the main difficulty faced by purchasers in the NHS in deciding what health-care activities are most worth buying?

■ That we currently know very little about the benefits or the costs of most health activities, making it hard to assess value for money.

☐ In the examples given by Williams, what two pieces of information are required in order to measure the health gain from, for instance, a Coronary Artery By-pass Graft (CABG)?

■ In order to measure the health gain, it is necessary to have information on the improved *length* of life from the intervention, and the improved *quality* of life.

In arguing in favour of the use of a QALY framework to aid decision-making in health care, advocates such as Williams acknowledge its crudity, but claim that a sketch map is better than nothing when you are lost in a fog. More generally, the QALY framework is commended by some on the grounds that it makes difficult moral choices and rationing decisions explicit and more consistent, and counters the tendency of some doctors to 'shroud-wave', that is, to make an emotional appeal that, unless they get their way, patients will die.

However, there are also many criticisms of the QALY approach, which go far beyond technical doubts about measurement. For example, as Williams acknowledges,

---

[12]For example, see Table 9.4 in Chapter 9.

[13]*Health and Disease: A Reader* (revised edition 1994).

individuals and groups of the population do not always agree on the valuations of particular health states, raising the question of whose valuations should prevail. The approach does not take account of the number of dependants a patient has, although many would claim that this could be relevant in making rationing decisions. The QALY framework suggests that a treatment that extends one person's life by 20 years is equivalent to a treatment extending 20 people's lives by one year, or 2 000 people's lives by a few days—an equivalence that many people might find hard to accept. Some people have even doubted whether there is obvious merit in making all decisions explicit and coherent, arguing instead that idiosyncratic and opaque decision-making by doctors may be more humane and democratic. And the fact that such issues have been fiercely debated in TV programmes, the medical press and elsewhere, illustrates that rationing of health care has many political and moral as well as technical dimensions.

Resolving the dilemmas

The Oregon experiment

Perhaps the most extreme application to date of an explicit rationing system for health care has been devised in the State of Oregon in the USA. There, the commissioners responsible for administering the Medicaid public insurance scheme (for those on low incomes) had insufficient funds to give the full range of available medical treatments to everyone in the state who had no private insurance. In the late 1980s they decided that, rather than letting the poorest sections of the community receive little or no health care, it would be better to ration the types of treatment available. Taking a wide range of the most common diseases, they decided that if they could rank the treatments provided according to their cost, improvement in quality of life, and treatment effectiveness, then they could start at the top of the resulting list and work down until the available money was used up, thus ensuring that the largest number of people gained access to the most cost-effective services.

The initial results of this exercise were criticised widely: for example, headaches appeared as a much higher priority for treatment than cystic fibrosis. However, a revised list was prepared, backed up with surveys of public opinion towards health-care rationing. Table 3.2 gives some examples of the kinds of conditions that appeared at the top and bottom of the list.

Table 3.2 Health priorities in Oregon

Top ten health priorities	Bottom ten health priorities
pneumococcal pneumonia, bronchopneumonia, influenza with pneumonia	gynaecomastia (benign swelling of the breast)
tuberculosis	kidney cyst
peritonitis (an inflammation of the abdominal cavity)	terminal AIDS-related disease (with less than 10% survival rate at 5 years)
foreign body in pharynx, larynx, trachea, bronchus, oesophagus	chronic pancreatitis (untreatable inflammation of the pancreas)
appendicitis	superficial wounds without infections
ruptured intestine	constitutional (inherited) aplastic anaemia
hernia with obstruction or gangrene	prolapsed urethral mucosa (a minor urinary tract condition)
croup syndrome or acute laryngitis (upper respiratory ailments)	central retinal artery occlusion (blockage)
acute orbital cellulitis (inflammation of tissue around the eye)	extremely low birthweight babies (under 1.3 pounds) and under 23 weeks gestation
ectopic pregnancy (embryo implanted outside the uterus)	anencephaly and similar conditions in which a child is born without a brain

Source: Oregon Health Services Commission quoted in *The New York Times* (1991), February 22, p. A11. (Explanation of some medical terms has been added.)

Some features of the table are fairly predictable: top priority to life-threatening emergency conditions such as acute appendicitis, choking or a ruptured intestine, for which there are known to be effective remedies. At the foot of the list are some conditions which many people would expect to see there: very severe birth defects, extremely premature babies, very superficial injuries.

However, even at these extreme ends of the ranking many problems arise: for example, are people with terminal AIDS-related illness to be offered no treatment or even palliative care? Has *humane* care been sacrificed to cost-effectiveness? Such difficulties multiply in the middle of the ranking, where all the most uncomfortable decisions arise about who to treat and who to turn away. It should also be recalled that the Oregon plan is still confined to the Medicaid scheme which is only used by the poor: it could be argued that it simply represents a different way of rationing health care to the poor, which would not be acceptable to the wider population. And finally, at the time of writing in 1992, the plan had still not been fully implemented, despite several years of discussion.

Lessons for rationing British health care?

Nevertheless, the Oregon scheme has excited a great deal of interest in many countries, and it seems certain that the questions it asks, if not the remedies it proposes, will continue to be heard. This is certainly true of the United Kingdom, where the whole issue of rationing has been brought into focus by the NHS reforms of the 1990s. GP fund-holders, for example, have been made much more aware of the costs of the services they are purchasing and of the health outcomes they are meant to be pursuing. And purchasing authorities now have to make explicit

plans for the type and quantity of services they wish to buy within their resource constraints, and some have already reached towards the QALY framework as one possible tool to assist them in making these difficult strategic decisions.

This takes us back to the discussion of health-care management in Chapter 2: in the past, rationing decisions in health care have often been hidden from sight, but in the future it seems inevitable that they will become much more publicly visible as decisions are taken increasingly by NHS managers in accordance with strategies set by central government. As Chapter 2 pointed out, the question of accountability and democracy in health-service decision-making is sharpened when the power to influence 'who gets what' rests primarily with managers employed for their business acumen.

OBJECTIVES FOR CHAPTER 3

When you have studied this chapter, you should be able to:

3.1   Explain what is meant by need, demand and supply, and the relationship between them.

3.2   Outline some of the main ways in which rationing of health care takes place.

3.3   Discuss some of the problems in defining 'equal opportunity to benefit' from the NHS, and describe the policy steps that have been taken to improve equity.

3.4   Outline the method and application of cost-effectiveness analysis in health care, and comment on the strengths and limitations of the QALY framework.

QUESTIONS FOR CHAPTER 3

Question 1 (*Objective 3.1*)

In 1985 the *Guardian* newspaper carried a story headlined 'lack of cash "killing" transplant

patients', which stated that a confidential report on the future of heart transplants had shown that 68 patients had died while waiting for the operation, which had become available only during the early 1980s (Andrew Veitch, *Guardian*, 28 January 1985). Describe this story in terms of need, demand and supply.

Question 2 (*Objective 3.2*)

Why is rationing inevitable in any system of health care? In what way is health care rationed in the NHS?

Question 3 (*Objective 3.3*)

What aspects of equity did the RAWP formula attempt to improve, and how successful was it?

Question 4 (*Objective 3.4*)

'If only we could accurately measure changes in life expectancy and quality of life from a particular treatment, we could see if it was sufficiently cost-effective to be worth doing.' What faults can you find in this line of reasoning?

4 The evaluation of health care

This chapter includes a discussion of certain methods of evaluation of health-service activity (such as performance indicators and medical audit) which were introduced briefly in Chapter 2. It also builds on the general description of randomised controlled trials (RCTs) in an earlier book in this series, Studying Health and Disease.[1] During your study of this chapter, you will be asked to read two articles in the Reader:[2] the first is by Archie Cochrane, entitled 'Effectiveness and efficiency', and the second is a series of articles and letters from different sources under the collective title 'Ethical dilemmas in evaluation', which relate to neural tube defects (also known as spina bifida).

This chapter was written by Clive Seale, a medical sociologist and Lecturer in the Department of Sociology, Goldsmiths' College, University of London.

Evaluation and decision-making

The provision of health care through a large organisation such as the NHS involves a continuing process of decision-making by health-care workers (doctors are the most influential), health-service managers on both the purchasing and providing sides of the internal market, and politicians who formulate policies affecting the nation's health. In all these decisions there is the chance that self-interest, prejudice and the search for personal or political power will influence matters, particularly where there is strong pressure for or against a particular policy from service-users, the media and the wider community.

In theory, evaluation—the subject of this chapter—helps create a rational decision-making process to replace such irrational influences. This is because systematic evaluation may be able to provide an objective assessment of the degree to which different treatments, policies and programmes of care are successful.

The search for rational methods for making decisions about health care has been an aim of numerous policy initiatives during the history of the NHS. The 1974 reforms in particular[3] can be interpreted as a major effort to help managers make more rational decisions. Chapter 3 described the efforts of health economists to produce cost-effectiveness studies. These are, fundamentally, an attempt to produce information that will increase the rational basis of decision-making, even if purely rational decisions are beyond our competence or aims.

In addition, the evaluation of medical therapies has a long history.[4] A large part of the authority of the modern medical profession rests on the claim to have treatments of proven effectiveness: for example, systematic evaluation led to the final rejection of blood-letting as an effective practice; dramatic proof of the effectiveness of the smallpox vaccination lay behind its widespread adoption.

□ What objections have been raised to the claim that modern medical practice is based on scientifically evaluated treatments?

■ Critics claim that much medical practice has not, in fact, been evaluated—particularly in surgery. Clinical judgement may also be subject to trends in fashion.[5]

[1] Studying Health and Disease (Open University Press, 1985, Chapter 6; revised edition 1994).

[2] Health and Disease: A Reader (1984; reprinted in revised edition 1994).

[3] See Caring for Health: History and Diversity (revised edition 1993), Chapter 7.

[4] This was discussed in Medical Knowledge: Doubt and Certainty (Open University Press, revised edition, 1994).

[5] Also discussed in Medical Knowledge: Doubt and Certainty.

Nevertheless, the scientific methods used for evaluating the effectiveness of medical treatments have had a profound influence on thinking about the evaluation of health-care policies and programmes of care. It will be one of the tasks of this chapter to assess critically the extent to which these methods can be transferred to the policy arena. Scientific methods emphasise proof of *cause and effect*, and are often impractical and inappropriate when considering the evaluation of policies and programmes of care, rather than specific medical treatments. The place of *qualitative* methods in such evaluations will be highlighted.

The discussion then turns to the measurement of *health status* in evaluation studies, which will be shown to reflect competing objectives in health care of different people and interest groups. Lack of consensus about the aims of health care needs to be reflected in the design of evaluation studies. Some of these controversies will be illustrated by means of a case study of the evaluation of equity in general practice consultations. The chapter concludes with an assessment of initiatives that the health-care professions (mainly doctors and nurses) and health-service managers have taken to evaluate health-care programmes and policies.

Evaluation is not always helpful in solving the problems of decision-makers. It is, of course, sometimes possible to prove that one treatment is better than another at achieving aims which most people agree to be worthwhile. More often, however—and particularly in relation to health-care policies and programmes of treatment—evaluation does not reveal a clear-cut answer about the best course of action. Sometimes, the best that an evaluation can do is to show that two courses of action involve different trade-offs between advantages and disadvantages. In this sense, evaluation may occasionally reveal more dilemmas than it solves.

The relationship between the results of research and the process of decision-making is not always straightforward. In 1969 Donald Campbell, an American psychologist with a long-standing interest in methods of evaluation, provided a light-hearted guide to people threatened with such scrutiny.

Advice for trapped administrators

Human courtesy and gratitude being what it is, the most dependable means of assuring a favourable evaluation is to use voluntary testimonials from those who have had the treatment. If the spontaneously produced testimonials are in short supply, these should be solicited from the recipients with whom the program is still in contact. The rosy glow resulting is analogous to the professor's impression of his teaching success when it is based solely upon the comments of those students who come up and talk with him after class...

Another dependable tactic bound to give favourable outcomes is to confound selection and treatment, so that in the published comparison those receiving the treatment are also the most able and well placed. The often-cited evidence of the dollar value of a college education is of this nature—all careful studies show that most of the effect, and of the superior effect of superior colleges, is explicable in terms of superior talents and family connections, rather than in terms of what is learned...

(These examples) remind us again that we must help create a political climate that demands more rigorous and less self-deceptive reality testing. (Quoted in Bynner and Stribley, 1978, pp. 106–7)

The only way to detect self-deception such as this is by gaining a thorough understanding of the principles of evaluation, which we can outline in this chapter. The first principle of evaluation must be to establish criteria against which the outcome of health care can be evaluated. But this raises several dilemmas, not least about definitions of 'good' care.

Conflicting definitions of good health care

Different interest groups—for example, politicians, managers, doctors, or health-service users (often referred to as *consumers* in the 1990s; the subject of Chapter 5)—may have differing views about what counts as a 'good' outcome. To judge the value of health care, we must first agree on what might indicate success. You have already been introduced in earlier chapters to a number of criteria that might be used to define good health care.

☐ What were they?

■ Effectiveness, efficiency, equity and humanity. Effectiveness (divorced from the issue of cost) may be defined as the extent to which policies or treatments succeed in improving peoples' health. Efficiency refers to whether health-care resources are being used to get the best value for money. Equity concerns the fair distribution of resources in relation to need. Humanity involves placing value on the subjective perceptions and feelings of health-service users and workers.

All four of these criteria may not be met at the same time by any one policy or treatment. Sometimes the criteria conflict, as examples earlier in this book have shown (for example, it may be possible to provide a more efficient service at the cost of equity or humanity). Further, the criteria may each be open to varying interpretations in relation to specific policies. For example, some people believe that *effective* health care should concentrate on restoring physical functions; others argue that overall quality of life—which may or may not be dependent on bodily capacity—should be the aim. How can the best course of action be decided? Remember that a dilemma is an uncomfortable choice between conflicting alternatives. This underlines the need for analysis of the various *aims* of health-care programmes if evaluation is to be useful.

You will also recognise by now that decision-making in health care occurs at a variety of levels (strategic, operational and clinical), each with consequences for evaluation design. The point we are making here, is that all these decisions can—or should—be based to some degree on an evaluation of the need for health care, the various options for meeting that need and their predicted outcomes. Evaluation can aid rational decision-making.

Decision-making step by step

The role of evaluation in helping to make decisions more rational can be illustrated as a series of steps. First, the problem must be identified, along with known options for coping with it. Second—and this is where evaluation plays the largest part—the costs and benefits of each option need to be identified and measured. In theory, at least, the third step should then be easy. This simply involves selecting the option that yields the most favourable ratio of benefits to costs. This is an idealised model, and the real world is unlikely to be as perfect as this, but the ideal remains something to which many aspire, including Alan Williams whose article 'Priority setting in the NHS' you studied with Chapter 3.

An example quite close to this ideal model, showing rational decision-making based on the results of evaluation, is provided in a study published in 1978 by a British epidemiologist, Michael Adler. He investigated the effects of discharging patients from hospital early after operations to repair an inguinal hernia (a weakness in the muscular wall of the abdomen in the groin, through which internal organs may protrude). He and his colleagues compared two randomly allocated groups of patients spending different amounts of time in hospital after the operation. The measures of success were: the incidence of major post-operative complications, the length of time it took to convalesce, and the rate of

Table 4.1 Complications recorded up to seven days after operation in an evaluation of length of stay for inguinal hernia patients

Type of complication	Long-stay[1] (49 patients)	Short-stay[2] (56 patients)	Total (105 patients)
wound infection	2	2	4
chest infection	2	2	4
blood-filled swelling	0	1	1
stitch abscess	0	1	1
breathlessness due to anaesthetic	1	0	1
accumulation of fluid in scrotum/penis	0	1	1
total with complications	5	7	12

[1]6–7 days. [2]48 hours. (Source: Adler, M. W., Waller, J. J., Creese, A. and Thorne, S. C., 1978, Randomised controlled trial of early discharge for inguinal hernia and varicose veins, *Journal of Epidemiology and Community Health*, **32**, Table 2, p. 139)

recurrence of hernias. Some of the results are shown in Table 4.1.

□ Which group had more complications, in absolute numbers and as a rate per patient in each group? What do these results lead you to conclude?

■ The short-stay group had the higher number of complications (seven, as opposed to the long-stay group who had five). But there were more short-stay patients (56) than long-stay (49), so the two groups had a roughly equal *rate* of complication (about 1 in 10 patients in either group). This would suggest that early discharge was as successful as later discharge—at least as far as 'success' can be judged in terms of post-operative complications.

No difference between the two groups was found on the other measures, and early discharge costs less. Adler then told the doctors concerned about his results and they decided to shorten the length of stay for this type of patient as it appeared to make no difference to recovery. Adler later reported changes that occurred in the hospitals as a result of the study, showing a drop in the average length of stay for the operation.

□ Which of the four criteria for successful health care are addressed in this study and which have been left out?

■ Medical effectiveness and efficiency are included. Equity was not addressed, and the humanity of the discharge policies was not a priority for the researchers. (In fact, the report stated that the relatives of those with short stays were *less* happy about the policy than relatives of longer-stay patients.)

However, although it is possible to find successful examples such as this one of rational decision-making based on step-by-step evaluation, many areas of health care have not been evaluated. Agreement on the aims of health care may be difficult to achieve. Those with the power to make decisions—whether clinicians deciding on treatment strategies, or managers and politicians formulating plans and policies—may have a variety of reasons for ignoring the results of evaluation, or indeed commissioning evaluations only when it suits them.

Ignoring the results or 'muddling through'

A notorious example of decision-makers ignoring the results of evaluation is that of the British Admiralty, which in the nineteenth century took 50 years to act on the finding that citrus fruit relieved scurvy, during which time countless sailors perished unnecessarily.

Even where evaluation exercises *are* commissioned at the strategic level, they are sometimes overtaken by the pace of events. Thus the Resource Management Initiative (RMI), whereby doctors became responsible for the management of their own budgets, was evaluated by a team of researchers from Brunel University (Buxton *et al.*, 1991). However, before they could report, decisions had been taken at the political level to extend the RMI. The researchers observed:

> The extent to which the NHS can learn from pilot initiatives such as this is vastly diminished if the pace is such that reforms follow each other without an intervening opportunity to assess their independent impact. With hindsight the original initiative (RMI) was grossly optimistic...(Quoted in Rue, 1991, p. 1 292)

Faced with examples of irrational decisions it is easy to feel a sense of despair and cynicism about the motives of planners. Such a feeling led one writer (C. E. Lindblom in 1959) to describe decision-making in large organisations like the NHS as the 'science of muddling through'. Lindblom felt that managers, or other policy-makers, were more interested in balancing the rival interests of power groups than in scientifically assessing the outcomes of policy options (a view which resonates with some of the points made earlier in Chapter 2). Some argue that to expect planners of health services to behave purely according to the dictates of reason is very naive. David Allen, writing about the 1962 *Hospital Plan* to provide every district with a general hospital, notes that subsequent evaluation of these new hospitals showed that hoped-for savings through economies of scale were not realised in practice. Rather than regretting the decision to build, he writes:

> To ask why hospital building rather than another alternative was chosen as the appropriate thing to do, is to ask the wrong question. It conceives the decision-making process far too abstractly, as though decision makers choose the best solution from a selection. Policy makers are busy people, they are confronted by many things to do, by conflicting pressures for action and conflicting information about the alternatives available to them. Hospital building presented an opportunity to be grasped, it was acceptable to the NHS employees, to the medical profession, to the Ministry of Health, it was an improvement over the current circumstances and above all the Treasury was not against it; it was financially feasible. There was consensus about the initiative with no evidence of any conflict. An opportunity too good to be missed. (Allen, 1981, p. 15)

□ According to Allen's analysis, what led the planners to invest in the hospital building programme?

■ It was politically and financially feasible at the time. Allen reveals his doubts about the practicality of rational decision-making in the NHS.

There have been attempts to break out of the complex process of decision-making that is necessary when a variety of interest groups are allowed to have a say in policy-making. This was one of the aims of Roy Griffiths, when he proposed the 1983 management reforms in the NHS. Griffiths felt that *consensus* management in the health service produced decisions of the 'lowest common denominator' since everyone involved in a decision had the power to veto it at any stage. Griffith's analysis, however, exposed a tension between democratic values and efficiency—a dilemma that is difficult to resolve in a way satisfactory to all.

'Muddling through' may be more characteristic of national and local politics than of decisions that clinicians make about medical treatments. Indeed, some treatments *must* be evaluated before doctors are allowed to use them; new pharmaceutical products are required by law to meet certain safety standards before licensing for use (this is covered in more detail in Chapter 7 of this book). However, innovations in surgery are not subject to such requirements and the conservatism of the medical profession has been responsible for some irrational treatment practices. Thus, for decades, surgeons trained to treat breast cancer by mastectomy (removal of the whole breast) ignored research evidence that less radical surgery (lumpectomy) was often just as effective. But, on the whole, the technical problems of evaluating biomedical treatments are fewer than in the evaluation of health-care policies and programmes of care. Clinicians like to believe that they have a better record than managers and politicians in applying the rational model and this sometimes leads to tensions. One of the key elements of the BMA's campaign against the 1991 NHS reforms was the cry that the internal market had not been evaluated.

The randomised controlled trial and health-care evaluation

In 1971 Archie Cochrane, an epidemiologist, published a book called *Effectiveness and Efficiency* in which he presented powerful arguments for the more widespread use of the **randomised controlled trial** (**RCT**) in health services. This, he felt, would open up 'a new world of evaluation and control which will, I think, be the key to a rational health service' (Cochrane, 1971, p. 77). An extract from this influential book is provided in the Reader[6] and you should now read it.

☐ According to Cochrane, what are the key features of the RCT?[7]

■ The RCT is an experimental design, in which people are allocated to two groups at *random*, with one group receiving the new treatment that is being evaluated, and the other (the control group) receiving either no treatment, some inactive substance known as a *placebo*, or the old treatment for the

condition. Random allocation should ensure that the two groups are the same in all respects, except for the fact that only one group is receiving the new treatment. Thus any differences in outcomes for the two groups can be attributed to the new treatment rather than any other characteristic of the people taking part.

☐ Cochrane cites several reasons why many aspects of health care have not been subjected to RCTs. What are they?

■ His reasons are that:

(a) Ethical objections are sometimes raised.

(b) There is a lack of *objective* outcome measures for assessing the effectiveness of many health-care activities. (If he were writing now, this judgement might be reversed—see the section on measuring health status later in this chapter.)

(c) Resistance by those who feel threatened by RCTs.

We shall look at the ethical objections in more detail. They can include the fact that many people feel it is wrong to withhold a treatment (as is done for control groups in RCTs) that *might* be effective, even if its effectiveness has not been proved. (To counter this, supporters of RCTs would no doubt argue that doctors should not be administering treatments whose value is unproven.) There is the further dilemma that since health care is rationed, is it ethical to 'waste' money on testing a new treatment that would otherwise have been spent on an established treatment of proven worth?

An ethical debate that took place prior to the setting up of an RCT to assess the effectiveness of vitamin supplements in preventing neural tube defects is presented in a collection of articles and letters in the Reader under the title 'Ethical dilemmas in evaluation'.[8] You should now read the following from this collection: *The Lancet* editorial of 17 May 1980, the letter from Peadar Kirke published in *The Lancet* on 14 June 1980, and the two *Guardian* articles and a letter published (respectively) on 10, 13 and 14 December 1982.

☐ On what grounds did some people oppose the RCT?

---

[6]'Effectiveness and efficiency' by A. L. Cochrane, in *Health and Disease: A Reader* (1984; reprinted in revised edition 1994).

[7]These were also discussed in *Studying Health and Disease* (1985; revised edition 1994).

[8]These articles were set reading for *Studying Health and Disease* (1985; revised edition 1994) and can be found in *Health and Disease: A Reader* (1984; reprinted in revised edition 1994).

- On the grounds that 'to deprive women of a totally harmless vitamin cocktail seems unethical', to quote John Lorber. In other words, even though the benefits of vitamins are not proven, the possibility of *some* benefits makes it unethical to withhold them from the control group of women.

☐ On what grounds did people support the RCT?

- On the grounds that the benefits of vitamins were not proven and there was a possibility that vitamins could cause some harm to some foetuses. To prescribe vitamins without first carrying out an RCT would, in the view of one correspondent, be 'sanctioning what amounts to a situation of uncontrolled experimentation on mothers and babies'.

Limitations of the RCT

The RCT was developed initially as a method for assessing the effectiveness of agricultural technology in promoting crop growth, and in the medical field it has probably been most widely applied in the assessment of new drugs. Thus its origins lie firmly in the disciplines of the *natural* (and particularly the biological) sciences. Cochrane's argument for its more widespread application would extend the method to cover evaluation of levels of health care that have usually been regarded as the province of

the *social* sciences: strategic and operational policies and care programmes, rather than clinical decisions about treatments. At one point in his book he even argues the case for conducting RCTs of social work. It is undoubtedly the case that the record of social scientists in establishing clear proof of cause and effect has been poor, but the claim that the RCT can solve this dilemma for decision-makers at all levels requires careful examination.

First, it is very much more difficult to control all the experimental conditions in a health-care *programme* than it is in evaluating the use of a particular medical treatment or drug. For example, in 1984 a group of American researchers led by a physician, Robert Kane, reported an RCT of hospice care in which terminally ill patients were randomly allocated to a hospice or to ordinary hospital care. Hospices specialise in the terminal care of cancer patients. The hospice philosophy involves not performing 'heroic' attempts at 'rescuing' terminally ill people from death with treatments whose side effects may be very severe, such as chemotherapy or major surgical interventions. The emphasis is on easing symptoms, such as pain, and on helping patients and their families cope with anxieties.

Kane and his colleagues interviewed patients and their relatives in both settings. They found that measures designed to test whether hospice care was successful, such as control of pain, depression and anxiety, were not significantly different between the two groups, suggesting that hospice care was no more successful than hospital

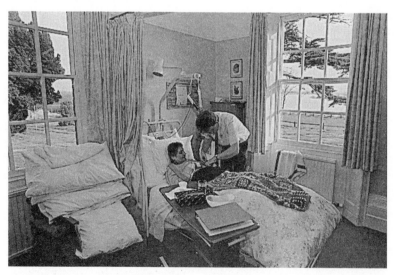

The Hospice of Our Lady and St John at Willen in Milton Keynes. Illuminative studies of the process of health care may be able to throw light on subtle differences between, for example, hospital and hospice care for people with a terminal illness. (Photo: Mike Levers)

care. However, some further results concerning the treatment and care received by the two groups are shown in Table 4.2. In interpreting these results note that, on average, the patients in both treatment (hospice) and control (hospital) groups took part in the study for the same length of time. Intermediate care and general medical wards are both locations within the hospital.

Table 4.2 Use of services in a randomised controlled trial of hospice care

Service	Average number per patient	
	Hospice (128 patients)	Hospital (102 patients)
Total in-patient days	51.0	47.5
general medical wards*	13.2	20.7
hospice	29.2	–
intensive care unit	0.2	0.3
intermediate care wards*	8.3	26.5
Nursing-home days*	1.0	11.4
Days at home	44.8	37.9
Surgical procedures	0.51	0.31
major surgical procedures*	0.09	0.01
minor surgical procedures	0.42	0.30
Radiation treatments	7.4	7.7
Chemotherapy treatments*	1.3	0.49

*$P < 0.05$ (i.e. the difference between hospice and hospital patients is statistically significant). (Source: Kane, R. L., Wales, J., Bernstein, L., Leibowitz, A. and Kaplan, S., 1984, A randomised controlled trial of hospice care, *Lancet* (**i**), Table 2, p. 892)

□ Were the two groups described in Table 4.2 treated differently or the same?

■ Hospice patients spent fewer days on general medical and intermediate care wards and in nursing homes. They had more major surgical procedures and chemotherapy treatments than hospital patients. There were no significant differences in the other measures, such as days spent in intensive care, minor surgery and radiotherapy.

Clearly, the hospice philosophy of non-intervention was not pursued in the hospice that Kane studied. In practice, the hospice patients had experienced very similar treatment regimes to the patients in the hospital, even

receiving care from the same doctors at times. Because the care given to the treatment and the control groups was not clearly separated, statements about the effectiveness of one form of care over the other were not justified. This type of problem in an RCT is known as a **contamination effect**.

The second major limitation of RCTs is that practical and ethical difficulties in achieving random allocation increase when evaluating care programmes rather than medical treatments. Kane's trial of hospice care was possible because the hospice was a part of the hospital concerned in the study, so getting patients to agree to be randomly allocated to hospice or hospital care was relatively easy. Other researchers have not been so fortunate. If we consider the highest level of decision-making, that of national policy-making, the practical difficulties of evaluation multiply.

□ For example, what problems might occur in attempting to set up an RCT of the 1990s internal market in health care?

■ There would need to be areas of the country where the internal market was *not* operating in order to provide a control group. Areas would have to be randomly chosen for allocation to a market system (the treatment group) or a non-market system. This would be likely to be politically unacceptable.

A third limitation of RCTs as applied to care programmes relates to the *placebo effect*. In drug trials, the people receiving the drug that is being evaluated normally do not know whether they are receiving the active ingredient or a dummy placebo pill. This is to make sure that the psychological effect of knowing that a treatment is being given does not of itself produce an improvement, which would then be impossible to disentangle from the pharmacological effects of the drug. However, this *'blind'* effect (or indeed the *'double blind'* effect where even those administering the treatment and the placebo do not know who is in which group) is not possible to achieve in the evaluation of health-care programmes. People entering, for example, a specialist geriatric unit, or receiving visits from a social worker, normally know that these things are happening.

Quasi-experimental designs

Practical and ethical problems like this have led researchers to consider evaluation designs which are less adequate than the RCT for proving cause–effect relationships, but which are more feasible. You will recall from your reading of the correspondence in the *Reader* about neural tube defects (NTD) that John Lorber, at the end of his letter to the *Guardian*, proposed an alternative to the RCT that he felt would surmount the ethical problems involved. Designs of the type Lorber outlines have been called **quasi-experimental** designs. A fully experimental design is the RCT, where *all* variables except the 'treatment' being tested are (to use the jargon of experimental science) *controlled for* by random allocation of subjects to treatment or control groups. A quasi-experiment compromises on the control of variables, controlling only for *some* that might be expected to influence the outcome, and which can be readily measured given the constraints on the study design.

□ What did Lorber propose, and why might it be termed a quasi-experimental design?

■ He proposed to give the vitamin supplementation to *all* women at risk of giving birth to an NTD baby. If the incidence of NTD infants born to women at risk dropped below the known rate of 5%, he would conclude that the treatment was successful. This is only a quasi-experiment (in this case a *'before–after'* study) because other factors that might influence the result have not been controlled for. For example, some systematic change in the diet, behaviour or environment of the women during the period under study could account for any change in the NTD rate. Such factors could not confound the outcome in an RCT as women in both treatment and control groups would experience them equally.

Another example of a before–after study is the evaluation of the introduction of the breathalyser in Britain in 1967. Accident statistics showed a decline in the weeks after its introduction, compared with the weeks before. Similarly, there was a drop in abortion-related death in women after the introduction of the 1967 Abortion Act.

□ What objections might be raised to the conclusion that these policies were successful?

■ In the first example, there are problems in proving cause and effect in a quasi-experimental design because other factors have not been ruled out. Driving behaviour might have changed for other reasons—perhaps the weather changed during the period concerned. The second major objection concerns disagreement in defining what is meant by 'success' (an objection that also applies to the outcome of RCTs). Some people regard the introduction of the Abortion Act as an unmitigated disaster for the life of the 'unborn child'.

Threats to validity

Designing a good quasi-experiment is very much like constructing an argument so that it is proof against threats from counter-arguments. These have sometimes been called *threats to the validity* of the quasi-experiment. For the most part, such threats concern the extent to which cause–effect relationships are proven (known as **threats to internal validity**). An example of a threat to internal validity is the objection you have just seen to the conclusion about the breathalyser policy. Here, the objection is that some third factor, such as the weather, might have caused a spurious appearance of a causal relationship between the policy and the accident rate.

The RCT generally avoids succumbing to such threats to internal validity because random allocation is so effective at ruling out other possible causal factors. In the quasi-experiment, a degree of control may be achieved by a procedure known as **matching**. Here, people are not allocated to two groups at random, but people receiving treatment are matched to people not receiving treatment on a number of criteria thought to be relevant to the outcome of the programme. For example, a test of the effectiveness of social work might ensure that the age, sex and social class of a group receiving social work services was the same as a control group that did not receive these services.

There is another type of validity called **external validity**. This concerns the extent to which the results of an evaluation can be reliably generalised. If an evaluation shows conclusively that threats to internal validity have been overcome, and that a particular health-care programme has been successful, will the same success be achieved by others who try to repeat the programme in other settings? On this issue the RCT may have fewer guarantees to offer. This is because the RCT is always, to a greater or lesser extent, an artificial exercise. A great deal of attention is normally paid to ensuring random *allocation,* but the random *selection* of people to enter the trial is usually given less attention.

□ What uncertainty does this create about generalising from the results of the RCT?

■ It raises doubts about whether the people in the trial are typical of those whom it is hoped to treat should the treatment be proven successful. People may refuse to enter the trial. Those who agree to take part may be special in some way that affects the outcome.[9]

[9]Bias due to voluntary participation is examined in relation to screening tests in Chapter 9 of this book. The importance of representative sampling is discussed in *Studying Health and Disease* (1985; revised edition 1994).

Lastly, the programme of care being evaluated may differ in all sorts of subtle ways from others bearing the same name. Imagine that an RCT has shown that a programme for rehabilitating people who have suffered a stroke is successful in one hospital. There is no guarantee that a programme with the same name will be similarly successful in another hospital unless all the features of the original are the same. This may be an unrealistic expectation, as physiotherapists and others involved in such care usually have different ways of giving treatment, even though they may be trying to apply the same principles.

Illuminating the process of care

Given the complex demands of evaluation design, Raymond Illsley, a sociologist concerned with the evaluation of health care, has suggested that:

> Successive partial evaluations and reforms are superior to perfect trials which demand such stringent conditions that they cannot be carried out. (Illsley, 1980, p. 129)

His alternative approach to evaluation is called an **illuminative approach**, in that the aim of the evaluator is to throw light upon the processes going on within health care. The illuminative approach calls into question the over-riding emphasis put by those conducting RCTs and quasi-experiments on proof of cause–effect relationships.

To understand the illuminative approach it is important to distinguish between two things in evaluative studies of health care: **outcome** and **process**. The outcomes of health care may be measures of improvements in health, and the process of health care consists of the activities of people providing and receiving care as it proceeds. Another way of thinking about this distinction is to consider processes as being the means by which ends are reached, the ends being the outcomes.

☐ Here are five features of health care. Identify which are measures of process, and which are measures of outcome. Which processes might influence which outcomes?

(a) The rate at which appendicectomies are carried out

(b) The number of questions asked by patients during consultations that lead to explanations by the doctor

(c) The death rate from appendicitis

(d) The number of patients with high blood pressure who comply with doctors' advice in taking pills regularly to reduce blood pressure

(e) The death rate from stroke.

■ (a) is a process, which leads to (c) as its outcome (i.e. a high rate of appendectomy might be expected to reduce the death rate from appendicitis). (b) is a process, which is likely to influence (d). However, although compliance may be thought of as an outcome of the extent to which doctors explain the reasons for their advice to patients, it is *also* an example of a process, since in this case it influences (e), the death rate from stroke, which can be thought of as the *eventual* outcome.

From this you will see that a chain of cause–effect relationships may be involved in health-care activity. The distinction between process and outcome is useful for analysing this causal chain, but a process may stand between another process and the eventual outcome, as does compliance in the example above.

Setting standards for the process of care

Standard setting involves reaching agreement on the process that represents a high standard of care (known as a *care standard*). For example, good practice in care might be that the people providing care should offer patients explanations of their condition and the options available for treatment. Box 4.1 (*overleaf*) shows another example of a *standard of care statement*, developed by nurses, concerning access to respite care, a form of hospital care for dependent people designed to give the people looking after them at home a period of respite. The standard is used to evaluate practice.

When standards for the process of care have been set, it may be that all the evaluator need do is to establish whether the standards have been achieved. This may be a routine and relatively simple exercise: for example (from Box 4.1), checking to see that an information booklet is available. On other occasions, and especially in illuminative evaluation, it may need to be more elaborate.

Using qualitative and observational methods

The qualitative and observational methods routinely used by social scientists in their research are useful tools in evaluation studies.[10] To illustrate these methods, consider an illuminative evaluation of the *process* of hospice care (which contrasts with Kane's RCT, described earlier). In 1976, Robert Buckingham—a doctor who also trained as an anthropologist—and a number of colleagues, published an evaluation of hospice care using the technique of *secret participant observation*. With the agreement of

---

[10]See *Studying Health and Disease* (1985; revised edition 1994) for a discussion of these methods.

Box 4.1   Example of standard setting in nursing: a standard of care statement on access to respite care

All carers of dependent people (who are suitable for hospital admission) are able to arrange respite care with the hospital for a maximum of two weeks at any one time.

Structure criteria (structures necessary to achieve the above aim)

1   Two beds set aside for respite care.

2   Diary system for 'booking' patients.

3   GPs accept that any carer can refer to the hospital although initial acceptance has GP approval.

4   Hospital's operational policy reflects this use of beds.

5   Criteria for what constitutes 'suitable hospital admission':

(a)   Has GP in the area (unless cover is arranged through a GP in the area)

(b)   Only one severely dependent patient admitted at one time.

(c)   Does not exhibit overt antisocial behaviour (at senior nurse's discretion).

6   Information booklet available.

7   Development of a respite care assessment form that recognises both the patient's life-style and the carer's needs.

8   Nursing knowledge of carer's needs (resource file).

9   Patient always assigned to the same primary nurse.

Process criteria

1   Nurse will check availability of bed and book patient onto diary.

2   Patient's GP informed (if referral not through GP) of need for hospital admission.

3   Primary nurse will visit patient and carer at home (if considered appropriate) prior to first respite care admission.

4   Respite care assessment form sent to carer prior to admission.

5   Primary nurse will use the assessment form as a basis for discussing care with carer, to plan and give care.

6   Primary nurse will assess how the carer is coping to identify need.

Outcome criteria

1   Carer obtains relief of care.

2   Patient's normal life-style is minimally disrupted.

3   The carer is confident about the relative coming into hospital.

4   The carer has coping resources identified and met to enable more effective coping at home.

5   The carer's role as prime carer is recognised by feeling involved in the care process.

6   The carer indicates satisfaction with care.

(Some technical terms have been 'translated' into everyday language.) (Source: Johns, C., 1992, Developing clinical standards, pp. 156–171 and Figure 10.1, p. 159, in Vaughan, B. and Robinson, K. (eds) *Knowledge for Nursing Practice*, Butterworth Heinemann, Oxford)

the hospital authorities, he posed as a terminally ill patient with cancer of the pancreas, preparing himself for the role by, amongst other things, dieting to lose weight over a period of six months and preparing false medical documentation. He reports that he entered the role so effectively that he began experiencing phantom symptoms of pain, exhaustion and restlessness at night.

Buckingham spent four days and nights in a hospital surgical ward, and a similar period in the palliative care (hospice) unit attached to the hospital, making observations of the process of care that he and others received. Some of these were of a quantitative nature, recording the length and frequency of interaction between patients and staff. Some of his data are shown in Table 4.3.

Table 4.3 Verbal contact of Buckingham with staff in the four-day periods in the surgical ward and palliative care unit

	Surgical ward	Palliative care unit
contact time (minutes)	164	512
number of contacts	30	27
mean number of minutes per contact	5.5	19.0

Data derived from: Buckingham, R. W., Lack, S. A., Mount, B. M., Maclean, L. D. and Collins, J. T. (1976) Living with the dying: use of the technique of participant observation, *Canadian Medical Association Journal*, **115**, Table 1, p. 1 212.

Other data were qualitative:

> On the surgical ward, doctors rarely entered the patient's room alone. Ward rounds were typically made…in groups of two or three. This practice fostered discussion…between the doctors but completely prevented doctor–patient communication on any but the most superficial level…Frequently staff, including doctors, went in and out without any recognition, by word or look, of the people in the room…(By contrast) in the palliative care unit the doctors made rounds alone, thus providing the patient with this essential opportunity for communication. (Buckingham *et al.*, 1976, pp. 1 212–13)

These observations led him to conclude that:

> The active treatment wards under study in this hospital, geared as they are to aggressive therapy and prolongation of life, do not offer an optimal environment for the dying. There is a need for comfort, both physical and mental, for others to see them as individuals rather than as

hosts for their disease, and for someone to breach the loneliness and help them come to terms with the end. These needs may be better met by a unit specially designed for this purpose. (Buckingham *et al.*, 1976, p. 1 215)

☐ How does Buckingham's illuminative evaluation differ from Kane's study of hospice care?

■ Kane assessed the effectiveness of care by *asking* patients and their relatives about anxiety, depression and other aspects of mental and physical health. He only incidentally presented the data in Table 4.2 which describes the process of care. Buckingham, on the other hand, did not interview patients to discover the impact of care upon them, but described *from observation* processes of care that differed between the two settings. The amount of time staff spent with patients might be expected to have a particular outcome, but Buckingham leaves that inference to the reader of his report. Thus his is a study of the process of care, and its implied humanity.

Measuring health status

Although studies of the process of care may use qualitative methods, it is often important for effectiveness to be assessed by the *quantitative* measurement of people's **health status.** You should recall that in 1971 one of Cochrane's explanations for the limited use of RCTs in the NHS was the lack of outcome measures. This is no longer the case. The production of questionnaires and checklists to measure health status has become a small industry, for the most part led by American researchers. These measures are so numerous, and concern so many different aspects of health, that reference books have been devoted to helping evaluators choose appropriate ones. In one of these (Hersen and Bellack, 1988), 286 were listed: these included measures of functional ability, psychological well-being, social activity, life satisfaction, morale and self esteem.

Choosing between these measures poses a number of difficulties for evaluation design. It was noted earlier that different interest groups may have different criteria for judging whether health-care policies and programmes are successful. Choice of a measure of health status has to reflect this variety of aims. Consider the measurement of mental health: if a measure that simply records the absence of symptoms is chosen, this would exclude attempts to record feelings of well-being. In cancer chemotherapy, the avoidance of death might be considered the crucial outcome measure; others might

Box 4.2 The Barthel Index

The observer chooses the score for each activity. When summed, the score for a person with no disability is 100.

	With help	Independent
1 Feeding (if food needs to be cut up = help)	5	10
2 Moving from wheelchair to bed and return (includes sitting up in bed)	5–10	15
3 Personal toilet (wash face, comb hair, shave, clean teeth)	0	5
4 Getting on and off toilet (Handling clothes, wipe, flush)	5	10
5 Bathing self	0	5
6 Walking on level surface (or if unable to walk, propel wheelchair)	10	15
[* score only if unable to walk]	[0*]	[5*]
7 Ascend and descend stairs	5	10
8 Dressing (includes tying shoes, fastening fasteners)	5	10
9 Controlling bowels	5	10
10 Controlling bladder	5	10

Source: Mahoney, F. I. and Barthel, D. W. (1965) Functional evaluation: the Barthel Index, Maryland State Medical Journal: Annual Meeting, p. 62.

Box 4.3 The Nottingham Health Profile (extracts)

(Respondents are asked to answer Yes or No to each statement or question and a numerical value is assigned to the response.)

I'm tired all the time

I have pain at night

Things are getting me down

I have unbearable pain

I take tablets to help me sleep

I've forgotten what it's like to enjoy myself

I'm feeling on edge

I find it painful to change position

I feel lonely

I can only walk about indoors

I find it hard to bend

Everything is an effort

Source: Hunt, S. M., McEwen, J. and McKenna, S. P. (1986) Measuring Health Status, Croom Helm, London.

The Barthel Index was constructed by nurses involved in the care of elderly hospital patients, and the questionnaire is designed to be filled in by a professional who knows the person concerned. The scores are added up so that a person with no disability scores 100. The Nottingham Health Profile was designed so that people could answer the questions themselves on paper. It was developed from interviews with 768 people who were asked how they felt when they were ill or well. The scores that result from it are not summarised in a single number, but are given separately for the different dimensions of health involved—pain, sleeplessness and so on.

□ What differences are there between the two questionnaires?

■ The Barthel Index focuses on physical functioning and a limited range of self-care skills. The Nottingham Health Profile includes physical functioning, but also includes subjective perceptions of well-being, pain, sleeplessness, social isolation and personal relationships. The Barthel is based on a professional definition of health; the Nottingham Health Profile is based on lay peoples' perceptions of how illness affects them.

wish to trade this against quality of life. Disability is thought of by some as simply a matter of limited physical function; for others, the effects on social activity and contact are more crucial.

To illustrate the difference in approach, examine the two questionnaires reproduced in Boxes 4.2 and 4.3.

The type of questionnaire chosen, then, can reflect the differing aims of those giving and receiving health care. Health status measurement is an important technique for assessing the effectiveness of health care, just as studies of the process of care may be more appropriate for assessing its humanity. Process studies could also shed light on cost-effectiveness by illuminating whether resources were being used effectively. In addition, health status measures can help in assessing the cost-effectiveness of health care.

☐ Which health-status measure, intended for the assessment of cost-effectiveness, were you introduced to in Chapter 3?

■ The Quality-Adjusted Life Year (QALY).

Equity: the case of the GP consultation

The importance of the distinction between process and outcome in health-care evaluation can be demonstrated by considering the evaluation of *equity* in the GP consultation.

Achieving equity in the distribution of health-care resources, and in access to them, was one of the founding principles of the NHS. Policy initiatives, such as RAWP[11] and efforts to ensure an even geographical spread of GPs, have been designed to promote equity in resource allocation. Discovering the extent of inequalities between social classes has also been the focus of a sustained research effort. For example, it is well established that there are social-class differences in the use of many preventive services. Differences have been found in the use of, among other things, ante-natal care, family planning services, immunisation and dental services, with people from lower occupational groups in every case having lower rates of use.

An important aspect of equity in the use made of services is the way in which people are treated once they gain access. There is plenty of evidence to show that people from lower occupational groups have shorter consultations with GPs and ask for, and are given, fewer explanations. One such study was done by two social psychologists, David Pendleton and Stephen Bochner, who tape-recorded consultations and identified within them single 'units' of information and explanation.

[11]Discussed in Chapter 3 of this book, and in *Caring for Health: History and Diversity* (revised edition 1993), Chapter 9.

Box 4.4   Examples of units of information and explanation identified in GP consultations

1   *Volunteered information*

Dr A: I don't expect those little crusty bits to come back again.

Dr B: It will clear up by itself in a few months.

2   *Volunteered explanation*

Dr A: You have an infection in there which has made the skin scarred and hard and that's why it hurts because its in a very tender part of the finger.

Dr B: The ligaments around your shoulder joint have become inflamed and this is why it's giving you so much pain.

3   *Information in answer to a question*

Patient A: Isn't there anything else I can do?

Dr A: No…if it goes niggling on you sometimes get a deformed nail.

Patient B: Should I wear a sling?

Dr B: It's better to move your arm around.

4   *Explanation in answer to a question*

Patient A: Why does it seem to be a source of infection?

Dr A: Because you've obviously got a gap between the edge of the nail and the nail fold and things get in there.

Patient B: Why can't you give me an anaesthetic before the steroid injection?

Dr B: Because the anaesthetic injection would dilute the steroid and reduce its effectiveness.

Source: Pendleton, D. and Bochner, S. (1980) The communication of medical information in GP consultations as a function of social class, Social Science and Medicine, 14a, p. 670.

Examples of the units are given in Box 4.4 and the results of the study are shown in Table 4.4 (*overleaf*).

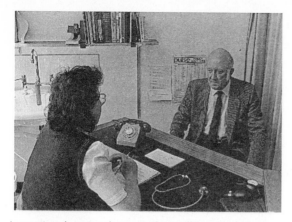

Interactions between doctors and patients is an important area for evaluation. (Photo: Mike Levers)

☐ Look at Table 4.4. To whom do doctors volunteer most information, and what happens when people from different social classes ask questions?

■ Doctors volunteer more to patients of higher social class and less to patients of lower social class, even when they ask questions.

It would be tempting to stop this account of equity here, and conclude that more needs to be done both to educate patients and train professionals in communication skills,

Table 4.4 Mean length of consultation and mean number of health-related statements given by the GP

	Social class of patients (female)		
	High	Medium	Low
average length of consultation in minutes	7.6	7.0	5.0
average number of 'units' of information and explanation volunteered by the doctor per consultation	5.3	4.0	2.2
average number of information and explanation 'units' per consultation in response to a question by patient	4.6	2.5	1.0
Total health-related statements per consultation	**9.9**	**6.5**	**3.2**

Source: Pendleton, D. and Bochner, S. (1980) The communication of medical information in GP consultations as a function of social class, *Social Science and Medicine*, 14a, Table 1, p. 671.

as many researchers have done. However, the results of another study of general practice consultations carried out by a sociologist, Mary Boulton, and her colleagues, suggest caution in adopting this view. Note, first, that studies such as those of Pendleton and Bochner are studies of the *process* of care. Mary Boulton's study demonstrates the value of examining *outcomes* too.

She starts by observing that individual consultations are only one moment in a continuing relationship between patients and their doctors. Other consultations, and indeed the discussions that patients have with other people about their doctor, will influence patients' thinking about their health. Further, a simple count of the number of questions and explanations that occur may say little about their quality. Boulton and her colleagues analysed the transcripts of 405 consultations with 16 different doctors. Like Pendleton and Bochner, Boulton *et al.* categorised the conversations into four strategies (see Box 4.5).

Figure 4.1 shows the strategies used by patients which the researchers classified into three social classes: workers, intermediate and service class (the highest).

Box 4.5   Examples of patients' strategies in a consultation with their GP

1   *Indicating a lay diagnosis*

I've had a few problems with my arm. I don't know whether I've torn some tendons or not.

2   *Requesting a further explanation*

How long have I had it [thrush]?…Is that why I have a bloody discharge?

3   *Requesting clarification of instructions*

We've got penicillin to last until Thursday. Shall we continue with that?

4   *Doubting or disagreeing*

Dr: I think this is highly likely to be a pulled muscle rather than anything awful.

Patient: I see. But wouldn't that make my knee hurt as well?

Source: adapted from Boulton, M., Tuckett, D., Olson, C. and Williams, A. (1986) *Social class and the general practice consultation*, Sociology of Health and Illness, **8**, p. 333.

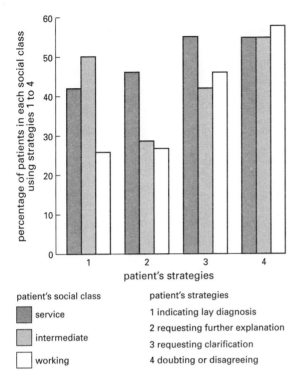

patient's social class

service

intermediate

working

patient's strategies

1 indicating lay diagnosis

2 requesting further explanation

3 requesting clarification

4 doubting or disagreeing

Figure 4.1 *Patients' strategies in consultations with GPs, in relation to the patients' social class, based on a sample of 328 patients. (Source: adapted from Boulton, M., Tuckett, D., Olson, C. and Williams, A., 1986, Social class and the general practice consultation,* Sociology of Health and Illness, **8**, Table 1, p. 338)

☐ What does Figure 4.1 show about social-class differences in patients' behaviour?

■ Service-class patients were considerably more active than working-class patients in indicating their own (lay) diagnoses, and requesting further explanations. The difference was not so marked in requesting clarification of instructions, and was roughly equal between the classes on doubting or disagreeing.

The findings about interaction were broadly what would be expected from a knowledge of studies like those of Pendleton and Bochner (see Table 4.4). However, Mary Boulton was also interested in what she called the *cognitive outcomes* of the consultations. Did all this extra talk for the service-class patients lead to a better understanding of the doctors' views, or being more committed to doctors' interpretations of their illness? To test this, the patients were interviewed after the consultation and

Box 4.6   Examples of patients' cognitive outcomes

1   *Misinterpretation*

Mr D., a 45-year-old bus driver, complained of stomach pain which had been diagnosed as a stomach ulcer. The doctor recommended Tagamet tablets, which 'stop you producing acid', and were to be taken continuously for 3 months. He also advised a week off work in order to 'eat regularly'. When interviewed, Mr D. said he was to have a week off work because his stomach pain broke his concentration when driving. He was also to have a course of Tagamet tablets, which he understood would disperse the poison in his stomach and dry up his ulcer. He did not recall anything about 'eating regularly'.

2   *Lack of commitment to treatment*

Mrs F., a 24-year-old woman, consulted the doctor about a pain down her leg. The doctor decided that the pain was a 'muscular pain' and recommended rest and aspirin. When interviewed, Mrs F. rejected the doctor's diagnosis, saying it felt more like a nerve pain—'a toothache in the leg'—because it had a 'shooting' sensation. She therefore also rejected the treatment advice as inappropriate. She thought a nerve was pinched by a displaced leg joint and wanted to have the leg 'whacked back into place'.

Source: adapted from Boulton, M., Tuckett, D., Olson, C. and Williams, A. (1986) Social class and the general practice consultation, Sociology of Health and Illness, **8**, pp. 336–7.

these outcomes were categorised. Examples of two of the categories are given in Box 4.6. The results of the study are shown in Figure 4.2 (*overleaf*).

☐ What does Figure 4.2 show about class differences in the cognitive outcomes of consultation?

■ Working-class patients are slightly more likely to misunderstand at least one important element, but commitment to treatment seems roughly equal across the classes.

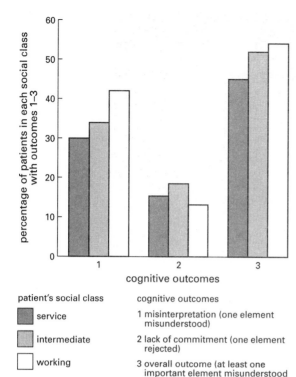

patient's social class

■ service
▨ intermediate
□ working

cognitive outcomes

1 misinterpretation (one element misunderstood)
2 lack of commitment (one element rejected)
3 overall outcome (at least one important element misunderstood or rejected)

Figure 4.2 *Cognitive outcomes of patients' consultations with GPs, in relation to the patients' social class, based on a sample of 328 patients. (Source: adapted from Boulton, M., Tuckett, D., Olson, C. and Williams, A., 1986, Social class and the general practice consultation,* Sociology of Health and Illness, **8**, *Table 2, p. 339)*

In fact, several of the large differences between the classes in Figure 4.1 are statistically significant, whereas none of the differences in Figure 4.2 are large enough to be significant. This suggests that although there are strong differences in behaviour during the *process* of consultations, these are not matched by strong class differences in their *outcome*. The authors conclude that:

> These findings suggest that the distinction between process and outcome is an important one, and requires more attention in research on the consultation...the contribution of the social sciences must follow trends in medical practice where emphasis is increasingly upon the evaluation of the outcomes of procedures (cf., Cochrane, 1971) as well as on the processes of care themselves. (Boulton *et al.*, 1986, p. 346)

□ In Mary Boulton's study, understanding the doctors' explanations was thought of as an outcome of consultation. In what circumstances might this be thought of as a process?

■ If the study had been trying to discover whether patient's health status changed as a result of consultation, their level of understanding could be thought of as a means to that end, and therefore a process on the way to the eventual outcome of change in health status.

Initiatives by practitioners

It is costly to set up research exercises to provide one-off judgements about the success of particular policies or treatments and doctors working in related areas may feel the results are not relevant if the conditions they face are in some way different from those that applied in the original evaluation. An alternative to formal evaluation exercises is to change the *culture* of clinical practice, so that the practice of medicine, nursing or other health-care occupations come to involve systematic and routine appraisal by practitioners of the success of their own activities.

□ What advantages and problems might there be in practitioners assessing their own activities rather than being assessed by outside agencies?

■ Advantages: the relevance of results will be directly evident to the decision-makers, as these will be the practitioners themselves. Thus evaluation results are likely to be acted upon.

Problems: practitioners' definitions of success may be at variance with those of recipients of care. Topics might be selected to suit the interests of practitioners. Self-criticism is never easy.

Medical audit

One method that has been adopted by practitioners, particularly doctors, to assess the success of their activities is known as **medical audit**. The method comes from the USA, where audit has been imposed externally upon doctors by insurance companies concerned about the high cost of medical care, and wanting to reduce unnecessary intervention. Medical audit may take a variety of forms, but a useful definition in the United Kingdom is given in the Department of Health's paper on the subject:

> Medical audit can be defined as the systematic, critical analysis of the quality of medical care, including the procedures used for diagnosis and treatment, the use of resources, and the resulting outcome and quality of life for the patient. (Department of Health, 1989b, p. 3)

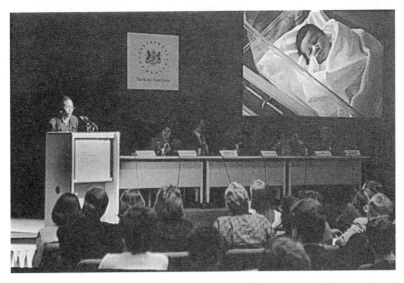

Case management guidelines and treatment protocols have been developed for some conditions by discussion and agreement between large groups of professionals at consensus conferences. Here participants attempt to develop guidelines for the management of maternity care in the NHS (London, 1993). (Photo: Mike Levers)

One of the most popular methods of medical audit is the **case-note review**, which involves discussion of selected patients ('cases'), sometimes involving one group of doctors assessing the work of another group (also known as **peer review**). These cases may be selected in a variety of ways: at random, according to specific conditions, or according to specific outcomes such as post-operative complication or death. The aim is to learn from the critical analysis of past practice. Agreed criteria for the management of particular cases may be applied, or may indeed be the product of such discussion exercises. Treatment policies may gradually change as a result of the adoption of **treatment protocols**, which are descriptions of a set of procedures considered to represent the best clinical management of a particular disease or condition.

They are basically the medical version of a nursing care standard (see Box 4.1 earlier).

This type of evaluation need not be restricted to private discussions by groups of local professionals. In 1987 a report of a *confidential enquiry into peri-operative deaths* (CEPOD) was published. This involved analysis by specialist assessors of the case notes of people who had died within thirty days of an operation, in order to identify the contributory factors. The enquiry was done for two medical associations, of anaesthetists and of surgeons, and involved looking at the work of consultants in health authorities that had volunteered to participate. Some of the results are given in Table 4.5, which lists surgeons from the most junior grade (Senior House Officer, SHO) to the most senior (Consultant).

Table 4.5 Surgeon assessors' opinions about the causes of peri-operative death, according to the grade of the surgeon who did the operation

Grade of surgeon	Number of deaths	Percentage of deaths with avoidable elements	Percentage of cases for which operation was inappropriate	Percentage of cases with inappropriate pre-operative management
Senior House Officer	124	27.4	8.1	22.6
Registrar	885	25.6	12.8	14.4
Senior Registrar	329	22.8	9.7	10.9
Consultant	1 312	20.2	8.6	7.7

Derived from Buck, N., Devlin, B. and Lunn, J. N. (1987) *Report of a confidential enquiry into peri-operative deaths*, Nuffield Provincial Hospitals Trust, London, Table 4.64, p. 101.

☐ What do the data in Table 4.5 show about the causes of peri-operative deaths?

■ The most junior grade of surgeon doing appreciable numbers of operations (SHOs) have the highest rate of deaths with avoidable elements (27.4%) and this proportion decreases as the seniority of the surgeons rise, with consultants having a rate of 20.2%. The rate of doing inappropriate operations does not drop with grade of surgeon, but the rate of inappropriate pre-operative management does, with the most junior grade having the highest rate (22.6%), and consultants having a rate of 7.7%.

☐ What might explain these differences?

■ Junior doctors have less experience, so make more mistakes. Alternatively, the assessors might have been influenced by their expectation that the more junior surgeons would make more mistakes.

In fact, the assessors knew the grade of surgeon doing the operation when they made their judgements, so the second explanation cannot be ruled out. Nevertheless, the report was critical of the fact that junior or inexperienced surgeons were too often involved in certain operations, and the authors also observed that

> General surgeons doing non-urgent brain surgery...and orthopaedic surgeons doing bowel surgery are examples that are difficult to defend. (Buck et al., 1987, p. 37)

Among other things, the CEPOD evaluation has contributed to arguments for the funding of more specialist centres for certain surgical procedures. The report did much to encourage the medical profession and the government in promoting medical audit.

Clearly, case-note review is dependent on the quality of information in the medical notes, or in the case of the CEPOD enquiry, the quality of doctors' replies to the survey. Massive amounts of information about activity in the health service is collected routinely, for administrative purposes. It is tempting to want to use this in auditing medical practice, but the interpretation of such data can present special difficulties. Consider, for example, using re-admission rates to hospital, which are routinely collected and computerised, as an indicator of the quality of medical care. In theory, if there is a high rate of re-admission in a hospital, it may be possible to conclude that the medical care that patients received there was ineffective.

☐ What might threaten the internal validity of using re-admission rates as an indicator of the effectiveness of medical care?

■ Other factors than the quality of medical care can affect the rate. Some re-admissions are planned, and some that are not planned are not avoidable by good medical care. To get a valid indicator you would need to know the *proportion* of re-admissions that were due to an *avoidable* outcome.

In fact, records kept for administrative purposes would need to be far more detailed before they could be used to make firm judgements about the relationship between medical care and outcome.

Medical audit under medical control?

Audit has been better established in hospitals than in primary care, but the expansion of audit in both areas was encouraged by the publication of the 1989 White Paper, *Working for Patients* (Department of Health, 1989a) and the subsequent working paper on medical audit (Department of Health 1989b). DHAs were required to set up medical audit advisory committees to advise on audit in the hospital and community services, and Family Health Services Authorities were required to set up similar groups of GPs. On the whole, central government relied on the medical profession to take the initiative. However, the White Paper gave managers the responsibility to check that adequate audit systems were being implemented in their area, the right to instigate an audit if they felt it necessary, and suggested that the general results of audit should be made available to managers. As Chapter 2 pointed out, this process can be expected to bring clinical activity more under the influence of operational managers.

Doctors have been keen to set up audit arrangements. The *British Medical Journal*, in cooperation with the King's Fund Centre, began in 1990 a regular weekly section describing audit initiatives throughout the country. The focus and detail of medical audit are very much the province of the medical profession, and fears have been expressed that focusing on narrow medical criteria for judging success may lead to faulty judgements. Jane Mallett, a research worker based at the Royal Marsden Hospital in London, in an article arguing for 'client and population-centred' audit rather than a 'profession-based philosophy' provides a hypothetical example of how narrow definitions of success can mislead:

> The surgeon operates proficiently on a fractured neck of femur, but the nurse does not encourage or give confidence to the patient who does not mobilise well. The physiotherapist does not

teach the patient to walk up the stairs, and the occupational therapist fails to check that the patient can get around at home. Surgical audit suggests good treatment; the bone has healed well, and the patient is beginning to walk. But, the patient gets home, is inadequately mobilised, gets stiffer, sits in a chair, does not eat and catches pneumonia. (Mallett, 1991, p. 24)

Mallett feels that audit should be multi-disciplinary if it is to reflect patients' total experience of health care.

☐ Earlier in this chapter you were introduced to another form of professional self-evaluation. What was it and which health-care occupation practised it in that example?

■ Standard setting by nurses, an example of which was given in Box 4.1.

Both medical audit and standard setting can be included under the general heading of **quality assurance**. This term, derived from theories of business management, has been imported by health-service managers. Initiatives under this heading have not solely been the province of those who provide direct care. There have also been management initiatives to promote and evaluate quality in health care.

Management initiatives: the case of performance indicators

One of the most important ways in which managers have attempted to evaluate health care has been through the use of **performance indicators**. These consist of routinely collected statistics about various aspects of health-service provision, most commonly rates of specific activities, such as hospital admissions and length of stay. Performance indicators are supplied to health authorities by the Department of Health (and its equivalent in Scotland, Wales and Northern Ireland) in computerised form, so that local managers and others can get information relevant to their own concerns, asking, for example, how their authority compares with others on a specific performance indicator. Some examples are given in Table 4.6, which shows where Coventry DHA stood in 1989–90 in relation to the national picture for a number of performance indicators relevant to gynaecology.

Table 4.6 Health-service performance indicators relating to gynaecology in Coventry, 1989–90

	National average	Coventry average
gynaecology day cases for people aged 16–64, expressed as a percentage of what would be expected given national rates	100	121.7
hospital day-case episodes for people aged 65+ concerning gynaecology, expressed as a rate per 1 000 people in the population (national or district)	0.450	0.660
cervical cancer annual SMR for females aged 16–64	99.6	171.5
average length of hospital episodes for gynaecology (days)	2.5	2.45
number of patients awaiting admission for gynaecology, per 1 000 people in the population (national or district)	4.75	7.03
number of gynaecology consultants per 100 000 people in the population (national or district)	3.02	2.28
number of women aged 35–64 who have had a cervical smear in the last 5.5 years, divided by the number of women in the population (national or district)	68.21	85.37

Derived from *1989–90 Health Service Indicators package*, Department of Health. (For further details contact the Health Services Indicators Section at the DH.)

☐ On which indicators does Coventry have a high score in comparison with other districts?

■ The Standardised Mortality Ratio (SMR) for cervical cancer, the cervical smear rate and the waiting list for gynaecology are high in Coventry. The day case rate is also somewhat above average.

☐ How does Coventry compare on the other indicators?

■ The length of stay in hospital for gynaecology is about average, but the number of consultants in the specialty is below average.

The difficulties in interpreting performance indicators begin when attempts are made to make causal statements about sets of indicators such as those for Coventry. One interpretation might go like this: 'Coventry has below average resources for gynaecology (reflected in the number of consultants), yet the medical staff nevertheless maintain a rate of activity comparable with the national average, measured in day cases and length of stay. However, demand is such that medical activity cannot keep up with it, so waiting lists are long'. The most contentious step in this flawed line of reasoning would be to say that this failure to keep up with demand is the reason for the high SMR from cervical cancer.

□ Why is this line of reasoning flawed?

■ The number of consultants is not a complete measure of resources available to gynaecology, as the numbers of more junior medical staff, nurses, beds and so on may alter the overall resource picture. Medical staff other than consultants may be responsible for the day-surgery activity. We would need to know the proportion of the gynaecology waiting list consisting of women with positive cervical smears to know if activity was keeping up with need in this area. There is a variety of factors causing high SMRs from cervical cancer, among which the accessibility of preventive medical care may be relatively unimportant.[12]

Difficulties in interpreting performance indicators do not, however, mean that they are useless. Armed with a set of indicators, a local manager (or indeed doctor should one be so motivated), can begin to enquire into the local conditions that cause variation. Performance indicators are also potentially useful to managers who wish to influence clinical decision-making: doctors, when confronted with evidence that local performance is markedly different from the national average, normally feel constrained to consider why.

The main problem with indicators of activity, however, is that there is no guarantee that the national average level is the right one to achieve good health outcomes. There are only a few indicators that can be interpreted as outcome measures, and these normally refer to mortality rather than morbidity. Linking activity to outcome is fraught with threats to internal validity, as the flawed attempt (above) to link gynaecology waiting lists to cervical cancer SMRs showed. It is perhaps for this reason that

[12]See *World Health and Disease* (1993), Chapter 9.

doctors have shown little interest in performance indicators, and managers have only had limited success in using them to influence doctors.

It is also the case that not all of the potential users of performance indicators are proficient in reasoning about several of them in combination. You should be better at doing this if you have understood the main ideas of this chapter.

Conclusion

You will have gathered by now that evaluation is an exercise that has many pitfalls, requiring careful planning, time and resources. Its effect on the decision-making process is limited, although there are some examples of its usefulness, but it has the potential to contribute to a more rational decision-making process at all levels of the health-care system. However, it is important to recognise that methods such as the randomised controlled trial that have proved so successful in evaluating the effectiveness of medical treatments may not be feasible or appropriate at other levels of health care. The methods of the social sciences are often necessary to assess the process of care, rather than focusing solely on outcomes.

At the same time, developments in the field of health measurement offer the chance to assess success using a wider range of criteria than was the case twenty years ago. Initiatives such as medical audit, the use of care standards and treatment protocols, hold out the prospect of cheaper and more immediately relevant feedback on the success of health care, thereby increasing the potential for evaluation to affect the practice of those providing care. In spite of their technical problems, performance indicators can encourage health-care providers to question their patterns of activity intelligently.

In the last analysis, evaluation can only succeed if people are prepared to examine their practices critically and objectively, and then act upon the results. However, it may be unrealistic at the policy level to hope for the direct linkage of results to decisions in the way that the rational, step-by-step approach suggests. The results of research may often influence policy makers in a more diffuse way, seeping into their thinking, in a manner that eventually provides enlightenment.

OBJECTIVES FOR CHAPTER 4

When you have studied this chapter, you should be able to:

4.1 Discuss the ways in which evaluation may enhance rational decision-making, and understand some of the difficulties in achieving this.

4.2 Assess the extent to which the logic of the randomised controlled trial is applicable to the evaluation of different aspects of health care, and comment on the value and limitations of the quasi-experimental approach.

4.3 Understand what is meant by threats to internal and external validity in evaluation design.

4.4 Distinguish between process and outcome in evaluative studies, and describe the illuminative approach to studying them.

4.5 Give examples to show that different measures of health outcome reflect the different priorities of interest groups with a stake in health care.

4.6 Comment on the role of practitioner-based self-evaluation, such as medical audit, in improving the quality of health care.

4.7 Appreciate the advantages and difficulties in using performance indicators to judge the effectiveness of health services.

QUESTIONS FOR CHAPTER 4

Question 1 (*Objectives 4.2 and 4.3*)

Electroconvulsive therapy (ECT) is a controversial treatment that involves giving electric shocks to the brain of an anaesthetised patient. Many psychiatrists feel that it alleviates depression in severe cases. How would you design a randomised controlled trial of the effectiveness of ECT for alleviating depression, that would show if a *placebo* effect

was occurring? What threats might there be to the internal and external validity of the trial?

Question 2 (*Objective 4.4*)

You have been asked to evaluate a programme of community care for people with mental illness, covering its effectiveness, efficiency, humanity and equity. What would you need to define before you began, and what might a study of (a) the process of care and (b) the outcome of care tell you about these four elements of the evaluation?

Question 3 (*Objectives 4.1 and 4.5*)

A group of hospital consultants providing maternity care in a district general hospital is keen to prove that the birth of babies in the hospital is better than in other places because it is safer. The local Community Health Council wants to encourage the use of maternity units run by GPs, where technical procedures, they feel, are less intrusive; they also want to maintain home delivery as an option. Both interest groups commission an evaluation that will prove their point. How might each side choose outcome measures that will reflect their concerns?

Question 4 (*Objective 4.6*)

The 1989 White Paper *Working for Patients* sought to encourage medical audit by the medical profession. How might medical audit work for patients' interests, and what might be the obstacles to it doing so?

Question 5 (*Objective 4.7*)

In one health authority there is a very high rate of hysterectomy per 1 000 women in the catchment population compared with the national average, and in another it is very low. What more would a manager need to know before raising the issue with the doctors concerned?

5 The consumer voice

This chapter builds on information about the role of Community Health Councils in *Caring for Health: History and Diversity, Chapter 7.* You are also referred to discussion of interactions between doctors and patients in other books in this series.[1] During your study of this chapter, you will be asked to read an article entitled 'Transferring power in health care' by Fedelma Winkler.[2] A television programme, 'Who calls the shots?', is also relevant to this chapter.

This chapter was written by Clive Seale, a medical sociologist and Lecturer in the Department of Sociology, Goldsmiths' College, University of London, who also wrote Chapter 4.

A personal dilemma

On my desk is a leaflet called 'The Patient's Charter', which outlines ten rights and nine national standards for the NHS. William Waldegrave, Secretary of State for Health, writes in the introduction that this charter came into effect on 1 April 1992, just nine days ago. Should I feel I am being denied any of the rights outlined in it I am told I can write to Duncan Nichol, Chief Executive of the NHS. I am even given the name and address of someone in the Department of Health should I wish to propose new standards. Box 5.1 contains an abridged version of the Patient's Charter.

[1]Presented to students of the Open University from 1994 onwards in *Medical Knowledge: Doubt and Certainty* (revised edition 1994). In 1993, students can consult a limited discussion in *Studying Health and Disease* and *Experiencing and Explaining Disease* (original editions, Open University Press, 1985).

[2]See *Health and Disease: A Reader* (revised edition 1994).

My first reaction is that these ideas look very attractive. Then a more critical thought occurs to me: do the existing rights really exist so unequivocally, and will the new ones really be achieved? Opponents of the government have been telling me all through the election campaign that, under the newly reformed system, my doctor may allow financial considerations to influence judgement of my clinical need. Surely this affects the first right that is said to exist already? I am aware that many millions of pounds have been spent in the past few weeks paying surgeons to operate on people who have currently been waiting for more than two years. This seems a good thing, yet some doctors have been saying that this has led to people with more urgent clinical needs being pushed aside.

Then my thoughts become more personal. Currently I have a small lump on my toe, which can be removed in hospital. If my GP tells me I must go to have this done, how will I tell whether the doctor who does it will be good at it in order to exercise my existing right 4? How can I tell whether the GP explained all the possible treatment options for my problem (existing right 5)? Furthermore, according to a report that I saw in the paper a few months ago: my Regional Health Authority was no longer planning to provide for the removal of non-malignant lumps and bumps (I hope it isn't cancer!), tattoo removal and cosmetic treatment of varicose veins. Other procedures were deemed to be of higher priority. What does this say about my first existing right—to receive health care on the basis of clinical need?

A number of thoughts occur to me. Will the Patient's Charter affect me? My newspaper tells me that it is a part of a larger initiative, the Citizen's Charter, inspired by the Prime Minister, extending beyond health care to matters like the compensation of passengers whose trains have been cancelled, as well as to other public services. What does it mean, anyway, to be thought of as a citizen-consumer of health care rather than just a plain old patient? Should I be trying to make myself a better-informed consumer? Why is the government making these changes anyway?

Box 5.1   Extracts from the Patient's Charter (1991)

Seven existing rights

Every citizen already has the following National Health Service rights:

1   to receive health care on the basis of clinical need, regardless of ability to pay;

2   to be registered with a GP;

3   to receive emergency medical care at any time;

4   to be referred to a consultant, acceptable to you, when your GP thinks it necessary and to be referred for a second opinion if you and your GP agree this is desirable;

5   to be given a clear explanation of any treatment proposed, including any risks and any alternatives, before you decide whether you will agree to the treatment;

6   to have access to your health records and to know that those working for the NHS will, by law, keep their contents confidential;

7   to choose whether or not you wish to take part in medical research or medical student training.

Three new rights from 1 April 1992:

1   to be given detailed information on local health services, including quality standards and maximum waiting times;

2   to be guaranteed admission for virtually all treatments by a specific date no later than two years from the day when your consultant places you on a waiting list;

3   to have any complaint about NHS services investigated, and to receive a full and prompt written reply.

In addition, nine aimed-for *National Charter Standards* are outlined. These cover issues such as respect for people's privacy, religion and cultural beliefs; access arrangements for people with special needs; maximum waiting times for emergency ambulances, out-patient clinic appointments and accident and emergency appraisal; limits on cancellation of operations; allocation of a named nurse, midwife or health visitor; and arrangements made for continuing health or social care before discharge from hospital.

Source: Department of Health (1991a) The Patient's Charter, HMSO, London, extracts from pp. 8–16.

Consumerism in health care

Consumerism is a system of ideas and values that has appeared in a variety of forms in the 1970s and 1980s, but that has only more recently arisen in health care. In economics, a consumer is a person who buys goods or services for his or her own personal use, and consumerism relates to the protection of the consumer's interests. In this chapter, we will explore how relevant these definitions are when applied to users of health and social services.

First, the origins and recent influences on consumerism in health care will be discussed. We examine the relevance of *private-sector consumerism*, and in

particular the key mechanism of *consumer choice*, in the public-sector health service. Then we discuss some different approaches to consumerism, beginning with the strengths and limitations of *management-led consumerism*. You will be invited to read a critique of this model by Fedelma Winkler, a leading campaigner for consumers' rights. Next, we turn to the avenues for *consumer complaint and redress* in the NHS, and assess their adequacy in producing a more responsive service. Finally, a more radical view of consumerism as *representation and participation* is discussed. The chapter ends by looking at the implications for consumer choice of the NHS reforms of the 1990s.

A key dilemma in any discussion of consumerism is the difficulty of balancing what is best for the individual against what is best for all of the people served by a health-care system. The tension between these two principles emerges repeatedly throughout the chapter.

Origins and influences

Consumerist ideals can be invoked by a variety of interest groups to further their ends. People who buy a product or use a service can appeal to the ideals of consumerism to get a better deal for themselves. Those who provide goods and services, or sell them for a profit, can make them appear more attractive when they claim to be meeting the demands of consumers. If politicians can persuade consumers of publicly-provided services that users' interests are paramount in policy considerations, they think they will gather votes. Professional associations also often justify their monopoly over the provision of a service by claiming that the exclusion of non-qualified practitioners best protects the interests of consumers.

Before consumerism entered thinking about public services, it was well established in private business. Modern industry has become increasingly sophisticated in developing an awareness of consumer preferences and—some would say—in manipulating them through advertising and other means. Market research has, since World War II, become an indispensable tool of the successful business. Customer relations departments in private enterprises have mushroomed, and acquire a particular importance in service industries, where training in interaction with customers has come to be seen as a crucial determinant of the quality of the product. The airline steward may therefore wish that we 'have a nice flight', the fast food waiter that we 'have a nice meal and do come back again', and almost anyone may unexpectedly want us to 'have a nice day'.

As some of the preceding examples suggest, consumerism blossomed first and foremost in North America. In the United Kingdom, the Consumers' Association was founded in 1957 to represent and campaign for consumer's rights. The original *Which?* magazine published by this organisation was, and still is, largely devoted to providing readers with information about the quality of high-street products, particularly those where evaluation of quality requires specialist knowledge beyond the resources of individual lay people. More recently, the magazine has spawned various offshoots focusing on particular areas, such as gardening or cars. In 1989, *Which? Way to Health* was launched, publishing, amongst other things, surveys relating to public

perceptions of the quality of medical care. Two such surveys in 1991 were reported in the national press:

GPs who refuse second opinions

One in 10 patients who ask to be referred for a second opinion by their family doctor is refused, a survey from the Consumers' Association says today. 'We think that doctors who refuse to refer patients for a second opinion are sometimes being illogical.' The Association says 'They need to stop thinking that doctor knows best'. (Mihill, *Guardian*, 12 February 1991)

Patients 'being left in ignorance'

One in five people leaving a hospital consultation with a specialist still do not understand what is wrong with them, according to a Consumers' Association report published today. 35% said there didn't seem time to ask the consultant questions, and 22% felt they were keeping other patients waiting. The Association recommends making a list of questions in advance of the visit, doing some homework in advance to find out about the possible condition, and taking along a friend or relative. (Mihill, *Guardian*, 7 February 1991)

☐ Which points in the Patient's Charter (see Box 5.1) concern the issues raised in these reports?

■ The first report concerns existing right 4 which covers second opinions. The second report is not covered by existing right 5 as this concerns explanations about treatments, not diagnosis. Existing right 6, if exercised, could lead to more information about diagnosis, though the records might not be in a form that most people could understand.

A host of pressure groups representing the interests of particular health-service users also exist. Age Concern, MIND, the National Childbirth Trust, the National Association for the Welfare of Children in Hospital, and the Patients' Association are a few of the better-known examples. In addition there are numerous support groups which also campaign for better services for people with particular diseases (for example, epilepsy, AIDS, autism, multiple sclerosis, schizophrenia, sickle-cell disease). These groups vary in their relationship with medical interests, some of them being critical, others devoting a large part of their fund-raising efforts to the support of medical research.

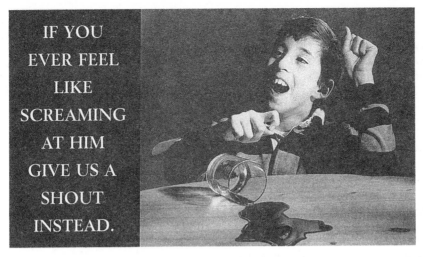

Pressure groups can provide practical help as part of their activities, as in the case of the Cerebral Palsy Helpline operated by The Spastics Society. (Source: The Spastics Society)

A distinctive feature of consumerism in the 1980s was its increasing application to public-sector services in Britain, where previously it had been very much a private-sector concern. This was associated with the free market political ideology of the so-called 'New Right', represented in the United Kingdom by the Conservative government under Mrs Thatcher. Broadly speaking, the New Right had an interest in countering what they saw as a 'dependency culture' encouraged by the Welfare State. There was new emphasis on individual choice exercised through the market place to improve the efficiency and quality of services. Associated with this was a desire to curb public expenditure and to assert authority over the activities of health professionals who, in the NHS, would otherwise determine expenditure by the cumulative effect of their clinical decisions. A constellation of forces came to bear on the public services, as pressure groups agitated for change, the broader public became more consumer conscious, and finally a government committed to assisting individuals to overcome their dependency on the services of a 'nanny state' was elected and then re-elected. Christopher Pollitt, a health policy analyst writing of this phenomenon in 1987, said:

> …'consumerism' has become an officially approved fashion. In hospitals, schools, housing schemes, advice and information services and many other aspects of public administration managers are being exhorted to pay more attention to consumer wishes, offer consumers wider choice, and develop techniques for 'marketing' their particular service. (Pollitt, 1987a, p. 43)

Relevance of consumerism to health care

But how relevant is consumerism to health care? We can approach this question by considering the similarities and differences between private-sector markets in goods and services, and the public-sector service of health care.

□ How is the consumption of supermarket goods different from the consumption of NHS medical care?

■ There are many differences that you may have thought of, but here are three:

• You pay for supermarket goods directly, whereas people pay for the NHS indirectly, through taxation.

• You can exercise more choice over what to buy from a shop, than over which NHS doctor to see and which treatment to have.

• You judge the quality of, say, apples by tasting them, but it is hard to judge the quality of medical advice because this needs a high level of medical knowledge.

The last two points were made by Margaret Stacey, a sociologist, who wrote an article in 1976 in which she analysed the position of the health-care user. On the one hand, she conceded that thinking of the patient as consumer might help patients assert themselves in the face of the overwhelming dominance of professional interests. But, she argued, the consumption of health care was not the same as the consumption of supermarket goods.

She felt it was important to distinguish between different types of patient. For some, such as long-term sick or disabled people, the patient's knowledge of their condition might exceed that of the professional, and 'patienthood' could become a way of life. For others, the patient role is much more temporary or intermittent. Because the importance of illness in peoples' lives varies, their investment in getting a good service also varies. Furthermore, certain patients are less able than others to articulate their preferences. Patients whose first language is not English, people with severe learning difficulties or some forms of mental illness, and certain elderly patients, may be in a weaker position than the otherwise healthy young adult consulting for a sore throat.

□ In the article we have just discussed, Margaret Stacey focuses on the consumer as the *current* user of the health service, following the logic that in the supermarket the consumer is the shopper. Who else but current users might claim to be consumers of health services?

■ You may have thought of the following:

• Carers of those who are ill may be profoundly affected by the services offered to those they care for.[3]

• Potential users of the health service, such as those in need of care but who have not sought it, or those who are likely to need care in the future, will be affected by decisions made by the providers of services. The accessibility of services, and decisions about preventive health care will be of particular importance here.

• Taxpayers who pay for the service but are not using it.

Unlike the private-sector consumer, in the public sector the people who pay for the service are not necessarily those who use it. In the private sector, if demand increases, supply generally expands to meet this. In the NHS, demand may be great, but (as Chapter 3 showed)

---

[3]See Chapter 8 of this book, which touches on the consequences for carers of community care provision; a more extensive discussion formed part of *Caring for Health: History and Diversity* (revised edition 1993), Chapter 7.

rationing decisions have to be made since those who pay for the service (and it is the government who speaks for them) may not wish to meet such a high level of demand. Thus, service-users do not have the right of unlimited access, and policy-makers or providers generally make decisions about rationing. One important focus for organised consumer demands is for the criteria on which rationing is based to be made more explicit. A variety of public outcries about the rationing of services such as kidney dialysis reflect consumers' uneasiness about the current situation.

This has implications for the principle of consumer choice, the key mechanism in the private sector for the exercise of consumer sovereignty, with all the assumed benefits that flow from this. In a system where there is rationing of scarce resources, quasi-political decisions are made about, for example, the priority groups discussed in Chapter 3. People who have learning difficulties may be deemed more deserving than people seeking cosmetic surgery, but less deserving than acutely sick children. Thus, a consumer in one part of the service getting a 'best buy' may disadvantage others who have then to settle for second-best. This sort of thinking led Rudolf Klein, a leading social policy analyst, to observe that the creation of the NHS

> ...represented the rejection of the market principle in favour of a collectivist solution... [which assumes] that there is a collective interest in the provision of health care over and above the self-interest of individual members of society. (Klein, 1989, p. 153)

On this thinking, the essence of a public service is that it involves some degree of *redistributive justice*. Clearly, unbridled consumer choice in health care, expressed through individuals with varying influence and wealth, could lead to an unacceptable and unfair distribution of resources. Those in most need might have little purchasing power under such a system.

The origins of consumerism in the private sector, then, raise important questions about its applicability in public-sector health services. This should remind you of the key dilemma outlined at the start of this chapter: the tension between the right of the individual to choose the best health care available, as against the rights of other consumers not to be disadvantaged by this choice.

However, consumerism is not just about the freedom to make personal choices.

□ Look at the Patient's Charter again (Box 5.1). Which aspects relate to enhanced consumer choice? What are other aspects concerned with?

■ Existing rights 4–7 could all enhance choice, as could the first new right. The third new right concerns the right of redress, and the other rights concern the availability of the service. Some of the standards concern patients' convenience and the respect offered by providers.

Consumerism therefore also concerns the responsiveness of providers to complaints, and the humanity with which the service is given. A service can, in theory, be responsive and humane without offering choice. There have been a number of government and management-led initiatives to improve these aspects of health care in recent years, to which we now turn.

Customer service in the 1980s

Management-led consumerism in the NHS received significant impetus in 1983 when the government received the Griffiths Report on management in the health service. Some years later Griffiths quoted three extracts from this report (see Box 5.2), saying that they 'give in effect my definition of consumerism'.

Management-led consumerism was promoted vigorously in the 1980s, and had a number of practical manifestations. Training in *customer relations* for health-authority staff and *mission statements* to help focus all staff on the common goal of public service are examples. Taking inspiration from market research in the private sector, **patient satisfaction surveys** multiplied. Such surveys were not a new phenomenon, having been done occasionally in the 1970s. Indeed the Royal Commission on the NHS which reported in 1979 had commissioned a survey of public perceptions of the NHS which showed widespread overall support for the service, coupled with criticism of specific aspects, such as the lack of appointment systems in hospital out-patient departments, and excessively early waking times for in-patients.

What was new about surveys of patient satisfaction in the 1980s was their relatively widespread usage, and their linkage to an overall management philosophy that stressed responsiveness to customers. (However, you will recall that the Audit Commission Report you studied during Chapter 1 firmly advocated an expansion of day surgery *before* learning the results of a patient satisfaction survey it had commissioned.) One of the challenges for those working in this field is to construct ways of routinely monitoring patients' views, at little cost, and to ensure that results are fed back into planning decisions. Too often in the 1980s surveys were done at some expense,

---

Box 5.2 Griffiths' definition of consumerism: the management-led model

1   The NHS Management Board and Health Authority Chairmen should ensure that it is central to the approach of management, in planning and delivering services for the population as a whole, to:

(a)   ascertain how well the service is being delivered at local level by obtaining the experience and perceptions of patients and the community: these can be derived from Community Health Councils and by other methods, including market research and from the experience of general practice and the community health services;

(b)   respond directly to this information;

(c)   act on it in formulating policy;

(d)   monitor performance against it;

(e)   promote realistic public and professional perceptions of what the NHS can and should provide as the best possible service within the resources available.

2   [The NHS cannot] display a ready assessment of the effectiveness with which it is meeting the needs and expectations of the people it serves. Businessmen have a keen sense of how well they are looking after their customers. Whether the NHS is meeting the needs of the patient and the community and can prove that it is doing so, is open to question.

3   Sufficient management impression must be created at all levels that the centre is passionately concerned with the quality of care and delivery of services at local level.

Source: Griffiths, R. (1988b) Does the public service serve? The consumer dimension, Public Administration, **66**, *p. 196.*

---

but reports ended up on managers' shelves without producing change in the service structure. One attempt at setting up a system for the routine monitoring of patient satisfaction is based on the questionnaire reproduced in Figure 5.1 (*overleaf*).

BLOOMSBURY HEALTH AUTHORITY

We are asking patients some questions about their stay in hospital to try to find out how we can make improvements. Please can you help by telling us what you thought about your care? Against the questions listed below, please join the dots like this ⊞ in the box underneath the face which best expresses your view. The faces range from very satisfied or pleased (number 4) to very dissatisfied or unhappy (number 1).

Please use a pencil or black pen like this ⊞ NOT like this ⊠ Other ways and other colours will not work.

Your completed questionnaire will be confidential — it will NOT be seen by the doctors and nurses who have treated you now or who may treat you in the future. This form is fed directly into a machine that only reads your answer marks.

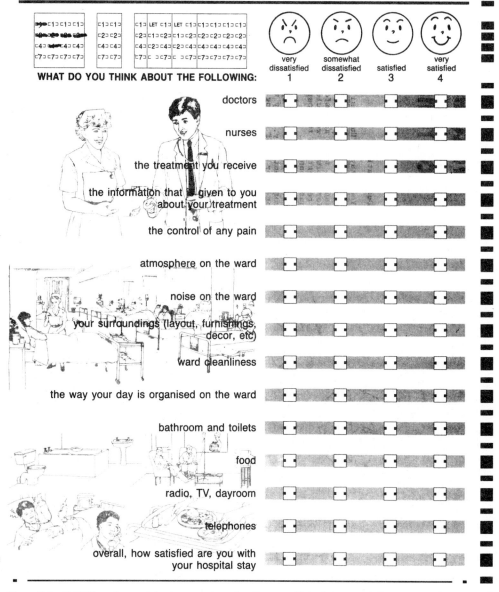

WHAT DO YOU THINK ABOUT THE FOLLOWING:

	very dissatisfied 1	somewhat dissatisfied 2	satisfied 3	very satisfied 4

doctors

nurses

the treatment you receive

the information that is given to you about your treatment

the control of any pain

atmosphere on the ward

noise on the ward

your surroundings (layout, furnishings, decor, etc)

ward cleanliness

the way your day is organised on the ward

bathroom and toilets

food

radio, TV, dayroom

telephones

overall, how satisfied are you with your hospital stay

Figure 5.1 *CASPE's patient satisfaction questionnaire. (Source: Clinical Accountability, Service Planning and Evaluation (CASPE), 1988, King's Fund, London)*

The questionnaire is designed so that results can be auto-matically entered into a computer. Patients are surveyed regularly, and the results collated each month, broken down by hospital ward, or by the consultant under whom the patient was admitted. This enables action to be taken should levels fall below agreed standards. Figure 5.2 shows how the result might vary over time between two wards.

   ☐ Which items on the questionnaire ask about the *effectiveness* of medical care?

   ■ Control of pain is the most directly relevant, although satisfaction with 'the treatment' received could include this, as might satisfaction with doctors.

In fact most of the questions in this and in other patient satisfaction exercises concern the quality of *hotel aspects* of care, such as cleanliness and food. This is largely because the people who plan such exercises feel that patients do not have the necessary expertise to judge technical aspects of the quality of medical care. At the same time, medical effectiveness is arguably the most important aspect of health care for consumers of health services.

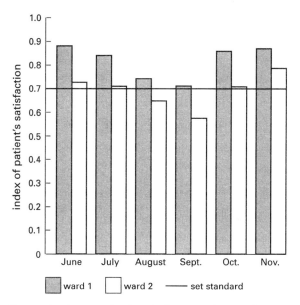

Figure 5.2 *An example of results from a patient satisfaction questionnaire. (Source: Green, J., 1988, On the receiving end,* Health Service Journal, *4 August, Figure 1, p. 881)*

The advantages of a survey such as the CASPE one include the ease with which the system is administered once set up, and its potential for feeding back into decisions about patient care. Traditionally, the NHS has had little incentive to improve the hotel aspects of care. In this respect private health care has a much better record. Such feedback, if institutionalised, could provide a stimulus for improvement.

   Management-led consumerism has a second aspect to it in addition to a concern with the quality of services. In *Listening to Local Voices in the NHS*, published in 1992, the NHS Management Executive argued that pur-chasing authorities should listen to local people's views on priorities for health care in order to legitimate the rationing decisions that they make (Sykes *et al.*, 1992). A variety of methods are being used to obtain such views, some of which were discussed in Chapters 2 and 3.[4]

Motives under suspicion

Management-led consumerism has been subjected to strong criticism by those promoting a more radical view of the proper role of the consumer. An example of such criticism is the article in the Reader,[5] 'Transferring power in health care', by Fedelma Winkler, a manager in a Family Health Services Authority and formerly chair of the Greater London Association of Community Health Councils. You should read it now.

   ☐ How does Winkler regard management-led consumerism?

   ■ With suspicion as to its true motives. She feels that managers in the NHS use consumerism as a weapon in their attempts to curb the power of doctors to make rationing decisions (a view explored in Chapter 2 of this book).

In the 1990s internal market, this may not be the only reason for suspicion. Think back to the audiotape 'Dilemmas in hospital management' that you listened to during study of Chapter 2. It contained a conversation between the hospital chief executive and a member of the local CHC.

   ☐ What attitude to the Patient's Charter did the hospital manager appear to have?

[4]See Chapter 2 and the study of health authority initiatives in England and Wales to consult local citizens on their plans, and Chapter 3, Table 3.2, on the Oregon health priorities experiment.

[5]*Health and Disease: A Reader* (revised edition 1994).

■ He seemed to view the attainment of targets mainly as points scored in the competition with rival providers in the area (he says he was converted to the Charter when he realised it was a 'beauty contest').

□ According to Winkler, what is the managerial response to challenge by consumers?

■ Direct opposition and hostility, as in their response to the women's health movement; neutralisation through diversionary activity, such as inviting users to participate in empty consultation exercises; and manipulating patient satisfaction surveys to their own advantage. Only occasionally do managers genuinely look for ways to share power.

□ What does she say about how consumerism can be made more effective?

■ Consumerism could be made more effective by the provision of statements of users' rights supported by a system that monitors abuse of rights; by providing the type of information that enables users to choose according to the quality of medical care; by supporting advocacy schemes that give individuals a voice in defending their rights; by encouraging an effective complaints procedure; by fostering informed and well-supported community representation; by bringing about a change in the culture of health-service institutions, from being 'provider-led', to 'user-led'.

Winkler's article represents a particular point of view, and you may not agree with her polemical approach. Contrary to Winkler's assumption, some patients do not want to participate in decision-making, preferring a more paternalistic style of health care.[6] You may also feel that her criticisms are unfair to managers. But her views are useful in pointing out that management-led consumerism reinforced by patient satisfaction surveys, is just one way in which consumerism may be manifested in health care. Another important avenue for consumerism she discusses is the development of an effective complaints procedure.

[6]Paternalism in interactions between doctors and patients is discussed in *Medical Knowledge: Doubt and Certainty* (revised edition 1994).

Complaint and redress

The right to return faulty products bought from shops is fairly well established. The equivalent to this in the consumption of services is the right of **complaint and redress**. Many private-sector companies use such experience as a way to get feedback on the quality of their service. In a consumer-conscious health service one might expect to see mechanisms whereby complaints could be heard and acted upon quickly, and where individual consumers were compensated in some manner for poor quality, accidents or negligence. Such mechanisms would become an important way of improving the quality of health care.

The experience of complaint and redress

Two examples from newspaper reports are given below of people who felt that they or their relative was treated badly by the health service, and wanted to do something about it.

Shortly before Christmas 1990, Jane Hanna's partner Alan died from an epileptic fit in his sleep. He was just 27 years old and a promising young barrister. He had been diagnosed as epileptic by his GP only seven months before. Not surprisingly, Ms Hanna was distraught. She was also very unhappy with how Alan's GP had treated him, so she made a formal complaint.

FHSA regulations laid down by the government state that complaints have to be made within 13 weeks. Despite her grief Jane Hanna met this deadline, only then to be told that the 13 weeks counted not from Alan's death, but from when the treatment from the GP began, seven months before. Ms Hanna protested, and eventually the FHSA waived the time limit, although it needed the GP's permission. A year after she complained she is still waiting for a hearing. (Berry, *Guardian,* 4 March 1992, p. 25)

Ten years ago Elsa Bentley, then 66, went into hospital to have her left hip replaced. Immediately after coming round from the operation she knew something had gone terribly wrong: she was in pain and her foot was numb with no sensation. Six weeks later she had an exploratory operation to find out what had happened. The verdict was permanent and severe damage to the sciatic nerve. Mrs Bentley has never walked more than a few yards since. Little did she realise but the failed operation was just the beginning of a ten year ordeal, still not over, to obtain redress. Injured by a medical accident, she was to be victimised all over again by the legal system.

Two solicitors and two barristers advised her she had little chance of proving the surgeon negligent…but she found a third solicitor and fought a two year High Court battle to allow her writ to proceed. Finally, last August a High Court judge ruled that her injury was caused by the surgeon's negligence. But with each side's costs estimated at £100 000, the fight is still not over. Bristol and Weston health authority has appealed, and she has yet to see a penny of the £85 000 damages. Russell Levy, her current solicitor, says: 'Mrs Bentley's case should have been concluded in 1986 or '87 at the latest. I've never understood why it has been so strenuously contested. They've made her fight every inch of the way. She stoutly declares: 'I'm not going to die before this is finished'. (Bunting, *Guardian,* 13 November 1991, p. 27)

These cases illustrate common difficulties in gaining redress and having complaints heard. Jane Hanna's case shows evidence of bureaucratic delay that has the potential to act in the interest of the doctor about whom she complained. Elsa Bentley's case shows even longer delay, this time caused by the legal system and the defensive action of the health authority.

□ What might the health authorities and doctors say to justify their decisions in these cases?

■ In Jane Hanna's case, it might be argued that it is difficult to investigate complaints made a long time after the event, recall of which may easy for the patient, but difficult for the doctor who sees many patients in a single day. In Elsa Bentley's case, it might be argued that until the judge's ruling it was not evident that negligence had occurred; the health authority was simply acting as a good employer in defending its employee's interests.

Defensiveness by the health service may be easier to understand if the impact of complaints on *providers* is considered. Dr Gerard Panting, head of GP services at the Medical Protection Society, has described this:

You can't imagine the anxiety a formal FHSA complaint causes a GP. It's often hanging over their heads for months, which can make their

clinical judgement erratic. Often the onus is on the GP to prove that he didn't breach his contract, rather than on the patient to prove that he did, especially if there is a death involved. (Quoted by Berry, *Guardian,* 4 March 1992, p. 25)

Who pays the bill for negligence?

In spite of the difficulties of obtaining legal redress in the United Kingdom, there was an increase in the frequency and severity of medical malpractice claims during the 1970s and 1980s, to the extent that one study by Robert Dingwall and colleagues at the Centre for Socio-legal Studies in Oxford, published in 1991, estimated that the total cost of medical litigation in England in 1988 was around £75 million. The cost to doctors in insuring themselves against such claims rose very quickly—by 70 per cent in 1986–7 and by a further 87 per cent in 1987–8 for example. Because this financial burden had become intolerable, responsibility for meeting the costs passed from individual doctors to health authorities in 1991, adding to managers' financial anxieties.

In the USA, where the population is generally less deferential to professional expertise, and also more willing to go to law to sort out disputes, fears have been expressed that medical practice has been distorted, becoming increasingly *defensive.* For example, there was a rise in the rate of caesarian delivery in the USA, from 5.5 per cent of births in 1970, to 20.3 per cent in 1983. It has been argued that this is because obstetricians have become increasingly concerned to avoid being blamed for neurological damage to babies. (There is, however, an alternative explanation, which is that caesarians have become safer over the years, so doctors may have become more willing to consider them.)

Complaints, too, have been rising. Between 1982 and the financial year 1990–1, written complaints to Health Authorities about hospital and community services more than doubled, as Table 5.1 (*overleaf*) shows.

□ Does the rise in complaints between 1982 and 1990–1 shown in Table 5.1 simply reflect a rise in the number of patients treated?

■ No, because the rate given for hospital care is 'per 1 000 patients treated', which adjusts for any increase in services provided between the two periods; similarly, the rate of community services is given 'per 100 000 population', which adjusts for any change in population size over time.

Table 5.1 Written complaints by or on behalf of patients in England between 1982 and 1990–1

	No. of complaints		Rate per 1 000 patients treated		Rate per 100 000 population	
	1982	1990–1	1982	1990–1	1982	1990–1
hospital	16 218	32 996	2.5	3.8	–	–
community	1 593	4 307	–	–	3.4	9.0

(Source: Department of Health, 1991b, *Return of Written Complaints by or on Behalf of Patients: England 1990/91,* Government statistics service and management information division, Branch SM12, Tables 2, 3 and 4, pp. 2–3)

It has been argued that one way to solve the unfairness, delay and stress to all parties involved in issues of medical accidents and negligence is a system of **no-fault compensation**. The proposed system would simply compensate people who had been damaged during medical care, without the need to prove the negligence of a particular doctor. In a sense, this would be a type of accident insurance. It is of interest to note that Arnold Simanowitz, the president of the Association for Victims of Medical Accidents, a body that exists to help people pursue negligence claims, has stated his opposition to no-fault compensation:

> A system that just gives money, not explanations, will not be good for patients or the Health Service. (Quoted in Millar, 1991, p. 16)

□ What other disadvantages might exist in such a system?

■ It could open the door to a flood of cases, resulting in a drain on health-service finances. It would still have to be proved that injury was the result of medical activity. Poor-quality medical practitioners would no longer have an incentive to practise safely.

The dilemma when considering redress and complaint can be summarised thus: on the one hand, it is right to compensate consumers who have received a bad or damaging service (and this can help providers assess the quality of their service too); on the other hand, the defensive medicine that this can involve may be to the disadvantage of other consumers, and the money spent on complaints and compensation would otherwise be spent on providing care.

Representation and participation

Earlier we introduced the supermarket analogy when discussing consumer choice. This can be carried further in order to explore a third approach to consumerism, **representation and participation**. This model of consumerism means that customers are not confined simply to deciding which product to take from the shelf, or complaining when the product is faulty. They are involved in decisions about what products should be on the shelf in the first place, or even where a new supermarket is to be built.

Representation and participation can occur at many different points in the health-care system, and involve taking part in decision-making. This can be done in a formal political way or informally at an individual level. People may represent themselves, or others. Essentially, these manifestations of consumerism are challenges to professional control over decision-making and may be at variance with the management-led model of consumerism. As in the earlier development of consumer movements in the private sector, there may also be spontaneous action on the part of local people, such as sit-ins at hospitals that are to be closed.

Community participation

The participation of representatives of local communities ('citizen representatives' as they were called in Chapter 2) in the formulation of local health policies is, in fact, an older tradition in health care than management-led consumerism. The creation of *Community Health Councils* (CHCs) in the 1974 reorganisation of the health service was, in part, an attempt to promote this.[7] As well as providing advice to individuals about the health service, many CHCs try to represent to health authorities the views of users about local provision, so that policy-makers can take these views into account. However, such user-participation has had a mixed record. In the USA, for example, in 1974, *Health Systems Agencies* (HSAs) were brought into being in some States. These were designed to enable the public to take part in the formulation of health policies. The first problem encountered by HSAs was in deciding which sections of the public were to be represented.

[7]The 1974 reorganisation of the health service in which CHCs were created is described in *Caring for Health: History and Diversity* (revised edition 1993), Chapter 7.

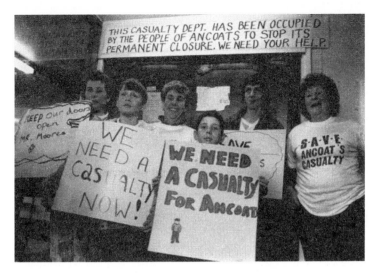

Members of the Ancoats Action Group during the eight-month occupation in 1987 by local people protesting at closure of the casualty department of Ancoats Hospital, Manchester.[8] The sit-in ended when a community clinic was promised, with local participation in its design and resourcing; it opened in 1989. (Photo: John Smith/Profile)

☐ Why do you think this was a problem?

■ Problems in deciding who should be represented mirror those of deciding who should be regarded as the consumer of health services. If patients are chosen, this would leave taxpayers and carers unrepresented. Some patients—for example those with learning difficulties—might be unable to represent themselves. A variety of voluntary groups might also claim a right to be represented.

HSAs also faced the problem of the weakness of the public interest in health matters, compared to the concentrated strength of service-providers. Because health issues tend to be intermittently important in peoples' lives, representation of the public interest was carried out by those who had a general interest in 'public affairs' rather than by consumers directly affected by health services. Providers of health services, on the other hand, had a continuing full-time interest in health care, and possessed resources and specialist knowledge of the system unequalled by community representatives. Thus, the outcome was weighted towards the interests of providers in the USA, just as the authors of Chapter 2 described for the United Kingdom.

[8]An image of Ancoats Hospital in 1952, by L. S. Lowry, appears as Figure 6.2 in *Caring for Health: History and Diversity.* The hospital is due to close completely by 1994.

In the article by Fedelma Winkler that you read earlier, the section headed 'Neutralisation through diversionary activity' provides graphic examples of how the odds may be stacked against user-representatives by managers and doctors. In an earlier article, she described the support that user-representatives require if they are to have an effective voice in health-service planning committees:

Lone user representatives on committees frequently get overwhelmed and feel unable to contribute. They can also become co-opted into the professional orbit and become supporters of the status quo. 'Your representative was present when the decision was taken' is a standard excuse by authorities to stop comment by a group at a later discussion.

To minimise the sense of isolation for the user representatives and to make sure their views are based on collective experience, it is important that they are held accountable by an outside community group that can provide them not only with support but with systematic background information.

This returns us to CHCs. City & Hackney CHC's representatives on Committees are never there as individuals. They must report back to a special interest group of the CHC. This group shares experiences and decides on policy collectively. The special interest group members come not only from the CHC but also from the relevant community organisations and interested individuals. Representatives go to Health Service Committees knowing that they have support, backing and information. They are not isolated. Each Group in turn reports to the full Community Health Council. (Winkler, 1987, p. 7)

Although there is a CHC in every health authority, there is great variation between them in the way in which they interpret their role. Indeed the role of CHCs has never been a very clear one, and their history has been marked by small budgets from the health service and periodic suggestions from central government that they are unnecessary. Thus, at the beginning of the 1980s, the Secretary of State for Health (Patrick Jenkin) suggested that CHCs might no longer be needed because DHAs were becoming increasingly responsive to community interests. Support from a variety of sources ensured the survival of CHCs, but official scepticism continued throughout the 1980s and into the 1990s.

In line with its scepticism about the role of CHCs, central government further weakened community participation under the *Working for Patients* reforms begun in 1989. As mentioned in Chapter 2, the boards that govern health authorities no longer had to appoint a certain proportion of members from the ranks of local councillors, and CHC members lost the right to attend board meetings. Paradoxically, then, central government initiatives in the 1990s became increasingly consumerist, encouraging responsiveness by local health-service managers ('supermarket consumerism' in Winkler's terms), but discouraged representation and participation—the more political forms of consumerism.

Any discussion of representation and participation at local level must also face up to the key dilemma of this chapter: the tension between the demands made by some consumers, and competing demands made by others. The requirements of a *nationally* planned service inevitably conflict with *local* demands for control over decisions about resource allocation. This is because redistributive justice requires central control if equity in health-service provision is to be achieved.

Patient participation

Representation, however, does not just have to occur at the level of policy-making. It has long been recognised that people who are seriously ill, or very elderly, and those with learning disabilities (previously known as 'mentally handicapped'), or whose command of English is weak, may have reduced ability to influence the care

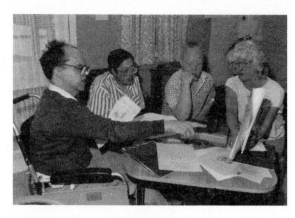

Support groups for people with disabilities, sometimes (as here) including an able volunteer, can empower members to identify and express their needs for health and social services. (Source: Leon Grech, The Open University)

they receive. **Patient advocacy** is a growing movement, in which users of health and social services provide each other with mutual support. Relying largely on volunteers who are independent from these services, advocacy involves the befriending of individual users of services on a one-to-one basis, with the advocate representing the patient's position to professionals at important decision points. **Empowerment** is a term frequently used to summarise the essence of advocacy, which *enables* the service-user to exercise some power over the care they receive.

Kate Butler and her colleagues describe the experience of one long-stay hospital patient, Robert, whose advocate was Doreen:

> Robert's advocate has become his appointee and successfully claimed backdated benefits which he had not received. She has also claimed Mobility Allowance on his behalf, and Supplementary Benefit for a period he spent on holiday. He regularly spends time outside the hospital with his advocate and her family. Doreen would often find Robert in bed when she arrived at the hospital to take him out, despite having made previous arrangements with staff. She raised strong objections and now staff help Robert get ready. Doreen has taught him to use the launderette, and also wash clothes at home. She persistently argues that if Robert wants to buy his own clothing, he should receive his share of the hospital clothing budget for this purpose. Robert now buys food and helps to prepare meals at Doreen's home. Doreen attends his case conferences and has

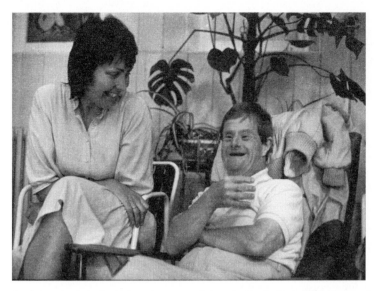

Advocacy can lead to rewards for both the advocate and those in need of a 'voice'. (Source: Leon Morris)

written to the National Development Team complaining about the lack of continuity of staff on his ward. (Butler *et al.*, 1988, pp. 9–10)

General practice is another arena where the consumer voice is beginning to be heard. A number of general practices have encouraged the formation of patient groups to advise and consult on the running of the practice. Patient groups have engaged in activities as diverse as the organisation of health education sessions, the coordination of voluntary schemes for the care of others, and participation in decision-making about matters such as appointment systems, the level of home visiting by GPs and prescribing in relation to antibiotics (Wood, 1984).

The empowerment of users of health and social services is clearly most appropriate in the case of vulnerable or disadvantaged groups. However, it is worth remembering that at this individual level, some people are better able to represent their interests to health-care professionals than others.

☐ What factors do you think might increase the ability of patients to influence the course of consultations?[9]

■ Age, social class, verbal fluency, medical knowledge and wealth. Adults are better able to influence

[9]Factors that increase the influence of patients in consultations with doctors are discussed in *Medical Knowledge: Doubt and Certainty* (revised edition 1994).

the consultation than children, and so are people from higher social classes, those who are articulate or who have a great deal of knowledge about their condition (e.g. someone who has been ill for a long time). Patients in private health-care settings are generally better able to influence the doctor for whose services they pay directly.

☐ What informal avenues may be open to the NHS patient whose views are at variance with those of the professionals?

■ There are several possibilities: non-compliance with instructions; use of alternative health care; use of private health care; reliance on self-medication.

Consumer choice in the 1990s

If the 1970s, broadly speaking, was the time for experiments with representation and participation, and the 1980s was the time for new initiatives in management-led consumerism, the 1990s may be the beginning of more substantial attempts to enhance consumer choice in health care.

☐ What objections have been raised so far in this chapter about a health-care system that allows total consumer sovereignty, exercised through choice?

■ Unbridled choice in a free-market system could result in imbalanced resource allocation since those with the most purchasing power, or the loudest voice, could consume resources at the expense of less powerful groups.

On the benefit side, there may be an incentive for providers to improve quality if consumers are allowed to choose where they go for care.

'Voting with their feet'

Politically-led initiatives to enhance consumer choice gathered momentum from the late 1980s onwards.The Patient's Charter with which this chapter began focused mainly on hospital care and was a sequel to earlier incursions of consumerism into general practice. The 1987 White Paper on primary care, *Promoting Better Health* (Department of Health and Social Security, 1987) contained the proposal that GPs should indulge in a limited form of advertising of their services by providing information in a 'practice leaflet', a leaflet showing what their practice has to offer. A larger proportion of the GP's pay became determined by the number of patients on his or her list, thus raising the incentives to be attractive to patients. Easier procedures for patients to change their GP were also introduced.

These measures encountered considerable professional resistance. Advertising, in particular, was viewed as a challenge to professional power, as it threatened to set doctors against each other, so restrictions were placed on the type of information that a practice leaflet could contain. Eventually, the new conditions of service were imposed on the doctors by the Secretary of State, against the wishes of the BMA. Thereafter, articles have continued to appear in the medical press predicting 'consumer inertia' over the matter of changing doctors. Some experience, however, suggests otherwise.

Barking and Havering FHSA (1991), for example, reported that 'as a result' of the easier procedures, changes of GP had doubled between the first quarter of 1989 (2 409 changes) and the same period in 1990 (4 882 changes). However, in the same paragraph in which these statistics were announced, the FHSA also stated:

> It is important that patients are given clear information to ensure that their choice is informed. (Barking and Havering FHSA, 1991, p. 37)

This identifies a key issue in considerations about patient choice: the adequacy of the information that is available to consumers of health care.

Making informed choices

☐ Earlier in this chapter it was noted that it is easier for patients to judge the quality of some aspects of health care than others. What were they?

■ Although patients can judge the quality of hotel aspects of care, or the quality of communication between themselves and professionals, specialist knowledge is generally required to judge the quality of clinical decisions.

Even beyond this, however, there is the issue of whether information about clinical performance exists within the NHS, where the evaluation of effectiveness is sparse (as the previous chapter showed). For example, the success rates of particular operations performed by different surgeons are rarely recorded. Even clinicians may have difficulty in exercising their judgement in the absence of such information.

☐ What major problem of interpretation might there be in examining the success rates of medical procedures (e.g. the number of patients surviving a risky operation)?

■ Concluding that one hospital is better than another because more patients survive does not take account of other factors that influence the outcome. The hospital with the lower survival rate may be treating more people at greatest risk from the procedure (for example, very young or very elderly patients).

However, this may not stop the development of 'league tables' in the NHS. In spite of similar objections, schools are now required to publish their examination results to inform parental choice. The CEPOD enquiry into postoperative deaths (described in Chapter 4) shows that such information is *potentially* available, although the enquiry was only feasible because surgeons were given strict guarantees that the report would not link success rates to particular doctors or hospitals. Once again, however, the experience of the USA may provide a pointer to future British developments; in 1986, the US National Association of Health Data Organizations released hospital-by-hospital mortality rates to an avid public reception and considerable disquiet (Pollitt, 1987b).

Methodological objections to such information are not the only ones, however. Doctors tend to argue that medical practice is impossible under such intensive scrutiny of results. There is considerable debate over who may be allowed access to the results of *medical audit* (see Chapter 4); some doctors are quite reluctant to share results with managers, let alone patients. Even if the facts were available in a way that allowed clear interpretation, the right time to present the facts to patients has to be chosen. It is clearly inappropriate to publicise the death rate from a procedure to a patient just as they are entering the operating theatre, whereas it may be right to make such information available at an earlier stage.

However, it is possible to present information in a way that helps the users of health services to make better decisions. In the Reader article you read earlier, Winkler provides examples from the USA where information about treatment options and clinical policies for particular conditions or events, such as breast cancer or childbirth, are made available to service-users. There may come a day when it will be possible for patients in waiting rooms to gain access by computer to information about the performance of the service they are waiting for.

One by-product of the NHS reforms of the 1990s, which separated purchasers and providers, is a powerful incentive to set up information-gathering systems. If the internal market operates as intended, data-bases will contain information about the quality of care, and will be used by purchasers to monitor the extent to which providers meet the standards set in contracts. Theoretically, at least, such information could be used by consumers to make informed choices.

However, for such a scenario to unfold several things are necessary. First, it will be necessary for purchasers to state the *expected* clinical and other quality-related standards to be achieved by providers. Concentrating on the *cost* of services alone will not be enough. Second, the information systems are only likely to achieve the necessary level of sophistication if there is a commitment to *monitoring* the extent to which providers meet the standards set. Third, there is a formidable array of technical and practical hurdles to be overcome in *agreeing* what information is relevant and making arrangements for its *collection* on a routine basis—a procedure that could be very costly.

Finally, there remains the issue of who should be given this information. Providers will have an incentive to keep both purchasers and the public in the dark about their failures, and to trumpet their successes. Purchasers will have a primary interest in getting the information, but have no strong incentive to share it with patients. As currently conceived, the internal market is one in which GPs and health authorities act as proxy consumers. Diane Plamping, a health policy analyst, welcoming the new system, has written optimistically in the *British Medical Journal* that

> Previously doctors have 'known what's best' for their patients, but now purchasing health authorities will become the people's advocates.

> A new group of professionals will act as discriminating purchasers of services by becoming expert in assessing health needs and in monitoring the quality and effectiveness of health care. (Plamping, 1991, p. 737)

This, of course, ought to solve the problem that consumer choice in health care is inhibited by a lack of medical expertise. However, the freedom to withdraw custom from providers should standards not be met will not be a freedom that is exercised by patients, but by this 'new group of professionals' standing between them and the provider. There is no choice of health authority, beyond moving out of an area.

In addition, many GPs who were *not* fund-holders complained, when the internal market was proposed, that the new arrangements would lead to *reductions* in the choices that they could make on behalf of their patients. This is because they would have to refer patients to hospitals with whom the health authority had already negotiated a contract, whereas previously GPs could refer anywhere in the country. It was planned that GPs would be able to make *extra-contractual referrals* to get around this problem, but only with permission from local-health-authority managers. In practice, although there have been examples of requests for such referrals being blocked, managers have more often been unable to stop GPs and consultants agreeing to treat each others' patients. GP fund-holders, of course, are able to refer wherever they wish, if the funds are available.

The creation of the information data-bases that the reforms require represents a significant step along the road to greater opportunities for better-informed consumer choice. Medical audit, interest in which has increased rapidly under the 1990s reforms, presents a further source of information. However, ownership of this information is likely to become a fiercely contested issue, with both managers and doctors defending their territory against each other and against consumer demands.

Conclusion

Consumerism originated in the private business sector, and is an approach that cannot simply be transferred to the NHS, where conditions are very different. For the *individual* consumer, advocacy schemes and the provision of clinically-relevant information may lead to more choice, but access by the consumer to relevant data-bases in the 1990s remains at issue. As we have suggested, however, balancing the needs of individuals against those of all of the people is a key dilemma in health care. One major difference between the private sector and the NHS is that private businesses can expand supply to meet demand, whereas in health care, demand from one set of consumers may, if met, disadvantage others. Management-led consumerism mainly avoids this dilemma by focusing on aspects of the quality of care, rather than on rationing decisions. Consumer representation and participation also do not resolve the dilemma, though they may at least ensure that certain voices are heard that would otherwise be drowned out. Increasingly, however, purchasing authorities are attempting to legitimate the decisions they make by asking local people about their priorities.

In the Reader article, Fedelma Winkler identified another aspect of consumerism within the NHS—the challenge it can present to professional power. It remains to be seen whether examples where local people or patients have a major impact on the way health care is provided represent a significant shift in the balance of power between lay and professional voices in the health field.

OBJECTIVES FOR CHAPTER 5

When you have studied this chapter, you should be able to:

5.1   Consider the extent to which users of health services may be thought of as consumers.

5.2   Assess the arguments for and against consumer sovereignty in health care.

5.3   Assess the strengths and weaknesses of management-led consumerism, and of current systems of complaint and redress.

5.4   Describe the type of information needed by consumers in exercising choice in health care, and the difficulties in getting information relevant to the quality of clinical care.

5.5   Assess the strengths and weaknesses of consumer representation and participation.

5.6   Assess the extent to which the internal market will enhance consumer choice.

QUESTIONS FOR CHAPTER 5

Question 1 (*Objectives 5.1, 5.2*)

To what extent can the principles of private-sector consumerism be applied in public-sector and social health services?

Question 2 (*Objective 5.3*)

The following is an extract from Sir Roy Griffiths' 1987 Redcliff-Maud memorial lecture (published the following year):

> One cannot do justice to the consumer dimension by a few superficial statements or by asking employees to wear the fixed smiles of Arctic winter towards the customer. When I talk about the consumer dimension I intend it to be seen as part of a total management and organisational philosophy…The interests of the consumer have to be central to every decision taken by the authority and its management—it is not a 'bolt-on' option to be used occasionally. (Griffiths, 1988b, p. 196)

According to Fedelma Winkler, to what extent has management-led consumerism achieved these ideals?

Question 3 (*Objective 5.5*)

What problems must be overcome to ensure effective consumer representation at the level of (a) the individual, and (b) the group?

Question 4 (*Objectives 5.4 and 5.6*)

Mrs Thatcher wrote in the foreword to *Working for Patients*, 'All the proposals put the needs of patients first…we aim to extend patient choice'. Which aspects of the proposals are likely to realise these aims and which are not?

6 Health work: divisions in health-care labour

This chapter builds on the discussion of the diversification and specialisation in health-care occupations which has taken place in the United Kingdom this century, and was a major theme in Chapters 5 to 7 of Caring for Health: History and Diversity.[1] *During your study of this chapter, you will be asked to read two articles from the Reader:[2] the first is entitled 'Food-work: maids in a hospital kitchen' by Elizabeth Paterson, and the second is an extract from the 'Second Report on Maternity Services' by the Health Committee of the House of Commons (referred to as the 'Winterton Report' after its chairman Sir Nicholas Winterton). You will also listen to an audiotape band called 'Health work: nurses' perceptions'. The television programme 'Who calls the shots?' deals in part with disputes between different groups of health-care workers about responsibilities for the care of acutely sick children, and also illustrates the extent to which health work in the 1990s is determined by purchasing authorities.*

This chapter was written by Gillian Pascall, a Lecturer in Social Policy specialising in health and women's studies, in the School of Social Studies at the University of Nottingham—a department noted for its research into the structure, organisation and history of health care—and Kate Robinson, Professor and Dean of the Faculty of Health Care and Social Studies at Luton College of Higher Education, who has published widely on key issues in nursing.

Dilemmas in health work

In this chapter we turn to the million or so people who experience the NHS as work. Doctors, managers, and health-service users have already been the subject of close scrutiny in earlier chapters of this book, so here we focus on the nurses, midwives, ambulance personnel, physiotherapists, pharmacists, caterers, cleaners, clerical workers, and others, who together make up the majority of health-service workers. Within this highly varied workforce, we give special attention to nurses and midwives. This is partly justified by their sheer numbers (roughly half a million, the largest group of workers in the NHS); partly by the social divisions within nursing, which make it in some ways representative of the workforce as a whole; and partly by the central role in patient care which nurses and midwives undertake in hospital and community settings. And, in furthering the aims of this book, dilemmas in nursing in the 1990s illustrate several of the key issues facing other groups of NHS workers.

The first dilemma is over who should do what? A complex division of labour in the NHS and a changing political and technological environment result in constant competition and negotiation over territory and work roles. Later we describe the disputed territory between obstetricians and midwives over maternity care; and dilemmas over boundaries between nursing and medical tasks.

The second dilemma concerns how such a large and complex workforce is to be organised and controlled. The traditional form of organisation has consisted of medical control of other occupational groups, reinforced by stratification within the workforce along lines of social class, gender and ethnic status which mirror those in the wider society beyond the NHS. Medical dominance has been at the expense of most other occupational groups in terms of status, conditions, pay and control over work. In the 1990s it is increasingly challenged by other groups in the workforce. Nurses, midwives and others claim autonomy over their work and the professional status that goes with it. In this they are often implicitly aspiring to the medical example. To some extent their challenge is supported by

[1] *Caring for Health: History and Diversity* (1984 and revised edition 1993).

[2] *Health and Disease: A Reader* (revised edition 1994).

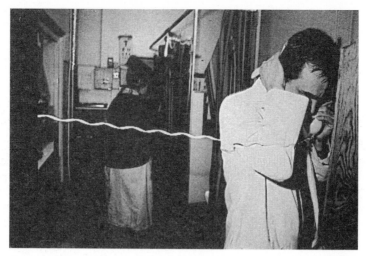

Junior doctors are one of many groups of NHS workers under stress in the 1990s. (Source: BMA News Review)

wider social trends—such as changes in expectations about women's work. But such a challenge is also pitted against attempts to control costs. Control of health care by 'the professionals' who give direct care to patients is also now challenged by managers, who have been given the task of sustaining the NHS in the face of limited public expenditure, rising costs and rising demands.

This leads to the third dilemma we discuss—the conflicts inherent in reconciling humane working conditions with strict budget requirements. Pressures on workers can be seen as a symptom of wider problems in the NHS: because health work is the major part of health costs, health workers are likely to experience the worst impact of public expenditure controls. A BMA report called *Stress and the Medical Profession* gives the following account of working conditions for all those employed in the NHS:

> Many staff are on very low rates of pay; training may be poor, and drop out rates among, for instance, nurses are high; the salary structure of most staff does not allow better pay for better performance; some groups work absurdly long hours in often poor conditions; career development is chaotic for some; sickness and accident rates are high, and occupational health services are often non-existent. (BMA, 1992, p. 21).

This may leave you asking how widespread are such poor conditions, and how do they vary between different categories of workers? Why should a health service submit any workers to damaging levels of stress? Divisions in the workforce may determine the gainers and losers from attempts to contain NHS costs.

To some extent, any developed health-care system will face the dilemmas outlined above: competition over the content of work roles and control over the diversity of skills employed, and efficient use of resources competing with good working conditions.

The chapter begins with an account of the scale and social divisions of the workforce; these data make it easier to understand the outcome of competition over work roles, control and resources. We then develop the argument about the dilemmas that emerge, using illustrations from the general health workforce and in particular from nursing and midwifery. The chapter ends by looking at some strategies adopted by nurses and managers—seen as key actors on this stage—to deal with the dilemmas as they appear from their own viewpoints.

Defining and counting the health-care workforce

Who are the health workers?

☐ How would you identify someone as a health worker?

■ This question has no single answer, but you should acknowledge that a definition confined to someone in paid employment in a health-care organisation is inadequate. Informal, unpaid lay care is also health work.[3] We would suggest an answer

[3]The extent of lay health care in the United Kingdom from 1500 to the present day forms a continuing theme in *Caring for Health: History and Diversity* (Open University Press, revised edition 1993).

that relates to health-care objectives: a person who contributes a substantial amount of time to health care, prevention of disease or promotion of health, or works for an organisation with these objectives.

Distinguishing health care from other forms of care is also problematic; delivering meals-on-wheels, for example, can be vital health and protection work. Here we simply draw your attention to the problems of setting boundaries around health work as well as to this chapter's limitations.

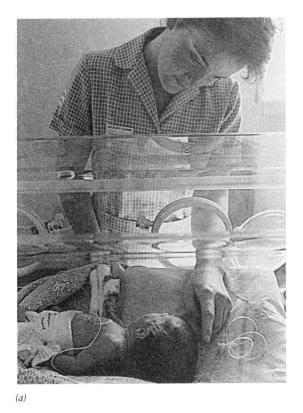

(a)

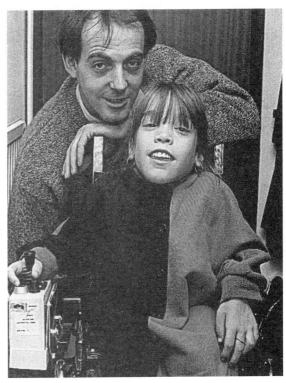

(b)

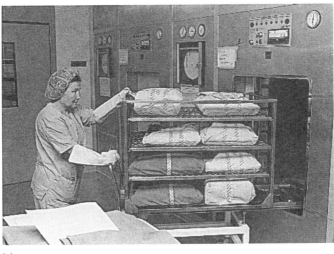

(c)

Would you identify these people as health workers? (a) Student nurse in a Special Care Baby Unit; (b) father and daughter at home; (c) ancillary worker sterilising surgical linen and instruments. (Photos: Mike Levers)

Our concern here is solely with paid work in the NHS. With this restriction, the counting of health workers depends largely on Department of Health (DH) definitions.

Numbers and trends in the health workforce

In 1990, the number of NHS workers in the United Kingdom—according to DH statistics—was approximately 1 million (actually 1 059 200; OPCS, 1992, p. 143). This includes NHS employees not directly providing patient care—caterers, cleaners, porters, etc.—whom you may or may not think of as health workers. It also omits the many who provide direct patient care outside the NHS in the private sector and at home. Table 6.1 shows how the number of NHS workers changed over the preceding decade.

□ What were the changes in the overall size of the NHS workforce between 1981 and 1990, as shown in Table 6.1?

■ There was a small decline (27 000) in the overall number of NHS workers during this period, but there was a larger fall in workers employed by health authorities (down 32 700) partly offset by an increase of 5 400 (10 per cent) in those working in family practitioner services.

These trends may be associated with some specific features of NHS policy, in particular the policy of **competitive tendering** for catering and cleaning services, which awards contracts to private companies who bid for work previously done by NHS employees. It has thus shifted some of this employment out of the NHS figures. The more detailed picture in Figure 6.1 shows contradictory trends between 1981 and 1990 in different sections of the workforce. (*Professional and technical* workers include radiographers, speech therapists and occupational therapists, physiotherapists and hospital pharmacists;

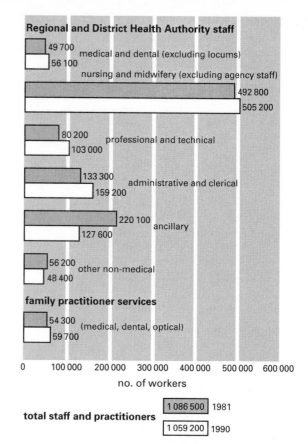

Figure 6.1 *The composition of the NHS workforce in the United Kingdom in 1981 and 1990 (numbers of family practitioners, all others in whole-time equivalents). (Source: OPCS,* Social Trends 22, *1992, HMSO, London, Table 7.43)*

ancillary workers include catering and cleaning staff, porters, gardeners, security guards, and assistants to professional staff in pharmacies, mortuaries, etc.)

Table 6.1 Changes in the number of NHS workers in the United Kingdom, employed by Regional and District Health Authorities or working in family practitioner services, 1981–1990

	thousands in:						
	1981	1984	1986	1987	1988	1989	1990
Regional and District Health Authority staff	1 032.2	1 030.4	1 011.0	1 008.3	1 001.0	1 000.0	999.5
family practitioner services (medical, dental, optical)	54.3	58.2	57.3	58.4	59.3	59.8	59.7

(Source: OPCS, *Social Trends 22*, 1992, HMSO, London, Table 7.43)

☐ Describe the main changes in categories of health authority workers as shown in Figure 6.1. Look first at changes in absolute numbers in each category, and then make a rough calculation of the *percentage* change over the decade.

■ The largest change in absolute numbers and in relative terms is in ancillary workers (down 92 500, a fall of 42 per cent). All workers directly providing care or technical services to patients have increased in number: hospital doctors and dentists have risen by 6 400, an increase of almost 13 per cent; professional and technical staff have risen by nearly 23 000, or about 29 per cent; nurses have increased by 12 400, but this represents a percentage rise of only 2.5—far less than the increase in administrative and clerical staff, who gained nearly 26 000 workers (a rise of 19.5 per cent).

This trend had been developing for some time. There was a 50 per cent increase in administrative staff during the 1970s and a 100 per cent increase in senior administrative staff during the 1980s; this may be related to the policy of shifting the balance of power towards managers (as described in Chapter 2).

The division of health-care labour

As you can see from looking back at Figure 6.1, *diversity* as well as scale is a feature of health employment. The variety of health work is traditionally seen in terms of occupational groups: doctors, nurses, physiotherapists, caterers, etc. But diversity can be expressed in other ways: gender and ethnic divisions are two more dimensions of the diversity of NHS employment. Income and working conditions are varied: employees range from among the lowest-paid catering and cleaning workers to the highest-paid consultants and managers. These several sources of division—by occupation, ethnic group, gender, income and status—intersect in complex ways. We turn later to dilemmas arising from these inequalities, but first we simply describe them.

Occupational divisions

During most of the twentieth century, a tendency to increasing *specialisation of labour* in health work has been detected. Margaret Stacey, a sociologist of health with a special interest in questions of work and gender, describes this process:

> Developments in medical knowledge, advances in technology and the conditions which pertain in advanced capitalist societies have all been involved in the increased number of divisions in health labour. Specialisms and

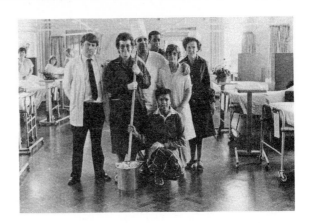

Workers in some of the occupations employed in an NHS hospital—porters, cleaners, catering and maintenance staff, and a nurse. Who is missing? (See Figure 6.2.) (Source: Gina Glover/Photo Co-op)

sub-specialisms have burgeoned in the last forty years, as have the number and range of non-medical workers, scientists and technicians—workers in the paramedical professions (the professions supplementary to medicine) upon all of whom doctors rely. (Stacey, 1991, p. 182)

Figure 6.2 (*overleaf*) shows the occupational divisions in some detail for England in 1990. Note that the categories used in these official tables are slightly different from those you saw earlier. The 'professional and technical' category in Figure 6.1 has been subdivided in Figure 6.2 into *professions allied to medicine* (known as PAMs, mainly radiographers and physiotherapists), and other professionals whose skills are variously described as 'technical', 'scientific' or 'works'; also, maintenance workers are given separately from other ancillary workers.

☐ What do you notice about the main occupational divisions shown in Figure 6.2? How is the workforce divided between those who directly provide some form of health care, and those who maintain the service in other ways?

■ Nurses and midwives make up almost half the total workforce. By contrast, the proportion of doctors and dentists is small (just over 5 per cent are hospital staff, with another 5 per cent in family practitioner services), and NHS opticians comprise less than 1 per cent of the total. Taken together, PAMs and the other scientific and technical professionals whose work has some direct relationship to health care contribute just under 10 per cent of NHS staff, and 2 per cent are ambulance personnel. The rest

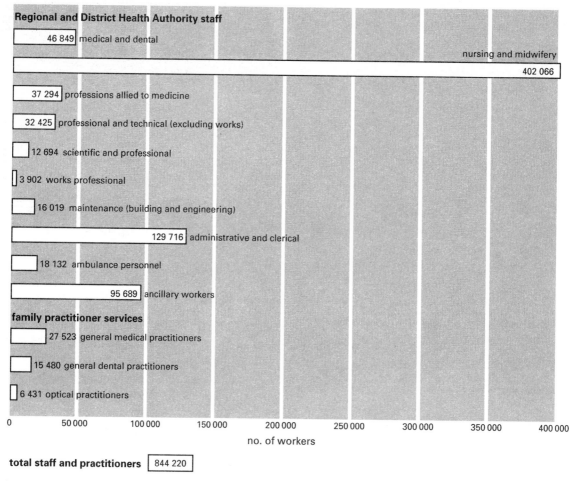

Figure 6.2 *Numbers in different occupations in the NHS in England in 1990 (numbers of family practitioners, all others in whole-time equivalents). (Source: Department of Health, 1992,* Health and Personal Social Services Statistics for England, *HMSO, London, Table 3.2)*

(almost 30 per cent of the workforce) are in occupations only indirectly concerned with patient care: despite competitive tendering, about half of these are employed in 'works', maintenance and ancillary jobs, and about half are administrative and clerical workers.

The high proportion of nurses and midwives in the NHS, most of whom are female, leads us to consider questions of gender in the division of labour, an issue which is addressed briefly on the audiotape band 'Health work: nurses' perceptions'.[4] The nurses we recorded also talked about their varied working roles and responsibilities, the

things they liked and disliked about their work, the status of nursing relative to the medical profession, and their commitment to patients. We suggest that you listen to the tape now—it gives an insight into the personal world of nursing, which illuminates the data that follow and illustrates dilemmas felt by many other groups of health workers. Questions about the content of this audiotape occur at several points in the rest of the chapter.

Gender divisions in the NHS

Historically occupations which have made successful claims to be professions, which have gained work autonomy and become dominant, have all been male occupations; those which have succeeded less well…have been female or female-dominated occupations. (Stacey, 1991, p. 80)

---

[4]'Health work: nurses' perceptions' has been recorded for Open University students, who should consult the Audiocassette Notes relating to this band before playing it.

The DH still provides a 'manpower summary', but the NHS is a major employer of women, who number approximately three-quarters of its workers. Women are more likely to appear in lower-paid occupations, for example they are a higher proportion of ancillary staff than of medical consultants. Within occupations they are more numerous at the bottom of power and status hierarchies than at the top.

Hospital doctors

Figure 6.3 shows staff grades within hospital medicine (house officers—often referred to as junior doctors—are in their first year of clinical practice after qualifying from medical school).

□ Describe the pattern of women's employment among hospital medical staff shown in Figure 6.3.

■ In 1990, women were approaching half the house officers, but contributed a decreasing proportion to the grades further up the hierarchy. Only 15 per cent of consultants were women.

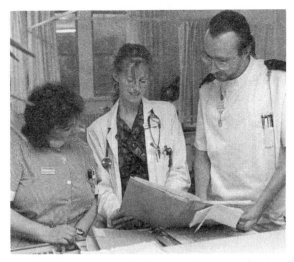

In the 1990s, almost half of all junior doctors are women, but the proportion of female doctors declines at higher levels of the medical hierarchy. Only about one in ten nurses are male, but they outnumber women in senior nursing posts. (Source: Mike Levers)

These figures partly reflect women's gradually increasing share of medical school places and junior jobs in the 1980s, and this may in time affect the higher grades. However, there is sufficient concern about women's careers in medicine for career progression to have been studied by a DH Joint Working Party which reported in 1991 (Department of Health, 1991c). It concluded that change was certainly necessary and suggested a number of actions, including enforcing good equal opportunity practice, monitoring gender balance and restructuring jobs.

Speech therapists and clinical psychologists

Gender divisions are felt in pay, as well as in status and control over work. For example, the Equal Opportunities Commission (EOC) reported that:

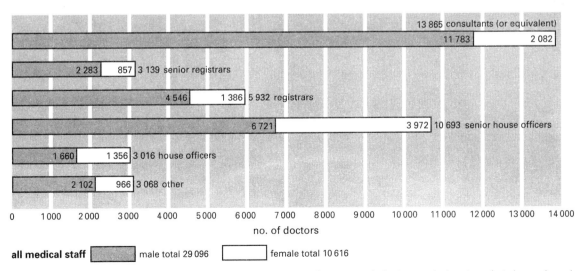

Figure 6.3 *Hospital medical staff employed in England on 30 September 1990 (whole-time equivalents): analysis by grade and sex. (Source: Department of Health, 1992,* Health and Personal Social Services Statistics for England, *Table 3.5, p. 38)*

Speech therapists (mainly women) have, with EOC assistance, challenged their pay rates under the Equal Pay for Work of Equal Value legislation, comparing their pay with that of higher paid, and mainly male clinical psychologists. (EOC, 1990, p. 33)

The clinical psychologists in this comparison were paid at rates about 60 per cent higher than the speech therapists. At the time of writing in 1992, the claim for equal pay had not been accepted in the United Kingdom, but awaited decision at the European Court. Its failure so far in British courts is instructive for the weight placed on professional divisions and has implications for the valuation of women's work in the NHS.

Nurses and midwives

It is a commonplace observation that most nurses are female—almost nine out of ten are. However men and women are not distributed in this ratio between specialties, as Figure 6.4 shows.

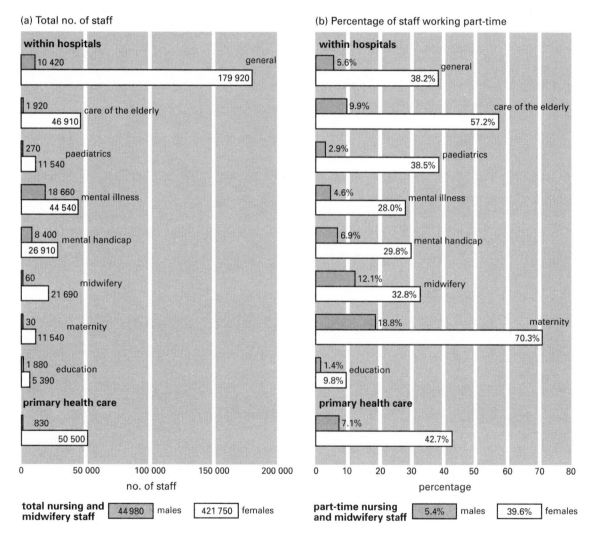

Figure 6.4 *Nursing and midwifery staff in England on 30 September 1989 (whole-time equivalents and percentage working part-time): analysis by areas of work and gender. (Source: Department of Health, 1990,* NHS Workforce in England, *pp. C1–4)*

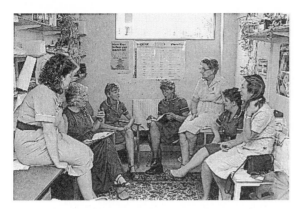

Almost nine out of ten nurses are women. Meetings between nursing staff typically take place in areas which 'double' as office space, interview room, stores, waiting room or cloakroom. (Source: Mike Levers)

□ Male nurses make up about 12 per cent of the nursing workforce in terms of whole-time equivalent posts. In which specialties are they noticeably over- or under-represented?

■ Male nurses are concentrated in the specialities of mental illness (45 per cent are men), mental handicap (33 per cent) and education (36 per cent). They are least represented among midwives and maternity nurses (fewer than 1 per cent are male), community nursing (2 per cent) and paediatrics (under 3 per cent).

The reasons are partly historical. The high proportion of men in mental-health nursing owes something to the need for physical strength in dealing with disturbed patients before the introduction of modern tranquillisers and sedatives. The feminine images of nursing associated with midwifery and paediatric care may deter male nurses, and it is only relatively recently that men have been trained as midwives. The prevalence of men in nurse education reflects the tendency of male nurses to leave the 'bedside' as their career progresses.

Men have an advantage in terms of promotion; they outnumber women in senior nursing grades despite being only about one-tenth of the nursing workforce. A study by Celia Davies and Jane Rosser published in 1986 found that men had been promoted to a senior nursing post in an average of 8.4 years, whereas women had taken 17.9 years; even women with no career breaks had taken 14.5

years. This is partly the consequence of part-time work among female nurses, on which nursing heavily depends (see Figure 6.4). Around 40 per cent of female nurses and over 30 per cent of midwives worked part-time in 1990, and in some specialties (care of the elderly and maternity nursing) the proportion is much higher. Much of this pattern of work is designed to fit around unpaid domestic labour and informal health care; note that two of the four female nurses on the audiotape had experienced long periods of part-time work when their children were young, and another began work as a nursing auxiliary only after her children were 'off her hands'. In general, part-time nurses tend to be older than their full-time colleagues.

A sociologist, Lesley Mackay, has documented nurses' feelings about discrimination against women with children, especially those who work part-time:

Part-time nurses are considered as very much second-class members of the team, given no opportunity or encouragement to embark on further studies or courses. This appears to be management policy. (Staff nurse, quoted in Mackay, 1989, p. 79)

The Royal College of Nursing (RCN) is aware of discrimination against women. Trevor Clay, when General Secretary, argued for increased provision of workplace nurseries and encouragement to return to practice after a career break:

But with [organisational changes] must go clear commitment for regarding these individuals, and encouraging them to regard themselves, as still having potential for promotion. In nursing this is not the case, and women who return to work part-time quickly lose their place on the ladder, being overtaken by other, usually single or male, nurses. (Clay, 1986, p. 22)

□ What other disadvantage of part-time working did the nurses on the audiotape identify, and what did it allow one of them to do in addition to combining her career with bringing up a family?

■ It interfered with their relationship with patients, which was fragmented by long gaps in the working week; but it also allowed one nurse to take a further training course and so enhance her career prospects.

Ethnic divisions in the NHS

The overt racism of nurse recruitment policies in the 1960s, described below, has left its mark on employment patterns, where ethnic minorities remain over-represented in lower paid work.[5] The nurse quoted here describes migrant nurses being recruited to the lower level State Enrolled Nurse (SEN), rather than the State Registered Nurse (SRN) category.[6]

> On the plane over, I got chatting to a woman who I found out was a nurse over here. I told her about the hospital I was going to, and she asked me whether I was going to be a pupil nurse or a student nurse. Well, I hadn't registered any difference at the time. Then she explained that SEN pupils were lower than SRN students and that Trinidad didn't even recognise the SEN qualification…
>
> The next day I had to be fitted for a uniform. Of course, the lady in the sewing room started measuring me up for an SEN uniform. She handed me this old, patched up uniform, and I thought, 'Have I come from Trinidad for this?' I told her no, I would be getting the starched, green uniform and she said 'But all the coloured girls are pupils'. That really got me going. I went to the Matron and demanded to change. They were taken aback, but there was nothing they could do about it because I'd passed the test. I didn't realise then that they thought that if you were Black, you were stupid. You learn quickly though. (Quoted in Bryan, Dadzie and Scafe, 1985, pp. 40–1)

In the late 1970s, sociologist Lesley Doyal studied the use of immigrant labour in a London hospital:

The NHS is one of Britain's largest employers of migrant labour. About one third of all doctors now working in the NHS come from overseas; so do some 20 per cent of all student and pupil nurses…local studies have shown that in some areas the number of ancillary workers from overseas is well over 50 per cent. Indeed our own survey of an acute non-teaching hospital in London showed that over 80 per cent of ancillary workers were from abroad—84 per cent of domestics and 82 per cent of catering workers. (Doyal, Hunt and Mellor, 1981, p. 54)

The same study showed two sources of division—gender and race—interacting to give the lowest paid jobs to ethnic minority women:

> In our survey the number of female workers from overseas was more than double the number of males, with overseas-born women accounting for 78 per cent of domestics and 55 per cent of catering workers. (Doyal, Hunt and Mellor, 1981, p. 59)

Official data in the 1990s do not give us an adequate account of ethnic divisions in the NHS; ethnic monitoring is new and not yet widespread, but anecdotal evidence of racism has been supported by findings from race relations tribunals. Small-scale research studies such as those in Manchester (Baxter, 1987) and South Derbyshire (Pearson, 1987) show black nurses over-represented within the Enrolled Nurse group, in unpopular specialties, within lower grades, and doing unpopular shifts: there is no categorical evidence of racism in this, but a pointer towards it, as one speaker on the audiotape suggests.

The King's Fund Equal Opportunities Task Force reported in 1990 that fewer black people are applying for nurse training and black nurses are leaving the health service in disproportionate numbers. The United Kingdom Central Council for Nursing, Midwifery and Health Visiting (UKCC, the body that oversees the training, registration and conduct of nurses) began ethnic monitoring of applicants in the early 1990s, and health authorities began building ethnic monitoring into training contracts. These practices will reveal whether discrimination against black Britons in the 1990s has become as widespread as the discrimination against immigrants of earlier decades.

[5] Migration of health-care workers from the Third World to Western industrialised nations is discussed in *Caring for Health: History and Diversity* (revised edition 1993), Chapters 8 and 9.

[6] The categories SEN and SRN were replaced in 1983 by EN (Enrolled Nurse) and RGN (Registered General Nurse), both of which were replaced in 1992 by a single category, RN (Registered Nurse).

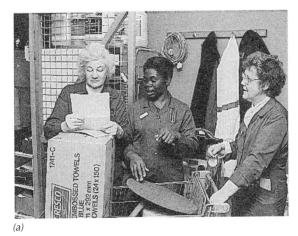

(a)

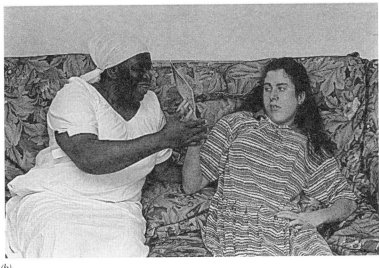

(b)

Ethnic monitoring of the NHS workforce in the 1990s will reveal whether black people (and especially black women) are over-represented in low paid jobs. (a) Cleaners in an NHS hospital; (b) community mental-handicap nurse with client. (Photos: Mike Levers)

Variations in income, working conditions and status

Income differences are a key feature of occupational hierarchies, and the NHS is no exception. The 1991 Review Bodies on Remuneration, covering doctors, dentists, nurses, midwives, health visitors (Department of Health, 1991d and e), and PAMs demonstrated some striking income differentials. They recommended that the lowest-grade hospital doctor (house officer) should earn approximately twice the lowest-grade nurse. But the recommended differentials were greatest at the top of the scale, with the highest-paid consultants earning well over twice the highest-paid nurses, and a few able nearly to double that with the top merit award (this refers to NHS salaries and excludes additional income from private practice).

As a result of competitive tendering, ancillary work may now be undertaken by firms outside the NHS on terms which give lower pay and less security than NHS contracts. The economic policies of central government and strategic changes in NHS management during the 1980s and 1990s have had variable effects on different parts of the workforce. Sociologist David Cox argues that the medical profession—whose autonomy and perceived lack of interest in cost-effectiveness the managerial changes were meant to challenge—have not so far felt the coldest blast of these policies (a view supported in Chapter 2), but for ancillary staff:

> Whether contracts go to internal or external contractors, the results have been job losses and reductions in earnings and hours, a narrow specification of duties and a weakening of trade-union influence. (Cox, 1991, p. 106)

For a range of people in the middle of this occupational hierarchy (including senior nursing staff) contracts have also become more insecure.

You should now read Elizabeth Paterson's account of 'Food-work: maids in a hospital kitchen', first published in 1981.[7]

☐ Contrast this hospital work and its social organisation with that of hospital doctors.

■ The work is clearly hard, routine, boring, sometimes dangerous, personally unrewarding and low paid. It is also highly controlled (in contrast to the 'autonomy' of clinical practice); separated from its end-product (the maids see the food, but not the people whose needs the NHS serves); and done largely by women.

☐ In what ways do the kitchen maids try to exert control over their work?

■ They work hardest on 'visible' tasks (like washing lettuce); take illegal breaks, act sullenly or answer back; and distance themselves from their work (this is not the real me, but something I'm paid to do).

Medicine provides the model for a high-status occupation marked by a high degree of control over its practice and training. Other health occupations have achieved some aspects of professional status, for example, the state registration of nurses, midwives and most recently (1960) PAMs—though this title suggests a range of occupations that work within a *medical* frame of reference, rather than defining their *own* work.[8] Professionalisation may describe part of the process of occupational change, but there are contradictory pressures to cheapen the labour process. Diversification of assistant grades—in nursing (as you will see later), clerical, reception, technical and scientific occupations—is also part of increasing labour specialisation, and for some of these workers, pay and conditions may be more serious concerns than professional status.

The contradictory pressures both to professionalise and to use cheaper forms of labour can be seen clearly within nursing. Patricia Owens and Howard Glennerster, social policy researchers who have studied nursing management, describe the tension between these strategies, where Registered Nurses (RNs) work alongside unregistered nursing staff:[9]

> Much of the day-to-day care in many hospitals, especially long-stay hospitals, is undertaken by unregistered nurses who have little or no training. About 50 per cent of all care is given by unregistered nurses particularly in the mental handicap and elderly sectors. At the same time, the need for highly trained and specialised nurses is growing as the specialised nature of medicine grows. Here the interests of educators, practitioners and service managers are often difficult to reconcile. (Owens and Glennerster, 1990, p. 36)

These authors argue that in the United Kingdom the respect accorded to nurses as professionals contrasts with inattention to unregistered staff.

☐ What does the nursing auxiliary on the audiotape you heard earlier have to say about her status?

■ She believes she is looked down on as 'second rate'.

Tensions over the division of work between different grades of nurse are a recurring theme in a more general debate in hospital management about the proportion of workers of different grades or types (in 1990s jargon, 'skill-mix') in the staffing of wards and other health-care settings. The debate includes the possible consequences for the quality of patient care, and for the educational and professional development of nursing—issues to which we return at the end of this chapter.

[7]In *Health and Disease: A Reader* (1984, and revised edition 1994).

[8]The circumstances resulting in certain health-care occupations (such as radiographers) being brought under medical control, while others (such as osteopaths) resisted incorporation are described in *Medical Knowledge: Doubt and Certainty* (revised edition 1994).

[9]Registered Nurses include all those approved by the United Kingdom Central Council for Nursing, Midwifery and Health Visiting (UKCC) to practise as nurses as a result of successful completion of a recognised training programme.
Unregistered nurses are often referred to as nursing auxiliaries or health-care assistants; their qualifications range from nil to a National Vocational Qualification (NVQ). The role of the UKCC in nurse registration and professional development is discussed later in the chapter.

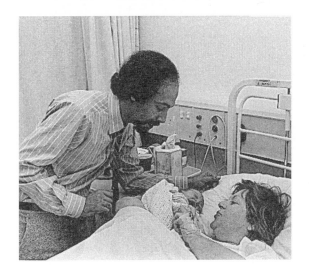

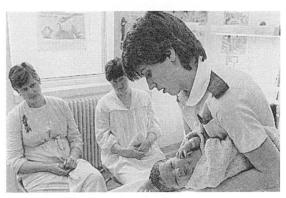

Who controls childbirth? Obstetricians, midwives or mothers? (Photos: Mike Levers)

Boundary disputes between occupations

It has been argued above that competition over work roles is an inevitable component of a complex health-care system with an elaborate division of labour and a changing social and technological environment. Work roles are not comprehensively defined in legal terms and overlapping responsibilities are common. Two examples follow, of contemporary areas of conflict over boundaries between different occupational groups.

Midwives and obstetricians

First read the extracts from the 'Second Report on Maternity Services' (known as the 'Winterton Report'), published by the House of Commons Health Committee in 1992.[10] Consideration of who should provide maternity care is at its centre. Then answer the following question.

☐ What does the Committee recommend about the boundary between midwifery and obstetrics and about their relative 'professional' status?

■ It concludes that maternity care in normal deliveries should become the province of midwifery rather than obstetrics (though it is not specific about what should be considered 'normal'). Its main instrument for bringing this about is enhancement of the professional status of midwifery. Notice the number of proposals concerning midwives' autonomy in practice and training.

If implemented, these proposals would provide a route for midwifery to achieve higher professional status and a model of practice resembling the current medical one. Enhanced training and research activity are allies in this process, although there are potential difficulties (see below).

You may have noticed that, with a focus on 'normal birth of healthy babies to healthy women', the Winterton Committee show some impatience with the professionals involved. They remark that discussions 'have been far too heavily influenced by territorial disputes between the professionals concerned for control of the women whom they are supposed to be helping'. And a number of their recommendations—for example the ending of 'shared care'—reflect a negative view of the impact of boundary disputes on the care of women and their babies.

☐ What part does gender play in the situation described by the Winterton Report and in its proposals for future practice?

■ What the report describes as the 'medical model of care' in childbirth has put it under predominantly male control. The proposals would shift 'normal' childbirth from male-dominated obstetric medicine to female-dominated midwifery. The committee also argue for an increase in the proportion of female consultants in obstetrics.

Doctors and nurses

A difficult boundary for nurses to negotiate has been that between nurses' and doctors' work. Some distinctions are clear: for example, doctors do surgical operations and theatre nurses work in support. However, at a psychiatric clinic the therapist could be a nurse, a doctor or a clinical psychologist. And at times when doctors may not be present on hospital wards, for example at night, nurses may substitute for them in some respects.

---

[10]See *Health and Disease: A Reader* (revised edition 1994).

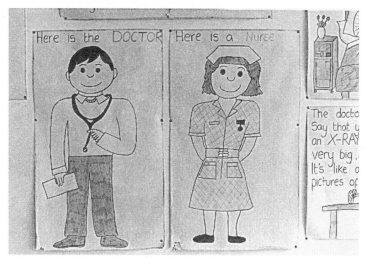

These stereotyped images of a doctor and a nurse were on the wall of a hospital waiting area, photographed in 1990, but the boundary between medical and nursing work is increasingly disputed. (Photo: Mike Levers)

☐ Think back to the audiotape. One of the nurses, a sister in a community hospital, talks about her attitude to calling a doctor to see a patient at night. How does this change when she is on a day-shift?

■ She takes more responsibility at night and frequently deals with situations which she knows she would call out a doctor to deal with during the day.

Financial constraints have given management an incentive to extend the nurse's role into the so-called 'lower' level medical tasks—nurses are cheaper than doctors. Such an 'exchange' of tasks between trades is possible because there are few legal constraints on the roles of doctors and nurses. An obvious exception is the prescription of drugs, but even here the law can be changed, as it was in 1992 when community nurses were in principle given powers to prescribe a range of drugs and dressings.

Martin McKee and Leila Lessof are doctors writing about policy issues in nursing; they argue:

> Changes in medicine have led some doctors to welcome the extended role of the nurse, notably in the context of the delegation of technical tasks. Because of an increasing concern about the excessive hours worked by junior doctors... several studies have demonstrated how many of the night tasks for which junior doctors are called could be equally well done by the nurse who calls them. (McKee and Lessof, 1992, p. 62)

They go on to discuss the bureaucratic obstacles which often prevent this happening; there are marked variations between employers in recognising certain tasks as appropriate for delegation to a nurse with a specific level of training.

> ...an experienced staff nurse may find herself calling a newly qualified house officer to the ward at night in order to explain exactly what needs to be done, or even a more senior doctor who has not previously performed a technically complex procedure, such as the insertion of a pace-maker. Patient care may suffer when an intravenous drug is given several hours late because the house officer was busy elsewhere, while in a neighbouring hospital the drug would be given on time during the nurse's drug round. (McKee and Lessof, 1992, p. 62)

Moreover, a study of the training of junior doctors found that nurses were playing a substantial role:

> In terms of nursing resources, two sisters suggested independently that supervising a new house officer in the house officer's first job might take them two or three hours in an eight hour shift and that such close supervision might be necessary for the first two or three weeks of a job. (Dowling and Barrett, 1991, p. 57)

An alternative strategy for nurses is to expand their role into new areas of patient care which have never been considered as 'doctor's work' (for example, promoting reminiscence therapy[11] with older clients or using complementary therapies with terminally-ill patients). This suggests developing a more characteristically nursing identity, rather than one as doctors' assistants.

☐ In general, how did the nurses interviewed on the audiotape summarise their present working relationship with doctors, compared with the past?

■ They seem optimistic that attitudes to nurses as 'doctors' handmaidens' are changing; one says 'there is not the hierarchy there used to be'.

Controversies about boundaries look set to increase in the 1990s. Managers of provider units are likely to want a more flexible workforce, with tasks and responsibilities pushed as far down existing hierarchies as possible. This is a feature of both the above examples, in which managers may well see midwives and nurses as more cost-effective caregivers. Operational changes such as these create opportunities for occupational development as well as inevitable conflict over the outcomes.

Controlling health workers

A complex division of labour invites questions about order. How is the workforce coordinated? Who is in control? What is the basis for their authority?

Medicine and managerialism

In the 1970s, the answer to these questions was clear and simple. Eliot Freidson, an American sociologist, argued persuasively that medicine controlled not only its own work and training, but also that of other workers: 'it is the physician's control over the division of labour that is distinct' (Freidson, 1975, p. 125). He located the source of power primarily in doctors' control over appropriate knowledge.[12]

In the 1980s, feminists contributed an analysis of the significance of gender within professional hierarchies.

For example, feminist sociologist Ann Oakley wrote sociological and historical accounts of women's experience of childbirth and of medical control (1980, 1984). Both works analyse medicine's control over midwifery as well as over women in their care.[13]

In the 1990s, the debate about professional power has been shifting and the view that doctors hold unquestioned leadership in health care is being undermined. Mary Ann Elston, writing in 1991, argued that the idea of medical dominance prevalent in the 1970s did not allow for the variety of the division of labour, or for differences between the national health systems of the United Kingdom and the USA (which informed Freidson's account). She describes a more contested and complex state of affairs than Freidson, though she concludes that medicine has not yielded control:

As yet, such changes that have occurred look more like uncomfortable adjustments than a major waning of either the medical profession's institutionalized technical autonomy or of their social and cultural authority. (Elston, 1991, pp. 83–4)

Medicine, then, continues to play a key role in the management of other health workers, but the challenge of managerialism is a serious one, likely to intensify with current NHS reforms (see Chapter 2), as is the challenge from service-users (Chapter 5) and other occupational groups.

☐ What obstacles might prevent the new role for midwives outlined by the Winterton Committee from being implemented?

■ Obstetricians may not be ready to surrender control of normal pregnancies and labour, or allow that any can be relied on to remain normal. Class and gender divisions may continue to be significant factors in maintaining the existing professional hierarchy.

Nurses and managers

Debates about nursing and management are high on the NHS agenda in the 1990s. How should nursing fit into the management of hospital and community services?

---

[11]A technique used with confused or withdrawn elderly people which encourages them to reminisce about their past and, in the process, regain confidence and lucidity.

[12]The professionalisation of medicine is discussed in *Medical Knowledge: Doubt and Certainty* (1984, and more extensively in the revised edition 1994); the historical development of medical power and influence is described in *Caring for Health: History and Diversity* (revised edition 1993).

[13]The feminist critique of the medicalisation of childbirth is discussed in another book in this series, *Birth to Old Age: Health in Transition* (Open University Press 1984, revised edition 1995). See also the case study on gender and medicine in the diagnosis and treatment of hysteria, in *Medical Knowledge: Doubt and Certainty* (1984, and revised edition 1994).

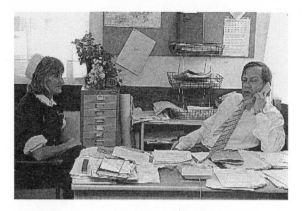

The management of nursing is a contested issue in the 1990s. Should nurses manage their own work or be subject to managerial control from outside nursing? (Photo: Mike Levers)

Should nurses manage themselves and others? Should they be managed by managers? Contrasting solutions to these problems have created upheavals to career structures and uncertainty about future directions.

Under the NHS management structure which followed the 1966 Salmon Report, nurses managed themselves; they were represented at every NHS level as nurses. The profession saw this as significant recognition, and it gave nursing (with half the NHS workforce) a substantial management role.[14] The Griffiths Report (1983) and the management changes that followed are generally assumed to have been directed at medical authority. But the challenge to nursing authority was more immediate; the ladder to the top of the NHS for nurses was effectively dismantled by the change to general management and the loss of the higher nurse-manager posts. After Griffiths, nurses could apply for general management posts, but as managers rather than as nurses. They have not been appointed in great numbers at the higher levels (look back at Table 2.1; in 1987, only 9 per cent of general managers at Unit level or above had a background in nursing), but they were appointed more frequently to management posts further down the hierarchy (for example, one of the nurses on the audiotape was a manager involved in the staffing of community nursing services).

These changes have left nurses facing uncertainty about the future direction of nursing. One possible scenario is for nurses to use their base in middle management to develop a larger role in general management at higher

[14] See *Caring for Health: History and Diversity* (revised edition 1993), Chapters 6 and 7.

levels in the NHS. Alternatively, nurses may see themselves as developing on more independent professional lines, within a clinical rather than a managerial framework—an issue to which we return later in this chapter.

In general, control of the NHS workforce seems more uncertain and contested in the 1990s than at earlier periods. Managers across the NHS are challenging medical authority and nursing's control over its own workforce. But neither doctors nor nurses have simply given way. Medical authority is entrenched so deeply that it will not easily be subject to managerial influence; and nurses have retained a place within general management. Curiously, the interests of nurses who wish to advance the status of the profession may coincide with those of managers seeking a more flexible and cost-effective workforce—as we note at the end of this chapter.

Resources for health workers

Public expenditure and health work

The pay of health workers is the major cost to the NHS—around two-thirds of its budget. The size of the health workforce makes it a significant part of the national economy, and in particular of the public sector. Pressures on public expenditure have been intensifying with government commitment to reducing the role of public authorities, while growth of the elderly population and innovations in medical technology have pushed up demand for health work (see Chapters 3 and 7). As a result, the health workforce now meets pressure from two sides: to contain the cost of health workers and yet do more health work. Strain on the working conditions and living standards of health workers is one result of these conflicting pressures.

The divisions in the workforce, underpinned as they are by divisions in gender, ethnicity and class, suggest lines of fissure that could be exploited under pressure to contain costs, by reducing the terms and conditions of the most vulnerable workers. Professionalisation by those groups who are able to achieve it can be seen as a strategy for protecting their working conditions in a contested environment. But the more that the better-placed occupations gain, the more likely it is that the costs will be borne by the less secure. Organisations representing workers may be torn between vigorous professionalising strategies on behalf of their better-placed members or a more defensive collective response which protects the rest. Recent studies of nursing illustrate the impact of these tensions at the workplace.

Nursing workloads and stress

Stress within nursing has received less publicity than the stress on junior doctors, especially those 'on call', for whom a weekly target of no more than 83 hours on duty was supposed to be enforced from April 1993.

> 1   There was times when I felt really guilty just sitting down and talking to somebody when there was so much to do—they obviously needed somebody to talk to. I found that really hard.
>
> 2   Because of staff shortages, if the staff see you sitting talking to a patient they will always come up and tell you to do something, whereas they don't really think that talking to a patient is doing anything—skiving the work really. (Quoted in Mackay, 1989, p. 25)

These two nurse recruits describe the painful gap between the nursing ideals of caring for patients and realities on the ward, which is echoed in other studies of nurses' working experience in the NHS, and in the audio-tape you heard earlier. Nurses in middle management were interviewed in another recent study and illustrate the point in a different way:

> When asked about their major focus of work in the previous week, no less than 63 per cent identified 'staffing the wards' as the principal task. Many complained that they were dominated by the day-to-day pressure to provide adequate nursing cover for their areas. The second major task was dealing with stress among nursing staff. (Owens and Glennerster, 1990, p. 121)

This pressure was illustrated in the audiotape 'Dilemmas in hospital management' (which was associated with Chapter 2); when a nurse called in sick, the nursing services manager had to put pressure on a Sister to release a nurse from her busy ward to cover the shortage elsewhere. The following account suggests reasons for the high stress levels in some units:

> In one sub-unit with many specialised services, there were 50 vacancies out of a staff of 172. The unit was characterised by high budgets, high dependencies and high staff ratios. This service was dogged by increasing levels of stress, expressed by staff who were constantly threatening to leave. The situation was exacerbated by the introduction of new medical techniques requiring more intensive nurse input, for example new dialysis procedures. (Owens and Glennerster, 1990, p. 125)

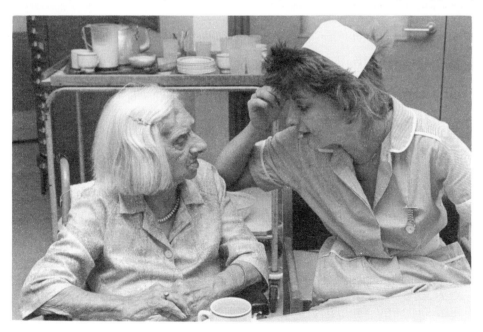

'...they don't really think that talking to a patient is doing anything—skiving the work really.' (Photo: Mike Levers)

The story of staff shortages and overwork is supported by more quantitative analysis. For example, a questionnaire study of 2 728 members of the Royal College of Nursing, found 53 per cent claiming to work hours above the official standard, amounting to 6.3 hours per week each. Among these nurses, 60 per cent reported working through meals and 34 per cent worked unpaid overtime without hours in lieu. By comparing results with their earlier research, the authors believe overtime is increasing (Buchan and Seccombe, 1991, p. 65–6).

An analysis of trends in British hospitals between 1962 and 1984 found that numbers of whole-time equivalent nursing staff rose by 47 per cent, but shortening of the basic working week and year reduced each nurse's hours by a fifth. At the same time in-patient admissions rose by 46 per cent and the average length of stay fell by nearly half. The overall result of these changes was calculated as a workload increase of 32 per cent (Moores, 1987). Although occupational stress is a routine claim for workers and their representatives, these studies lend weight to the nurses' case.

These studies take us straight from the squeeze on public expenditure and the drive for efficiency to the consequences for the humane aspects of health care. They show increasing activity levels, inadequately supported by increasing staff; improvements in working conditions (such as shorter basic hours) paid for in greater pressure on the job; and nurses feeling unable to carry out what they see as the core nursing task—patient care.

Dilemmas for health workers

These issues look different according to your standpoint. So far we have attempted to view workforce dilemmas from the outside, as issues of policy that would confront any health system, but which have particular relevance in the United Kingdom in the 1990s. Now we return to these issues from a new standpoint, that of two key interest groups—nurses and managers—who must develop strategies for operating within the system we have described.

Strategies for nurses

There have always been groups wanting to professionalise nursing, raise its educational standards and distance it from more menial roles by restricting entry. Throughout the 1980s these groups grew in power and prestige. They believed that gaining the same professional traits as doctors would give nurses a similar status.

The Nursing, Midwifery and Health Visiting Act 1979 was both an achievement for the professionalising movement and a base for further developments. This Act created the UKCC as an independent self-governing body, which controlled the entry gate and educational standards. By including midwifery and health visiting, which had formerly been separately-governed professions, it also generated a larger professional base. The UKCC registers practitioners, produces prescriptions for training, and defines the code of conduct to which practitioners must adhere, on pain of removal from the register. Governance of nurses, midwives and health visitors now resembles that of doctors in key respects of autonomy in registration, specified training and standards of practice.

The focus of nurse education had been on practical skills until the UKCC made a significant move towards professionalisation. A review of nurse recruitment, retention and training needs—known as Project 2000—was a major part of the UKCC's work in the 1980s. (You may recall from the extract of the Audit Commission report on day surgery, which you read with Chapter 1, that recruitment to nursing fell steadily throughout the 1980s—a source of growing concern in the profession.) The review proposed a number of changes in the preparation of nurses, principally a shift towards an academic framework for nurse training. It argued that nurses should receive training similar in academic level to that required for teachers and social workers. Institutional links should be made between Schools of Nursing (based within the NHS) and higher education institutions, in addition to the traditional links with hospitals, and more emphasis should be placed on working in the community.

The level of training recommended by the Project 2000 review was contentious. Nursing degrees had been offered since the 1960s, but produced only a tiny proportion of nurses.

□ Why might central government and the most senior levels of NHS management be reluctant to raise the level of nurse training?

■ Given the numbers employed in the NHS, you might suggest two reasons: the cost in salaries for better-qualified workers, and the problem of attracting enough recruits to nursing if entry standards were raised (which in turn would feed into staffing shortages in the future).

The profession wanted to increase the level of training, but the DH as primary employer needed to ensure adequate staffing of wards and clinics. A compromise was reached. The Project 2000 review opted for a Diploma in Higher Education, which is about two-thirds of the way to a degree. As it turned out, the severe economic recession of the early 1990s and shortage of employment for school-leavers reduced the expected recruitment problem.

Project 2000 also led to the end of Enrolled Nurse training. This again was intended to raise the standards and status of Registered Nurses by stopping the shorter, more practical training. It was supported by the Royal College of Nursing (RCN), as professional enhancement, but opposed by some nursing unions in defence of their existing Enrolled Nurse members.

However, within the same package of changes, the UKCC agreed to the establishment of a *health-care assistant* grade, receiving a training related to the specific practical skills needed by employers, but without a broader 'academic' framework. The role of the assistant would be to assist Registered Nurses in giving 'basic' nursing care. (The nursing auxiliary you heard on the audiotape was embarking on such a training course, and saw the qualification as giving her recognition for what she had been doing all along.) The more astute contemporary nursing observers suggested that the second-level (Enrolled) nurse had effectively been abolished and recreated (as a health-care assistant) at the same time. Whereas nurses hoped that they had secured a means to an enhanced registered workforce, the government and health-service managers hoped that they had achieved a reduced, but highly qualified, nursing élite, leading a less expensive army of health-care assistants.

Monica Baly, a nursing historian, observes:

The purists may fulminate, and legislation may change the legal position of the nurse, but whether she is village nurse, ordinary probationer, or enrolled nurse, it seems that nursing will always need some kind of two-tier system. Either there are not enough wholly trained people to undertake all the tasks, or there is not enough money to pay for them, or maybe all tasks do not require highly trained nurses, merely highly trained supervision. (Baly, 1987, p. 56)

The RCN recognised that fragmentation of the workforce into an élite 'core' and a 'peripheral' group of support workers threatened its claim to speak for nursing as a whole, as well as undermining its membership and income. The consequent debate on whether to admit health-care assistants to a form of subsidiary membership of the RCN was inconclusive. The UKCC, however, opted out of participation in developing the training of health-care assistants, and by implication firmly rejected them as 'nurses'.

Another strategy for professionalising nursing is to change the content and organisation of nursing work. A number of different approaches developed in the early 1990s,[15] with the common goal of reconstructing nursing practice from a fragmented, task-oriented activity, reminiscent of industrial work processes, and replacing it with professional models of work involving continuity of responsibility. Another linked strategy is to develop a nursing hierarchy on the medical model. This would replace the older bureaucratic hierarchy and allow nurses to become clinical nursing consultants.

These developments are at the centre of debate about nursing practice in the early 1990s. Contention centres on the relationship between improvements for nurses and improvements for patients. If there are fewer of the most highly-trained nurses overseeing an expanded corps of less-qualified staff, will the quality of patient care suffer? A report commissioned from the Centre for Health Economics by the DH on 'Skill mix and the effectiveness of nursing care' was published in 1992 and concluded:

…grade mix had an effect on the quality of care in so far as the quality of care was better the higher the grade (and skill) of the nurses who provided it, but the variation in the quality of care between different grades of staff was reduced when higher graded staff worked in combination with lower graded staff. (Carr-Hill et al., 1992, Summary, un-numbered page)

This is likely to be used by the RCN to argue that highly-qualified nurses not only deliver better quality care, but also:

Quality care can mean lower costs… Nursing skills can be employed in hospitals and in the community to prevent illness, to promote a quick recovery or an early discharge from hospital, to prevent people going into hospital in the first place, or to ensure patient satisfaction… in some settings a smaller workforce with a higher number of qualified nurses delivers better patient care and is more cost effective. (RCN, 1992, pages un-numbered)

The professionalisation strategy has had notable successes: the establishment of the UKCC, the enhancement of nurse training, the restriction of nurse registration to the fully qualified, and the creation of a clinical nursing hierarchy. But there are clear limitations to this strategy.

[15]For example, *primary nursing* in which each patient is assigned to a named primary nurse who assesses their needs and then prescribes and evaluates nursing care. The primary nurse normally delivers much of this care during her shift, but at other times associate nurses administer the care prescribed by the primary nurse.

Lack of room at the top, gender discrimination, educational requirements, the need for manual labour, and economic pressures, set limits on professionalisation. The dilemma for nursing representatives is whether to support such moves mainly to benefit an élite group of nurses, or to protect the interests of the wider membership. The nurses who are most vulnerable are women who work part-time, belong to ethnic minorities, or who are less well-trained. As you saw earlier in the chapter, this represents a very significant proportion of the workforce.

Strategies for managers

A rationale of both the Griffiths Report and the 1989 White Paper *Working for Patients* was to preserve the NHS under public expenditure constraints by more effective management. Managers must justify themselves within this framework or risk their jobs. In Chapters 2 to 4 we discussed the managerial strategy of evaluating and challenging medical decision-making to become more cost-effective.

□ Can you suggest another strategy for more efficient management of the workforce?

■ Given the size and relative vulnerability of the non-medical workforce, costs may also be contained by cheapening the labour process.

The first manifestation of such pressures came with the privatisation of laundry, catering and cleaning services on a wide scale in the 1980s (as Figure 6.1 revealed). In a period when public-sector employment was thought by central government to be too protected and less efficient than the private sector, many ancillary workers' jobs were removed from the NHS through competitive tendering exercises. The private contractors and their employees are still NHS-funded, but tendering reduces the number of directly-employed NHS staff and may produce savings, though not without costs to workers who have to increase productivity for lower pay and less job security.

Subsequent NHS reforms have intensified the pressure to contain workforce costs, to which nurses contribute a large proportion. Part of the agenda on every operational manager's desk is the reduction or containment of the nursing budget. To achieve a more flexible and cheaper workforce, managers may use short-term contracts, employ a higher proportion of less-qualified workers, and exert tight management control of the work undertaken.

Chris West writes as a District General Manager of the likely impact of the 1990 NHS reforms:

> I believe that at the end of this decade we may find that there has been a reduction, perhaps as high as 25 per cent, in the total labour force in the NHS and that some of that reduction will have occurred in the nursing profession. Just as nurses have been recruited wastefully, they have probably been deployed wastefully, and waste is something that no provider unit will be able to afford in the future...The successful implementation of the White Paper reforms may well lead to a smaller workforce working more flexibly, with a higher skill and knowledge base, working more productively and gaining higher personal rewards—and perhaps higher satisfaction as well. (West, 1992, p. 59)

Managers will argue that only with such strategies are they able to sustain acceptable standards of patient care within spending constraints and against a background of rising demand.

Conclusion

The health workforce, and nursing at its centre, are subject to contradictory forces. The pressure to professionalise involves increased accreditation for many workers and increased levels of skill and specialisation. This trend is reinforced by social changes beyond the NHS, such as increased expectations of women's employment. Opposing pressures may result in reduced numbers of better-qualified employees, and greater use of part-time, short-term, auxiliary workers to sustain levels of patient care within a political climate of public expenditure restraint.

Within such pressures, conflicts over work roles, control of workers and work processes and working conditions are intense. At present, the likely outcome seems to be an intensification of workforce divisions, with professional status won for some, while less well-placed workers suffer more occupational stress and less secure income and employment. The social class, gender and ethnic divisions in the workforce give an indication of where the gains and losses will be felt. There seems likely to be an increase in insecure and marginal work. But the relative fluidity of work roles and the gradual erosion of medical control may create space for rewarding occupational developments in the 1990s.

OBJECTIVES FOR CHAPTER 6

When you have studied this chapter, you should be able to:

6.1 Discuss the significance of the size and complexity of the NHS workforce for the effectiveness, efficiency and humanity of the health service.

6.2 Describe the division of labour within the NHS workforce in terms of occupational specialisation, gender, ethnicity, income and status.

6.3 Discuss areas of conflict over where boundaries are drawn between the tasks and responsibilities of midwives and obstetricians, and between nurses and doctors.

6.4 Comment on the major conflicts over control of the health workforce.

6.5 Discuss the dilemma facing the nursing profession as it seeks to protect and enhance its working conditions.

6.6 Comment on the strategies available to managers who are required to contain workforce costs.

QUESTIONS FOR CHAPTER 6

Question 1 (*Objective 6.1*)

Describe two consequences of the size and complexity of the NHS workforce for health workers in the 1990s.

Question 2 (*Objective 6.2*)

What does Table 6.2 tell you about changes in the ethnic and gender composition of GPs in England, and what does it fail to reveal? (Hints: begin with the most recent year and then look back for trends; then look at the totals for males and females and finally look at different places of birth).

Table 6.2 GPs in England: analysis of percentage by place of birth and sex, 1979–90

Place of birth		1979	1984	1985	1986	1987	1988	1989	1990
all places of birth	**total**	100.0	100.0	100.0	100.0	100.0	100.0	100.0	100.0
	male	84.7	81.6	81.0	80.1	79.1	78.2	77.2	76.2
	female	15.3	18.4	19.0	19.9	20.9	21.8	22.8	23.8
Great Britain	**total**	73.7	73.2	73.4	73.6	73.8	73.8	73.9	73.8
	male	62.7	59.7	59.3	58.6	57.9	57.0	56.3	55.3
	female	11.0	13.6	14.2	15.0	15.9	16.8	17.6	18.4
other UK or Irish Republic	**total**	5.3	3.9	3.7	3.5	3.2	3.0	2.8	2.6
	male	4.6	3.2	3.0	2.8	2.5	2.3	2.1	1.9
	female	0.7	0.7	0.7	0.7	0.7	0.7	0.7	0.7
elsewhere	**total**	21.0	22.8	22.9	22.9	23.0	23.2	23.3	23.6
	male	17.5	18.7	18.8	18.7	18.7	18.8	18.8	19.0
	female	3.5	4.1	4.1	4.2	4.3	4.4	4.4	4.7

Source: Department of Health (1991) *Health and Personal Social Services Statistics for England*, HMSO, London, Table 3.26.

Question 3 (*Objective 6.2*)

Predictions made for nursing in the next decade include:

- the total NHS workforce will decline;

- there will be increasing polarisation between highly qualified and less skilled workers;

- the proportion of male nurses will rise;

- part-time working will increase.

What might be the effect of these changes on (a) the proportion of men to women in senior nursing posts, and (b) the age profile of nurses?

Question 4 (*Objectives 6.3 and 6.4*)

Nurses will not only have to extend their clinical skills but also acquire a much wider range of managerial skills than they have had to hitherto. (West, 1992, p. 58)

Explain why nurses might have to acquire more clinical and managerial skills and who might advocate and oppose such moves.

Question 5 (*Objective 6.5*)

Describe some key elements of a professionalising strategy for nurses.

Question 6 (*Objective 6.6*)

What workforce strategies are open to managers, trying to sustain levels of service within tightening cost limits?

7 Innovations in health care

During this chapter you will be asked to look again at the extract in the Reader[1] from the 1990 Audit Commission Report, A Short Cut to Better Services, which discusses day surgery in England and Wales. As you read this extract in association with Chapter 1, it will only be necessary for you to skim through it again in order to refresh your memory and establish the relevance of the report to the present chapter. Some of the discussion in this chapter involves the use of technical terms with which you may not be familiar, but they will be explained when they are introduced.

This chapter was written by Nicholas Mays, a social scientist involved in health services research. He is Director of the Health and Health Care Research Unit at The Queen's University of Belfast.

The way of the new

All health services and health-care systems are in a constant state of change. This chapter looks at some of the sources of these changes, the mechanisms by which they are introduced, the obstructions they encounter, and their consequences for effectiveness, efficiency, equity and humanity in health care. The chapter concludes with a brief look at how health care may change in the future.

Change in the health service is not a random process. At all levels, individuals and groups attempt to shape that change and, in doing so, they encounter uncomfortable choices. Let us suppose that a pharmaceutical company discovers a new drug of great promise in the treatment of a serious disease: a promising scenario but one in which dilemmas appear at every turn. How stringent should the testing be of the drug? How should the present needs of suffering patients be balanced against the need for thorough scrutiny for possible side effects? To what extent

is it acceptable for present patients to act as guinea-pigs and perhaps contribute to the welfare of future sufferers? One step further back, is it ethical to test such a drug on animals using the justification that it will benefit humans? Let us further assume that the drug is proved to be both effective and safe. How does the pharmaceutical company set its price? It needs profits to satisfy shareholders and fund further developments. How does it weigh business interests against humanitarian concerns? Perhaps the drug is expensive. How does the health service balance the needs of this patient group against those in other groups? How does it balance present and future needs?

This is not an exhaustive list of the dilemmas associated with the introduction of a new drug and it would certainly require many additions if we were considering the wider field of technological change. However, it should provide some indication of the complexities involved in charting 'the way of the new'.

What is medical technology?

The development of the *welfare state* is most often explained in economic, ideological or social terms. It is less frequently analysed in terms of its technological basis. Technology is not just a source of the *wealth* and *economic growth* that enables resources to be spent on welfare. It is also one of the principal means of producing the range of *goods* and *services* which constitute welfare (a careful analysis of this relationship is given in Stephen Uttley's book, *Technology and the Welfare State*, 1991). If we want to understand health services fully, we have to understand the dynamics of the technologies that support and constitute them just as much as the particular political circumstances that have shaped them. These technologies include lasers used in surgery, genetic probes which help to identify defective genes, 'smart cards' which store diagnostic and treatment information, and animals which have been genetically engineered[2]

---

[1] *Health and Disease: A Reader* (revised edition 1994).

[2] The introduction of new genes into animals (including humans) is discussed in another book in this series, *Human Biology and Health: An Evolutionary Approach* (Open University Press, 1994).

to produce important human enzymes[3] such as α_1-antitrypsin (Figure 7.1).

From the examples given, it is clear that we are applying the term 'technology' to more than complex pieces of equipment. How widely should we frame our definition? What precisely do we mean when we talk of technology in the context of the health services (i.e. medical technology)? In one of the neatest general definitions of **technology**, the American writer Arnold Gehlen (1980) defines it as any substitute for, or enhancement of individual human capacities. He amplifies this definition to include machines that enhance our physical or mental activities, e.g. tools, robots, cars, computers, etc. At the time when these were first introduced they were all examples of **product innovations** (new products). But technology is more than the application of scientific knowledge to produce machines.

☐ How can we enhance our individual human capabilities without using machines?

■ By coming together in groups with a common purpose we can carry out activities that would be beyond the capabilities of a single individual. Social cooperation of this sort falls within Gehlen's basic definition of technology.

Human tasks are performed through organisations within which technical processes take place. These organisational and managerial structures themselves change and are deliberately changed (often with the aim of increased efficiency) and can, therefore, be seen as technologies in their own right. They are known as *process* technologies; new processes are described as **process innovations**. Changes in such technologies tend to attract less attention, particularly from the mass media, than product innovations, but their impact can be just as great, if not greater. In the NHS, 'resource management' (as described in Chapter 4) is a process innovation in which clinical teams in hospitals are made responsible for their own budgets in order to increase their awareness of the resource consequences of clinical activities and, thereby, improve the efficiency with which they use resources.

[3]An enzyme is a biological catalyst that enables a specific biochemical reaction in the body to proceed rapidly; without the enzyme the reaction would occur too slowly to be biologically useful. See *The Biology of Health and Disease* (1984) or *Human Biology and Health: An Evolutionary Approach* (1994).

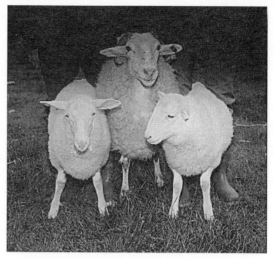

Figure 7.1 *Tracy is a very special sheep at the centre of a very special deal. Two years ago molecular biologists in Edinburgh gave her the gene to make human α_1-antitrypsin. Now Bayer AG, the German pharmaceutical company, is helping to finance a breeding and development programme by Pharmaceutical Proteins, the company that owns Tracy, in exchange for the right to exploit the α_1-antitrypsin produced by Tracy's offspring. In 1992 prices the potential market is about \$100 million each year. Tracy is shown here with female twin offspring: one inherited the human gene, the other did not. (Source: Pharmaceutical Proteins)*

Perhaps the best known definition of **medical technology** was given by the US Office of Technology Assessment in 1978:

> The drugs, devices and medical and surgical procedures used in medical care and the organisation and supportive systems within which such care is provided. (Office of Technology Assessment, 1982, pp. 200–1)

This definition includes both product and process forms of technology. Often, these are intimately related in that one technological change may facilitate another which, in turn, may lead to further opportunities or incentives for technological change. For example, the use of day surgery (a process innovation) is primarily a response to the need to make the best use of expensive hospital resources. However, it has only been possible because of the development of new anaesthetics (a product innovation) which allow patients to recover sufficiently rapidly to be discharged in a few hours. In turn, the spread of day surgery is encouraging surgeons to develop new, less invasive procedures, enabling new types of operation to be undertaken as day cases.

An international perspective on medical technology

There are substantial differences between countries in the availability and use of many technologies, even so-called 'essential' life-saving technologies. These differences cannot be explained away by corresponding differences in the levels of disease or age-structures of the population; nor can they be explained entirely by how wealthy a country is.

Table 7.1 shows the distribution in European countries of *lithotripters*, machines for pulverising kidney stones using shock waves. Table 7.2 gives the rate of treatment of people with irreversible kidney failure in the same countries.

☐ What do these tables indicate about the adoption of technologies in the countries listed?

■ It is abundantly clear that the pattern of adoption of the technologies is very different in the different countries. The availability of lithotripters in 1989 varied by a factor of nearly five, when population sizes per machine are compared. Even more extreme variations are evident in the numbers of patients treated by dialysis or transplant in 1975 when these techniques were fairly new.

Table 7.1 Number of lithotripters in Europe on 31 December 1989

Country	Population (millions)	Number of machines	Population per machine (millions)
Belgium	9.9	12	0.8
Denmark	5.1	3	1.7
France	55.2	36	1.5
Greece	9.9	10	1.0
Holland	14.5	11	1.3
Ireland	3.5	2	1.8
Italy	57.1	69	0.8
Portugal	10.2	4	2.5
Spain	38.5	50	0.8
Sweden	8.4	6	1.4
West Germany	61.0	72	0.9
United Kingdom	56.6	15	3.8

Source: Kirchberger, S. (1991) *The Diffusion of Two Technologies for Renal Stone Treatment Across Europe*, King's Fund Centre, London, Table 1, p. 7.

Table 7.2 The number of patients per million of the population either receiving kidney dialysis or with functioning kidney transplants in 1975 and in 1986

Country	Number treated per million in 1975	Number treated per million in 1986
Belgium	103	392
Denmark	132	262
France	102	303
Greece	48	225
Holland	90	318
Ireland	45	193
Italy	81	305
Portugal	4	269
Spain	27	337
Sweden	85	283
West Germany	88	333
United Kingdom	62	242

Source: OECD (1990) *Health Care Systems in Transition: the Search for Efficiency*, OECD Social Policy Studies, No. 7, OECD, Paris, Table 8, p. 96.

The scale of the differences in the availability and use of these technologies suggests that political, economic, religious, cultural, social or legal factors are as significant as the health-care needs of the population in determining whether and how quickly technologies are adopted. This observation is of more general validity. For example, the variations seen in Table 7.1 and 7.2 are also seen in the use of prescribed and over-the-counter drugs (Table 7.3, *overleaf*).

☐ Using the (limited) evidence in Tables 7.1 to 7.3, how would you describe the availability and use of medical technologies in the United Kingdom compared with other European countries?

■ The tables suggest that the United Kingdom tends to adopt these new medical technologies more slowly and in smaller quantities than in most other European countries. For example, the availability of treatment for irreversible kidney failure is low in the United Kingdom compared with most other European countries (Table 7.2).

Table 7.3 Consumption of pharmaceuticals in the European Community, 1987. The volume data are scaled so that UK consumption is defined as 100

Country	Volume of drugs consumed per person
Belgium	210
Denmark	91
France	292
Greece	74
Holland	75
Ireland	62
Italy	174
Portugal	65
Spain	105
West Germany	168
United Kingdom	100
European Community (average)	149

Source: Burstall, M. L. (1990) *1992 and the Regulation of the Pharmaceutical Industry,* IEA Health Series No.9, Institute of Economic Affairs, London, Table 2.1, p. 9.

The main reason why the United Kingdom tends to embrace new technologies less completely is the high degree of control exerted by central government over the total level of spending on health care. This is possible because the NHS is funded from general tax revenues and the government is able to fix a cash limit for health-care spending in relation to its priorities for other programmes such as defence, transport and housing. This is in contrast to the systems of social insurance which exist in most European countries where revenues are raised specifically for health care and the level of spending is driven in large part by the demand for health services.[4]

The differences in the consumption of prescribed drugs and in the use of technologies shown in Tables 7.1 to 7.3 are not just financially driven. They are also a reflection of cultural and national differences in both the perceptions that people have of their own health and the ways in which doctors and others respond to those perceptions. For example, in Germany, people, including doctors, regard low blood pressure (*hypotension*) as a medical problem requiring professional attention,

[4]See *Caring for Health: History and Diversity* (revised edition 1993), Chapter 9, for further discussion of alternative ways of financing and controlling health-care systems.

including medication. By contrast, hardly anyone in the United Kingdom is treated for hypotension. According to medical journalist Lynn Payer:

> Blood pressure considered treatably high in the United States might be considered normal in England; and the low blood pressure treated with eighty-five drugs as well as hydrotherapy and spa treatments in Germany would entitle its sufferer to lower life insurance rates in the United States. (Payer, 1988, p. 25)

The career of a medical technology

The rest of this chapter looks at the origins, introduction and effects of medical technologies. We begin by examining the early stages in the 'career' of a technology. The idea of a career was first put forward by John McKinlay, a medical sociologist who identified a series of stages in the life of a medical technology (see Box 7.1).

Box 7.1 The seven stages in the 'career' of a medical innovation.

1 A report identifies the new technology as promising (evidence from media reports).

2 The technology is adopted by professional bodies and health-care institutions (evidence from clinical experience).

3 The technology meets with general public approval and is recognised by the state as part of the health-care system.

4 The technology is accepted as the 'standard procedure' or most appropriate way of dealing with a particular problem (evidence from uncontrolled studies).

5 The technology may become the subject of a randomised controlled trial (evidence from controlled studies).

6 Professional denunciation of the RCT results if they question the 'standard procedure'.

7 Support for the 'standard procedure' erodes and it is eventually discredited, and replaced by a new procedure.

Source: derived from McKinlay, J.B. (1981) From 'promising report' to 'standard procedure': seven stages in the career of a medical innovation, Milbank Memorial Fund Quarterly/Health and Society, *59*, pp. 374–411.

However, in order to understand how change comes about, it is also necessary to consider the processes that *precede* the start of the career, the 'promising report'. Where do new technologies come from?

Invention and innovation

At first sight the title of this section may seem needlessly repetitious. Surely invention and innovation are the same thing? Not so! **Invention** is generally used by writers on new technology to refer to the generation of new knowledge from fundamental scientific research. By contrast, **innovation** refers to the deliberate *application* of inventions and scientific insights to produce goods and services (that is, the development part of the sequence of *research and development*, otherwise known as R&D).

There are two basic models to explain how a new medical technology begins its career. In the first, new ideas are seen as arising directly out of inventions in 'pure' science—that is, arising from scientific research carried out without immediate practical aims, but with the wish to obtain knowledge about the world. This model assumes that such research then leads to other more 'applied' developments (innovations), which exploit the new ideas or techniques and generate new products and processes to solve health-care problems. This is known as the **science-push model.**

In the second model, those engaged in health care—whether as clinicians, managers or manufacturers of equipment or drugs—identify needs or potential sources of profit which then result in the necessary research and development being *commissioned* and solutions devised. This is the so-called **market-pull model.**

In practice, neither model in its simple form offers an entirely adequate explanation of how medical technologies reach the stage of 'promising report'. On the one hand, the market may not know that there is a need until pure science has developed new knowledge. For example, few people would have seriously envisaged the possibility of looking inside the living human body without having to cut it open until the discovery of X-rays at the end of the nineteenth century. Furthermore, pure scientific advance may only lead to useful commercial exploitation after a lengthy delay.[5] On the other hand, even scientists engaged in pure research are not driven solely by intellectual interest. Modern scientific research is an expensive, professional activity, and scientists are dependent on funding bodies who display an ever-increasing interest in the possible application of the findings of pure research.

In reality most innovations emerge from a process in which both science-push and market-pull factors interact over time. Tracy, the genetically altered sheep, was the result of the interplay of scientific and commercial interests. The gene which contains coded instructions enabling living cells to make the human enzyme α_1-antitrypsin was isolated and introduced into sheep by scientists at the Agriculture and Food Research Council's Institute of Animal Physiology and Genetics Research. Their research was influenced by the knowledge that one in 2 000 people has a genetic deficiency of the enzyme leading in severe cases to emphysema (severe inflammation of the lungs) and liver failure. It was further stimulated by the existence of a company, Pharmaceutical Proteins, whose role is to act as a broker between scientists and the large drug companies in the field of genetically-altered animals.

Research and development

On the surface it may appear that *scientific* research that results in *product* innovations such as lithotripters is a very different activity from *social* research that results in *process* innovations such as giving GPs their own budgets to buy hospital care for their patients. Although lay people can still analyse and contribute new ideas about the organisation of health care (look at the recent history of the NHS to see the influence of politicians' beliefs on restructuring), natural science research is now almost exclusively the preserve of professional scientists. However, these differences are a matter of degree. For example, much social research in the health field requires high levels of funding and the application of sophisticated analytical methods, often similar to those used in the natural and physical sciences.[6]

Perhaps the most basic link between natural and social science research is their shared reliance on sources of funding. This obviously limits the amount of research which can be undertaken, but the source of funding also has important consequences for the choice of areas to study.

---

[5]For example, the identification of penicillin by Alexander Fleming in 1928 remained a laboratory curiosity for over a decade until techniques to produce the drug in bulk were developed.

[6]The methods used in research into health and health care are discussed in more detail in *Studying Health and Disease* (1985, and revised edition 1994).

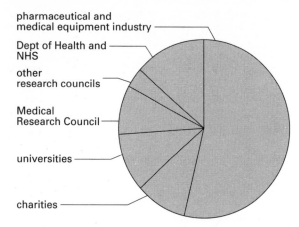

pharmaceutical and
medical equipment industry

Dept of Health and
NHS

other
research councils

Medical
Research Council

universities

charities

Figure 7.2 *Estimates of identified health research funding in England 1989–90, showing the proportion of funding by each major source (total £1.5 billion). (Source: Department of Health, 1991f,* Research for Health: A Research and Development Strategy for the NHS, *HMSO, London, Figure 1, p. 7)*

□ Looking at the data in Figure 7.2, can you identify the principal sources of funds for health research in the United Kingdom?

■ The most important source of funds for health research is the pharmaceutical and medical equipment industry, which provided over half the total funds in 1989–90. The DH and the NHS are the next most important source, followed (with similar shares) by charities, universities and the Medical Research Council.

As well as asking who funds research, it is important to ask what they hope to achieve from it and how the topics for research are chosen. We shall examine the three principal sources of funding—the state, industry and charities—with a particular emphasis on identifying their aims and the ways in which they influence the type of research that is carried out.

State funding

In the United Kingdom, the state funds research into health and social welfare through a number of channels; the Research Councils, the Universities, the DH in England and Wales, the Health Departments in Scotland and Northern Ireland and finally, the NHS itself.

The Medical Research Council (MRC), which is not part of any government department, though entirely dependent on government money, makes a major contribution. It spends most of its funds on laboratory science in

the so-called basic medical sciences (e.g. physiology, biochemistry and genetics), but it also supports work in public health, health psychology, medical sociology and health-services research. The MRC's priorities are set by scientists themselves by a process known as *peer review* (discussion between senior scientists who review research in progress and set future directions). However, there is an agreement with the various Health Departments in the United Kingdom that, in setting its agenda, the MRC will take account not only of scientific relevance but also of the health needs of the population.

□ This arrangement, in which the MRC rather than the government or the NHS is the main funding body, has been criticised periodically. Can you suggest why?

■ The assumption that scientists and researchers themselves can decide what research should be done through a system of peer review has been questioned on the grounds that the projects that result from this process may reflect the intellectual interests of the scientists rather than the needs of the country and the health services.

Supporters of the present arrangement counter this argument by asserting that the MRC is influenced by the broad social concerns of the day and responds to them. For instance, in its programme of research into HIV (human immunodeficiency virus), it has responded to an epidemic which is of major public concern.

The DH and the NHS (at different levels between the Management Executive and the health authorities) have priorities that are different from those of the MRC. They are generally less interested in advancing basic scientific knowledge than in commissioning health-services research—the evaluation of the effectiveness, efficiency and acceptability of health services. The DH funds several research units in universities concerned with topics such as child care and development, perinatal epidemiology, health-services management and so on.

In 1988, the House of Lords Select Committee on Science and Technology published a report entitled *Priorities in Medical Research*. It criticised the lack of a coherent mechanism through which the health service as a whole (as opposed to the DH) could make its research needs known and could ensure that the benefits of research—particularly research into the content, organisation and management of health services—was effectively communicated to and adopted by the NHS. The committee's report echoed long-standing concerns that innovations tended to be the result of the personal interests of scientists and clinicians and were often introduced into clinical practice without proper evaluation (a point made earlier, in Chapter 4). Furthermore, there was evidence that the best new techniques were not always adopted speedily in all parts of the NHS.

The government responded by creating a new top level post in the NHS in England, the Director of Research and Development, who was made responsible from January 1991 for developing, for the first time, a national R&D strategy for the NHS and for ensuring that the content and delivery of care was grounded in research relevant to improving the country's health. The holder of the post also became a member of the NHS Management Executive. The national health services in Scotland, Wales and Northern Ireland followed the lead with a similar series of initiatives. A distinctive feature of the R&D strategy is the emphasis given to the *development* of the results of basic research into new methods of care, followed by their experimental introduction, evaluation and eventual use throughout the NHS. There is also considerable weight given to the related task of ensuring that the results of all sorts of research are *disseminated* to those people in a position to act on them, such as managers and clinicians.

In the financial year 1989–90, about £225 million of the £1.5 billion spent annually on health research in England came from the DH and the NHS. To increase the priority given to R&D in the NHS, it is intended to move over a 5-year period to a target R&D expenditure of 1.5 per cent of the NHS budget. In 1989–90, this would have amounted to £317 million. Meeting the target would involve a considerable increase in the level of R&D expenditure in the NHS. It remains to be seen whether it will be reached when there is continual pressure for expansion in direct patient care.

Industrial funding: the case of the pharmaceutical industry

Industrial funding is concerned with product innovation. Many different types of industrial product are relevant to health and health services. For example, the design and durability of artificial hip joints and the skill of the surgeon unite to produce a good or bad outcome for the patient. Automated laboratory equipment developed by scientific instrument manufacturers has transformed routine work in pathology laboratories and made it far easier for a commercial company to set up in competition with a hospital laboratory. Computerised hospital record systems not only promise to help clinical staff of all kinds to audit the quality of their care, but are also big business for the firms that sell them.

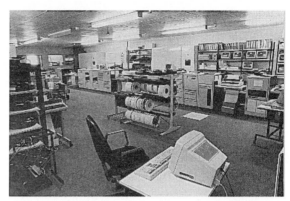

(a)

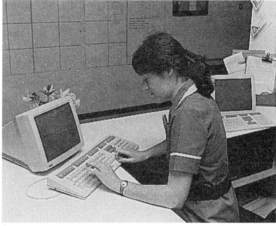

(b)

Computers now permeate the health-care system. (a) A large hospital computer-records room. (b) A nurse using a desk-top computer. (Photos: Mike Levers)

However, for several reasons, industrial research in product innovation in health care is best discussed in terms of the pharmaceutical industry. First, it operates on a large scale—in 1987, the United Kingdom consumed drugs worth £2 800 million, amounting to 11 per cent of total health spending. Second, unlike many other health-care innovations, new drugs have tended to come almost exclusively from the research activities of the drug companies themselves, although this situation is changing, particularly in the field of biotechnology, where the universities are increasingly involved through the setting up of their own commercial ventures. Third, the pharmaceutical industry has attracted a good deal of criticism for its pricing and advertising policies.

☐ What do you think would be the overall goal of the pharmaceutical industry?

■ Pharmaceutical companies, like other companies in the private sector, can only continue to exist by making profits, if not in the short term then over a reasonable period. Profitability has to be their underlying goal.

To pursue this objective, the industry has to be able both to produce and to market products that provide an adequate return on capital invested. At a fundamental level, therefore, the products are a means to an end rather than an end in themselves.

Given that there are almost 5 000 different chemical substances or compounds available or in general use, which act on human physiology, why should the pharmaceutical industry do research at all? The answer lies partly in the nature of the laws regulating the production and marketing of drugs. Any new drug is **patented** by the company that originated it. Only that company or its licensees have the right to produce and market it for a period of seventeen years. In other words, the company is given a monopoly by the Patents Office for a particular product and can in principle sell it at any price it wants. The chemical constituents of the drug may cost only a few pence to produce, but the company can sell it for many times that figure.

The purpose of patent laws, like copyright laws for published work, is to try to ensure that innovators are rewarded. This might not occur if everything were left to market forces and the skill of imitators. However, in the pharmaceutical industry, patent laws have had a profound effect on research: if other companies wish to share in the market for a particular drug that is protected by patent, then the only option, other than waiting for the patent to expire, is to engage in the intense research effort required to produce another drug that is as similar to the patented drug as possible but legally a different entity. The result of this process is that any successful drug is usually followed by several similar products, often referred to as 'me-too' drugs made by competitors. For example, Valium, one of the most commercially successful drugs of all time, gave rise to a vast range of similar tranquillisers. A variant of this strategy is the development of new products by combining existing drugs in new ways as in over-the-counter headache remedies which may contain muscle relaxants and even anti-depressants in addition to the conventional pain-killers.

Pharmaceutical companies have been responsible for developing most of the important new drugs since World War II, including tranquillisers, oral contraceptives, most anaesthetics, anti-malarial drugs and anti-histamines. In the 1980s they began to contract more work out to specialist research institutes, including universities, for the *genetic engineering*[7] of fundamentally new drugs. These techniques, which originated in academic research, offer new and cheaper ways of producing, on a large scale, substances such as hormones (e.g. insulin) and enzymes (the case of Tracy is a good example of this new relationship between industry and academic research).

Pharmaceutical companies make deals not only with universities but also with hospitals, in which they fund new research institutes to develop new drugs and to test them. They also offer academics well paid consultancies. The effects that these close industrial links may have on financially hard-pressed universities, and the issue of the commercial ownership of the results of such scientific research, continue to raise dilemmas about the quality, ethics and control of research.

□ How do you think the increasing dependence of universities on commercial funds for research could affect the way in which scientific work is carried out?

■ If commercial sponsorship is too prevalent, a situation might develop in which the only research areas that are pursued are those where there are clear opportunities for profit. Commercial funding bodies may also be tempted to try to secure an advantage over their market rivals by interfering with the traditional freedom of academics to publish the results of their research.

The government has to cope with this ambiguity in the relationship between the universities and drug companies in its system for regulating the pharmaceutical industry and licensing drugs for human use. After the thalidomide tragedy of the 1960s,[8] the regulations controlling new and old drugs were tightened up under the 1968 Medicines Act which established, among other bodies, the Committee on Safety of Medicines (CSM). The CSM is charged with ensuring the safety, quality and efficacy of any substance for human use and with monitoring the effects of drugs once they are on

[7]Genetic engineering of drugs, vaccines and other useful biochemical entities is discussed in *Studying Health and Disease* and *Human Biology and Health: An Evolutionary Approach* (revised editions 1994).

[8]Thalidomide was prescribed to relieve morning sickness during pregnancy, but caused malformation of the limbs of babies whose mother took the drug during the first three months of gestation. The manufacturer was forced to pay £millions in compensation after a series of court cases.

the market. The CSM is obliged to publish a register of its members' personal and non-personal (institutional) interests since most of the expert members receive either research grants or consultancies from the industry. Critics of the arrangements continue to argue that the members of the CSM and related bodies are likely to be insufficiently objective and impartial in their advice.

The drug industry argues that the lengthy licensing process in the United Kingdom and other Western countries leaves little time to recoup R&D expenditure before patents expire and is a disincentive to innovation. On the other hand, critics claim that the terms of reference of the CSM, for example, are still too lax in that drugs are only required to be safe and more effective than a placebo. There is no test in the United Kingdom of whether a drug is *medically needed*—this is required in some other countries.

Drug companies tend to be multinational industries. They try to operate a pricing structure for their goods which is geared to what each country can afford.[9] In turn, governments act to control prices and drug expenditure in a variety of ways. In the United Kingdom, the DH negotiates with drug companies each year a global return on capital based on several factors: their sales to the NHS, their investments, their research activities, and the long-term risks they face. As long as this rate is not exceeded, firms are free to price new products as they see fit.

This system produced an average trading profit for 1985 in the United Kingdom pharmaceutical industry of 30 per cent of turnover which is far higher than that in the rest of the chemical industry (Burstall, 1990). On this basis there are few more profitable industries than pharmaceuticals. The drug companies defend their pricing policies and their profits by pointing out that they have to bear the R&D costs of thousands of compounds which never reach the market. They also stress the fact that only the profit-orientated environment of private industry can generate so many new products. This still leaves unanswered the question of how many of them are necessary or beneficial.

Funding from charities and trusts

Charities and trusts are legally recognised non-profit-making bodies that are required by their charters to disburse money for defined purposes, which may be concerned with education, welfare or research. Charities rely on three main sources of income to varying degrees:

voluntary donations, investment income from trusts, and charges for services they provide. Medical and health charities are very popular and receive substantially more money in voluntary donations than any other area of charitable activity. Particularly prominent and successful charities are focused on cancers, physical disability and blindness (see Figure 7.3 *overleaf*).

Medical charities spend approximately as much on biomedical research as the MRC (look back at Figure 7.2). Two of the largest and oldest fund-raising charities, the Imperial Cancer Research Fund and the Cancer Research Campaign, dominate the funding of cancer research. Like most of the other charities that focus on particular diseases, they see their aims in military terms to 'win the war' on the disease and believe that this victory will largely be won through biomedical research in the laboratory and the hospital ward. The size and high profile of these charities obscures the fact that there are many other smaller charities working for innovation in the delivery of health care to people currently in need, for example the

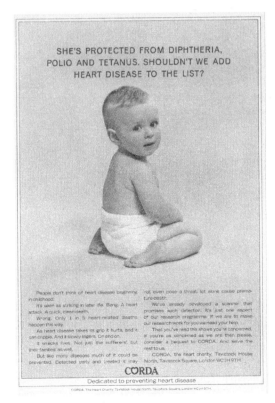

Charities campaign for donations to fund a wide range of activities, including medical research, as in this poster by the Coronary Artery Disease Research Association (Photo: CORDA, the Heart Charity)

---

[9] The international trade in pharmaceutical products and the impact of the drugs bill on health-care costs in developing and developed countries is discussed in *Caring for Health: History and Diversity* (revised edition 1993), Chapter 9.

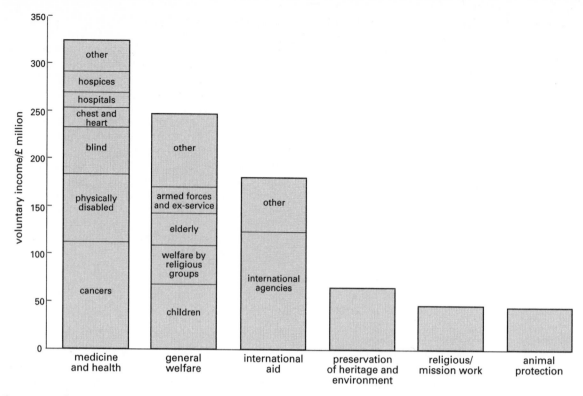

Figure 7.3 *Charities attracting the largest voluntary donations, 1987–8, based on the 200 charities with the largest voluntary incomes. (Source: Brophy, M. and McQuillan, J., 1989,* Charity Trends, *12th edn, Charities Aid Foundation, Tonbridge, Kent, p. 122)*

National Society for Cancer Relief, which funds the Macmillan terminal care nurses, and the Family Planning Association. In many cases, the example of the services provided by these charities has persuaded conservative statutory authorities to change or develop their services. Yet another group of charities such as the Spastics Society combines service provision with an emphasis on campaigning to influence public opinion and, thereby, government policy towards the needs of disabled people.

In this part of the chapter our focus has been on the agencies that bring about change. As the foregoing discussion illustrated, these agencies are motivated by a range of factors including intellectual curiosity, wealth creation and compassion. The importance of human and economic factors will be more apparent later in the discussion of the adoption and diffusion of technologies. But first, what creates a favourable climate for change?

The technological imperative

The urge to introduce new technologies has been dubbed the **technological imperative**: it is driven by a number of forces. First, medical equipment manufacturers are enthusiastic promotors of their wares to doctors and managers, and are constantly searching for innovations and for clinicians who will help to develop new technologies and champion them with colleagues. Second, most of the incentives in health research and medical practice (Nobel prizes, professional status, research grants, personal profit) encourage scientists and practitioners to expand the limits of what can be done to alleviate disease.

Third, there is the frequently observed reluctance of decision-makers to pass by any opportunity to acquire a new technology, even if they only have resources for a small investment, for fear that the one which they choose to forego will prove to be a great life-saver. They act to avoid the regret and criticism which they might face for denying patients the opportunity of treatment (in an article published in 1982, G. Loomes and R. Sugden referred to 'regret theory' as an alternative to rational decision-making). Following the same logic, clinicians may try a new technique before it has been evaluated, particularly in the case of incurable disease, out of a desire to act and to avoid the possibility of missing a positive outcome.

Although much of this activity can be beneficial in bringing the latest technologies into use at the earliest opportunity, it can also lead to the pressure to purchase equipment that is more expensive than the equipment being replaced and that has not been fully assessed in terms of the costs and benefits of its use in day-to-day as against experimental practice. Hospital managers may feel the 'imperative' of innovation in health care as a force outside their control, inexorably marching forwards and inevitably bringing higher costs. This underlines the need for regulation of innovation in the face of powerful commercial interests in the medical market, the so-called *medical–industrial complex* identified by Arnold Relman in 1980.

An example of how enthusiasm for a technological solution can overcome informed judgement has been provided by Howard Waitzkin, an American doctor and sociologist, writing in 1979. He discussed the proliferation of coronary care units in the USA in the 1970s (which occurred despite the lack of clear evidence at the time of their effectiveness) in terms of the profit-making objectives of a number of large corporations. They were involved at every step in the development of coronary care technologies and their interests coincided with those of leading cardiologists at prestigious teaching hospitals who acted as advocates for the new technologies. State agencies and private philanthropic foundations provided further encouragement by giving grants to clinicians and manufacturers and by undertaking market research to help identify export opportunities. Hospital managers felt compelled to invest. Without a coronary care unit, a hospital appeared to be falling behind the pace of medical progress. The result was the rapid spread of coronary care units and an increase in the overall cost of health care.[10]

The technological imperative plays a key part in the factors that promote the adoption and diffusion of new technologies, especially product innovations, in health care. In the next section we discuss these factors in more detail and in particular compare the careers of product and process innovations.

[10]Chapter 10 of this book discusses coronary heart disease in greater detail and provides fuller evidence of the complex forces that shape the response of health services to this common complaint.

Adoption and diffusion

The career of health technologies can be represented as a distinctive S-shaped curve in which extent of use is plotted against time (Figure 7.4). **Adoption** (the point at which the innovation is regarded as worthwhile), is followed by **diffusion** (growth of use), and then by a period of refinement and a slowing down in diffusion of the technology. Subsequently, in most cases, there is some degree of disillusionment leading to eventual disuse and the replacement of the technology by another innovation (look back at Box 7.1). The precise timescales and therefore the shape of the curve depend on the innovation.

Barbara Stocking, a British health policy analyst, identified three main factors that might influence the adoption and diffusion of a health technology (see Figure 7.5 *overleaf*):

1   The characteristics of the innovation itself;

2   The influence of the environment, and

3   The role of individuals and specific groups.

A given factor identified as influencing an innovation cannot always be assigned simply to one of these categories, but they do provide a useful framework. We shall explore each in turn.

First, relevant questions are provoked by considering the *characteristics* of the innovation. They include: how complex is it; how compatible is it with existing beliefs and working practices; how visible is it to public and professionals; how easy is it for people to see it in use before deciding whether to adopt it formally; and, finally, what perceived advantage does it confer over the existing technology (product) or organisation (process)?

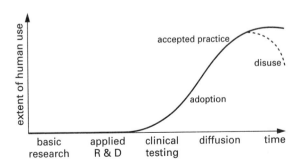

Figure 7.4 *The S-shaped curve of the development and diffusion of a typical medical technology. (Source: Office of Technology Assessment, US Congress, 1976, Development of Medical Technology: Opportunities for Assessment, U. S. Government Printing Office, Washington, D.C., p. 74)*

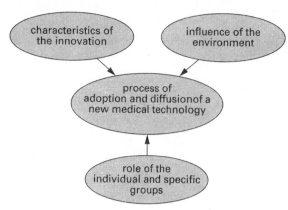

Figure 7.5 *A model of the main factors affecting the adoption and diffusion of a medical technology.*
(Source: Based on Stocking, B., 1991, Factors Affecting the Diffusion of Three Kinds of Innovative Medical Technology in European Community Countries and Sweden, *King's Fund Centre, London)*

In addition, the resources required to produce the technology are clearly important features since they affect future profitability and the commitment of the company to the development of the finished product. The obvious example is the pharmaceutical industry where development costs are high: about 1 in 5 000–10 000 compounds survive to reach the market, and it is 'guesstimated' that between £100 m and £170 m is spent on each active substance.

Second, consider the influence of the social, cultural and political *environment,* of which marketing is a part. Not surprisingly, companies spend large sums on advertising, but especially on the far more effective visits by sales representatives to doctors. In the United Kingdom, marketing costs are equal to approximately half the R&D costs of drugs and are probably up to three times higher than the average for other industries.

☐ Can you suggest some other major environmental influences on the adoption and diffusion of health technologies?

■ Environmental influences include: society's attitudes and expectations; the organisation of health care and its incentive structure; the physical environment of health-service buildings; and the level of resources available for new technologies. (Specific examples are given below.)

The influence of societal attitudes and expectations are revealed in life and death issues such as the availability of pre-natal diagnosis and abortion facilities in countries with different religious traditions, or the extent of high-technology care for very small newborn babies (Chapter 2), or the degree to which people are prepared to accept as legitimate a particular level of health-care rationing (Chapter 3 noted that the availability of certain forms of health care in the United Kingdom would be considered unacceptably low in the USA, but 20 per cent of Americans lack any form of health insurance).[11]

The influence of the organisation of health care on the diffusion of technology can be illustrated by the extent to which hospitals specialise. In the United Kingdom, the district general hospitals provide the basic range of acute services, but more advanced technology is found in other centres (mainly teaching hospitals) which offer more specialised treatment. The influence of the incentive structure of the health system is evident in the comparison of salaried practitioners with fee-for-service medicine; the latter encourages more intensive health care using more technologies in the form of tests and investigations.

The physical environment of health care, such as the lay-out of wards in hospitals, could influence the adoption of new working practices such as giving each patient privacy.

Finally, an obvious example of the influence of the level of resources on technology would be the ability of health-care providers to invest in the latest equipment. Providers with limited resources are more likely to wait to see if new technologies have proved cost-effective after evaluation before buying them.

The third set of influences on diffusion identified by Stocking concerns the role of *individuals and specific groups or agencies* such as doctors, pressure groups, funding bodies and the mass media. Individuals, particularly doctors, can play a crucial role not only in initiating change, but also in promoting innovations by acting as opinion leaders, lobbyists and disseminators of the latest techniques to the majority of their peers. The transmission of opinion by respected colleagues via the informal social networks that exist within the medical profession has been shown to be particularly important in the diffusion of innovations (see for example the study in Canada by Lomas *et al.*, 1991). The results of clinical trials, structured evaluations and medical audit are frequently given far less weight than the practice and views of respected colleagues, who can also play a crucial role in resisting innovation.

[11]A comparison of the structure and financing of the NHS and health systems in other countries occurs in *Caring for Health: History and Diversity* (revised edition 1993), Chapter 9.

Innovations in action: three case studies

The general arguments about the adoption and diffusion of innovations can be illustrated by three short case studies, which reveal the wide range of factors determining whether innovations are implemented quickly and widely and why it is that, in some areas, change appears incessant and disruptive and in others innovations are constantly frustrated by inertia in the system.

The first case study is of a process innovation involving the routine of hospital care; the second is of a product innovation—magnetic resonance imaging. The third case study takes you back to the Reader article you studied in Chapter 1, to identify obstacles to the diffusion of day surgery and possible ways of overcoming them.

As you read through the case studies, try to identify the factors that were most influential in leading to the adoption and diffusion of each innovation. Ask yourself:

- Who introduced the change and why?

- Who stood to benefit and who lost out?

- Who controlled the change?

- What social consequences did the change have?

- What were the economic consequences?

In addition, try to decide which model of research— *science-push* or *market-pull*—best fits each example.

Patient waking times in NHS hospitals

Attempts to change the time at which patients are woken in NHS hospitals may seem a straightforward, even trivial, example but it illustrates the difficulties of achieving even a relatively small change in established routines. Despite a recommendation in 1961 from a nursing committee of the Ministry of Health that patients should not be woken before 6.30 to 7.00 a.m., 76 per cent were still being woken before 6.30 a.m. when the Royal Commission on the NHS investigated in 1978. Early waking was the commonest cause of patient dissatisfaction (Table 7.4).

Why had later waking times not been adopted? In 1982, Barbara Stocking studied in detail four districts where there had been attempts to bring about change (Stocking, 1984).

□ Who do you think might have tried to promote change in waking times?

■ You may have suggested patients, who have most to gain; the Community Health Councils whose task is to represent the interests of patients; and staff, partly out of concern for patients, but also if a change would benefit their own work (e.g. night nurses).

Barbara Stocking found examples of all these groups trying to initiate change. In addition, individual nurse

Table 7.4 Aspects of hospital service with which more than 10 per cent of in-patients were dissatisfied. Percentages exclude people giving 'no answer'

Survey	Aspect of service	Percentage dissatisfied
700 adults	woken too early	43
	food	21
	washing and bathing facilities	19
	toilet facilities	15
	comfort of beds	13
	noise during daytime	12
	privacy during examination and treatment	11
797 people of all ages	information about progress of care	31
	difficulty understanding doctors (apart from usual medical terms)	15
	notice of discharge	12

Source: Royal Commission on the NHS, 1978, *Patients' Attitudes to the Hospital Service*, Research Paper No. 5, HMSO, London, p. 125.

managers, administrators, academics and the chairman of a hospital consultants' committee had also tried. They had all met a wide range of objections including inadequate nurse staffing levels, disruption of the relations between day and night staff, interference with the clinical management of patients (e.g. preparing them for morning ward rounds), effects on other staff such as cooks who would have to stay later and be paid for this if patients went to bed and rose later, patient expectations, and even ward design. For example, on long stay wards, it was found that patients were put to bed very early by the day staff because there were insufficient night staff to manage the process. This was felt to justify waking the patients early the following day. It was argued that, on open 'Nightingale' wards, it was impossible to wake some without waking all patients because of noise (Figure 7.6).

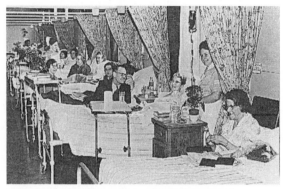

(a)

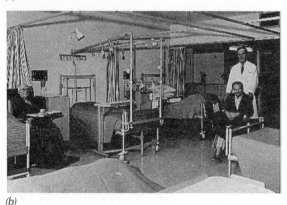

(b)

Figure 7.6 *Hospital ward design. The large 'Nightingale' wards (a) containing 20–30 beds have been replaced in many modern hospitals by (b) wards subdivided into single, two, four and six-bedded rooms or bays.*
(Source: Camera Press)

Despite these actual and supposed obstacles (depending on your point of view!), some hospitals did change and patients today are generally woken later than they were in the early 1980s. Stocking identified several factors that seemed to encourage permanent adoption of the practice: the simultaneous existence of a more significant change such as the opening of a new hospital; the persistent support of nurse managers; and consultants willing to question the need for routine early-morning ward-rounds and to conduct a round in a ward that had not been prepared specially for their visit. Introducing change on a trial basis did little to alter resistant attitudes and persuasion by managers was unsuccessful. In one hospital, managers responded with coercion which successfully moved the waking time but at the cost of antagonising the staff. This highlights an important aspect of organisational change—the need to balance the costs and benefits to both staff and patients. A more restful stay in hospital could mean more work for staff—a dilemma about the humanity of health care.

Magnetic resonance imaging

In contemporary medicine, diagnosis is heavily dependent on being able to ascertain the internal state of the patient. *Non-invasive methods* which avoid piercing the body are increasingly available, of which the best known is the X-ray, but more and more procedures (involving for example, ultrasound and radio-isotopes), have appeared in recent years. The machines used to see inside the patient's body are generally linked to computers to enhance the quality of the image. The information they produce *may* lead to more accurate diagnosis, more effective care and, finally, improved outcome for the patient. Unfortunately, the newer diagnostic imaging techniques are expensive, which raises the dilemma of how the investment of scarce resources on these innovations can be justified. Consider the case of *magnetic resonance imaging* (MRI).

The most important development in medical imaging, since the first X-rays, came in 1972 with the introduction of the *CT* (computed tomography) *scanner*. This is essentially an X-ray machine linked to a computer which analyses the data to produce detailed pictures of slices through, for example, the brain, spine or liver. By 1984, the USA had more than 2 000 CT scanners representing a capital investment of $2 billion[12] and operating costs of $1 billion per year (Institute of Medicine, 1985).

[12] thousand million.

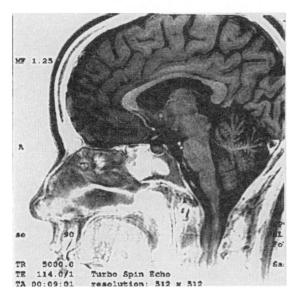

Figure 7.7 *An MRI image of a vertical cross-section through the brain of a normal person. (Photo: Siemens plc)*

In a CT scanner, the image is produced by the variable *opacity* of tissue to X-rays: bone, which is particularly opaque to X-rays, stands out in the image. MRI works on a different principle. If certain types of atom are placed in the field of a strong magnet and are exposed to energetic radio waves of appropriate frequencies, their nuclei 'resonate' (i.e. they respond by emitting radio signals that are influenced by the microscopic environments of the atoms). This is known as *nuclear magnetic resonance* or NMR. The technique was used extensively in chemistry and physics for analytic and structural investigations of matter before its application in health care. The medical potential of NMR relies on the ability to measure the resonance of atoms[13] in different tissues in the body and to use this information to produce magnetic resonance images (MRI) (Figure 7.7).

As the medical potential of this technique became apparent, new machines tailored to the investigation of the human body were developed. Medical adoption has been rapid in Western countries. Clinicians were attracted to MRI over CT scanning because multiple scans could be performed more safely (MRI does not involve potentially harmful ionising radiation) and because soft tissues showed up distinctly even when surrounded by bone (see Figure 7.7). By 1989, there were 1 300 MRI scanners in the USA compared with 4 000 CT scanners. The diffusion in the United Kingdom has been both

[13]especially the hydrogen atoms in water molecules.

slower and less extensive. While this difference may partly reflect a greater degree of scepticism among British doctors, another factor is probably more important.

□ What do you think is the main reason for these differences?

■ Cost—not merely capital cost, but maintenance and running costs.

In 1990, each MRI facility (Figure 7.8) cost approximately £900 000 to buy and about £250 000 a year to run; each test on a patient was costing between £100 and £300 depending on the number of patients scanned each year. Health-service managers in the United Kingdom are increasingly faced with deciding whether and how to introduce this expensive technology. What factors should they take into account?

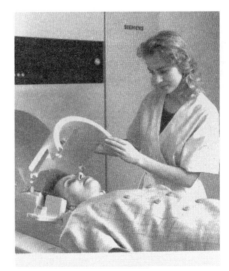

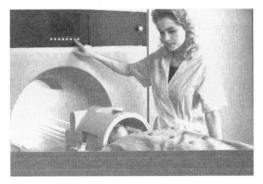

Figure 7.8 *An MRI facility. The patient is slid into a large coil-shaped magnet and held immobile during the measurement. (Photo: Siemens plc)*

Capital items such as medical equipment are no longer 'free goods' in the NHS. Since 1991–2 hospitals have been charged notional interest as if their capital goods had been purchased using commercial loans. This is to make managers and doctors more conscious of the need to use buildings and equipment cost-effectively. For example, it is usually the case that a centralised service treating a large number of patients is cheaper to run than a decentralised service, but this has to be set against the likelihood that centralisation makes it harder to ensure that all patients have an equal opportunity of using the service (a trade-off between efficiency and equity). In the case of CT scanning, the resolution of this dilemma was often taken out of managers' hands when machines were bought through charitable appeals, but had to be operated using NHS funds!

Apart from the cost of buying and running the facility, the hospital manager must also consider the possibility that the machine may become obsolete within a few years. CT scanning was rapidly followed by the development of MRI and there are now many new imaging methods which have advantages for certain purposes over MRI. Existing MRI systems need constantly to upgrade both hardware and software to maintain 'state of the art' performance.

The potential investor has to weigh carefully the potential costs and benefits of MRI. Will it duplicate, complement or replace other imaging tests? Does it improve the accuracy of diagnosis and does this, in turn, influence patient management or eventual outcome? According to an analysis by A. K. Szczepura, J. Fletcher and J. D. Fitz-Patrick (1991), MRI was widely introduced in Western health systems before its cost-effectiveness in improving patient outcomes was satisfactorily demonstrated.

There is also a tendency for new diagnostic techniques to be *added* to existing investigations rather than supersede them, so overall costs tend to rise even when the newer tests are cheaper than the older ones. Sometimes this happens out of habit when tests are ordered unnecessarily, but often it is found that new and old both have a place. The pros and cons of CT and MRI mean that the two techniques have become complementary. Doctors would argue that every major hospital should have access to both technologies and other newer, complementary imaging methods. In this case the arrival of MRI has not yet caused CT to move to that stage in its career described by McKinlay as erosion and discreditation (stage 7 in Box 7.1).

Day surgery

You have already studied extracts from the 1990 Audit Commission Report *A Short Cut to Better Services*, which appear in the Reader. The report is an attempt to foster the wider adoption of day surgery in England and Wales. This represents an important process innovation in health care, which exemplifies many of the points raised earlier about adoption and diffusion. You may find it helpful to remind yourself of the five questions posed at the beginning of the case studies in this chapter, before re-reading the Audit Commission report and answering the following question.

☐ Barbara Stocking suggested three general factors that influence adoption and diffusion of an innovation. Can you identify at least one example of each of these factors in the case of day surgery?

■ Many examples are possible—here are our suggestions. A particularly attractive 'characteristic of the innovation' was the potential for cost-saving, so the Report sought to hasten adoption and diffusion. The 'influence of the environment' is apparent in the link between the level of adoption and the existence of appropriate and properly staffed units. The 'role of individuals and specific groups' is equally prominent in the reactions of surgeons whose opinions are seen as crucial to successful implementation of day surgery.

The consequences of new medical technologies

You have now seen something of how new technologies are originated, developed, introduced and spread through the health system. They have a wide range of effects within health services and in society as a whole.

☐ Can you list some ways in which new technologies may have consequences beyond the boundaries of the specific tasks they were designed to fulfill?

■ There are many areas you could have highlighted such as the impact of new medical technologies on health work, on patient–doctor relations, on the experience of being a patient, on expenditure and on ethical questions.

A few examples will illustrate these areas. New technologies not only result in new types of health-care work and even categories of worker (for example, the artificial-kidney assistant who helps patients undergoing hospital haemodialysis), but also a reallocation of tasks and new opportunities for particular groups. For example, the advent of flexible endoscopes (instruments which can be introduced into the body without a major incision and which allow the operator to see and work within the body cavity) has led to the emergence of a new breed of *interventional* radiologists who undertake procedures that were previously the preserve of surgeons. Increasing diversification and specialisation of health work and boundary shifts between workers were discussed in Chapter 6.

One notable, long-term impact of modern medical technology on the relations between doctor and patient has been to downgrade the perceived importance of clinical evidence provided by patients themselves. Data derived from technologies (e.g. electrocardiograms, biochemical analyses) tend to take precedence in arriving at a diagnosis and monitoring the success of treatment. As a result, doctors spend less time talking directly with patients, particularly in hospitals.

For patients, new technologies can have complex consequences. On the one hand, it has been suggested that an over-zealous reliance on technology has de-humanised the experience of childbirth and even threatened the well-being of the infant;[14] on the other, technologies such as artificial knee and hip joints have transformed the quality of life of people who were previously immobile and in pain.

For patients, professionals and the public in general, new medical technologies can have profound ethical consequences. For example, the ability of modern medicine to keep the body biologically alive beyond the time when recovery is possible, has raised issues such as the patient's right to die, the costs of keeping patients alive artificially, the question of who, if anyone, should be permitted to take decisions to withhold life-sustaining treatment, and the validity of the distinctions between active euthanasia sought by the patient or imposed on him or her, and death brought about by omission of measures to prolong life.

New medical technologies have contributed to the real increase in health expenditure seen in all Western countries since the 1960s, both by enabling the old things to be done differently (and, it is to be hoped, better) and by widening the range of conditions for which some sort of response is available. Over time, this process has highlighted the need for society to regulate the introduction and diffusion of new techniques in the interests of having ethically acceptable, safe and effective technologies which are efficiently used.

However, even if resources are used efficiently, it is likely that there will be a gap between what we as a society are prepared to spend on health care and the cost of providing the range of beneficial techniques available

for which there is a need. In this situation, society needs to have some way of *rationing* health care, as Chapter 3 pointed out.

Conclusions

It is apparent that *product* innovations such as CT, MRI and lithotripters tend to be more readily adopted than *process* innovations such as day surgery or waking patients at a more acceptable time. We can use Barbara Stocking's framework to summarise why this is generally the case.

Some 'general characteristics' of product innovations, such as MRI, help their adoption: they offer supposed clinical advantages over existing technologies; they are compatible in their basic principles with existing thinking and the organisation of health-care work; and straightforward in operation. By contrast, many process innovations—like allowing parents to stay with their children on paediatric wards—are handicapped because they are incompatible with existing work regimes, involve complex changes to staff relationships, are difficult to test convincingly, and fail to produce obvious benefits to staff. It is interesting to note that product innovations frequently encounter adoption problems when they also involve related process changes.

An 'environmental factor' that is favourable to product innovations is their tendency to receive high profile coverage in the mass media. This is partly because they conform to the popular view of what constitutes 'progress' and partly because they tend to be identifiable tools with specific functions which can be explained easily in the time and space available. There is also a noticeable tendency to overstate the potential of new machines, which increases the pressure for their adoption.

☐ Finally, how do the 'individuals and groups' involved with the different types of innovation differ in their status and power?

■ Most product innovations, like MRI, are initiated and promoted through the interplay between manufacturers with money to spend on marketing and powerful clinicians in leading hospitals, all of whom have either professional or commercial interests at stake. In contrast, process innovations *may* have only the support of less influential groups such as Community Health Councils, consumer groups and professionals in less prestigious areas of health care. However, some process innovations are originated by central government, which may use financial incentives to promote their adoption (e.g. to encourage GPs to become fund-holders).

[14]See *Birth to Old Age: Health in Transition* (1985 and revised edition 1995).

Future prospects

Whatever else happens in the NHS in the future, we can be sure that there will be constant innovation of all types—of products, processes and organisations. Such change will continue to have major ethical, social, economic, professional and welfare consequences. Forecasting is a foolhardy task, but are any broad trends identifiable?

First, it seems likely that diagnostic and therapeutic machines will become ubiquitous in the health system, while being less physically invasive, less hazardous and easier to use. As a result, the role of large, acute hospitals will change. Day and out-patient therapy will probably increase and in-patients will spend shorter times in hospital.

Second, the centre of gravity of medicine could shift away from the hospital into primary care as more and more diagnostic and treatment technologies become available in forms which can be brought into the GP's surgery and the home. Already GPs have access to sophisticated desk-top blood analysers. The availability of technologies which patients can use themselves and which can be retailed directly to the public is also increasing.

Third, health care may become more decentralised and move away from conventional managerial and professional hierarchies towards network organisations held together by the interchange made possible by information technology.

Fourth, advances in biotechnology will be applied ever more widely. For example, it will become increasingly possible to detect people at risk of serious genetic diseases, or who are carriers of defective genes, or who have a genetic susceptibility which contributes to common diseases such as coronary heart disease.

Whatever the future holds in terms of innovation in either the products or processes of health care, they will inevitably create dilemmas as well as opportunities. The ethical, social and economic aspects of these dilemmas will require careful evaluation and informed public discussion.

OBJECTIVES FOR CHAPTER 7

When you have studied this chapter you should be able to:

7.1   Define the scope of what is meant by the term 'medical technology'.

7.2   Distinguish 'invention' from 'innovation', and 'product' from 'process' innovations, and assess the usefulness of these distinctions.

7.3   Summarise the 'science-push' and 'market-pull' theories of how innovation occurs.

7.4   Identify the main agencies involved in the fostering of innovation, summarise their general aims and discuss how they influence the types of innovation that occur.

7.5   Explain the notion of the 'career' of a medical innovation and use it to describe the trajectory of individual technologies from their early use to eventual abandonment.

7.6   Explain, using examples, why some technologies tend to be adopted and used more readily than others.

QUESTIONS FOR CHAPTER 7

Question 1 (*Objectives 7.1, 7.2, 7.4 and 7.6*)

The definition of medical technology used earlier in this chapter included drugs and organisational systems. Describe how each of these types of technology typically originates.

Question 2 (*Objective 7.2*)

Both product and process innovations played a part in the development of day surgery, but which came first?

Question 3 (*Objective 7.3*)

Was the introduction of magnetic resonance imaging brought about by science-push or market-pull?

Question 4 (*Objectives 7.5 and 7.6*)

At the same time as the Audit Commission was complaining about the slow pace of adoption of day surgery in the NHS, there was considerable pressure from doctors to purchase devices such as MRI machines. What lies behind these apparently different degrees of enthusiasm for change?

8 Care in the community: rhetoric or reality?

This chapter builds on the discussion of the history of community care policy and the shifting boundaries between formal and informal care since World War II, which can be found in Caring for Health: History and Diversity, *Chapters 6 and 7.[1] Chapter 9 of that book contains information about the different levels of expenditure on hospital and community services in England, Wales and Scotland, which is essential background to the present chapter. The television programme 'Who calls the shots?' concerns a hospital-at-home scheme and relates to this chapter, among many others in this book.*

The author of this chapter is David Hunter, Professor of Health Policy and Management and Director of the Nuffield Institute for Health at the University of Leeds. The Institute has an international reputation for research and training aimed at improving health and social care policy and management practice.

The community care conundrum

The term 'community care' has been in common usage for many years. Governments use it to refer to their policy of caring for people in non-hospital settings, usually in their own homes. The term is open to many interpretations, as you will see later in this chapter. The policy of care in the community, as pursued by successive governments since World War II, is beset by a number of persistent dilemmas or critical issues which it is the purpose of this chapter to consider.

[1] *Caring for Health: History and Diversity* (revised edition 1993).

As the chapter unfolds, a number of critical issues will appear, sometimes more than once since there is considerable overlap between them. The issues are as follows:

- The cost of community care—the evidence to date on whether community care is cheaper or more expensive than, or the same as, institutional (that is, hospital) care is equivocal and inconclusive.

- The term 'community care' is imprecise: it can mean all care provided outside hospital settings, including care in residential and nursing homes; or it can mean all care outside institutions of any kind and provided to a person living at home, either their own home or that of a relative or friend.

- Shifting nuances in the policy of community care from one of care *in* the community to care *by* the community have resulted in an increase in the burdens placed on families and/or on other so-called 'informal' carers such as friends and neighbours.

- The increasing burden on family carers is occurring at a time when many carers are themselves growing older and when potential (mainly female) carers are being encouraged to enter the labour market with the decline in the number of people of working age.

- Contrary to their stated policy to promote community care, in recent years the funding policies of central government have unintentionally created incentives to fund private residential and nursing home care rather than domiciliary care; these incentives were removed in April 1993 with the implementation of changes in the funding of community care which place the responsibility for assessing the need for care and its subsequent funding with local authority social services departments.

- Community care policy, particularly in England, has become confused with, and seen as inseparable from, the rundown and closure of long-stay hospitals for people with a mental illness or mental disability; a consequence of this is that community care policy has become discredited by claims that closure of hospital facilities is occurring before adequate community-based alternatives are put in their place.

You may already have encountered some of these problems or dilemmas either directly from your own experience of being a service provider, a carer or user of services, or indirectly from the experiences of friends or colleagues at work. There are very few people who are untouched in some way by community care. Indeed, it is quite possible to be a provider of services, a carer and a user of services all at the same time. The experiences of users and carers revealed by the quotations below give a vivid illustration of the problems and pressures they face.

Users

'I need flexible services so that I can be ill when I want to be ill.'

'Those who shout loudest get the attention and therefore get the most.'

'Having higher expectations (of services) brings more hassles.'

'You either have to give up or get bolshy.'

Carers

'Carers are taken for a ride.'

'We're not selfless dedicated people— we've got no options. It's like being flung into a prison.'

'I don't ever switch off completely. You're on duty 24 hours a day.'

'I only got help because I was determined to get hold of it. I can imagine someone who wasn't persevering and didn't mind kicking up a fuss could have a hard time.'

(Wertheimer, 1991, pp. 30–1; Brotchie, 1990, pp. 5 and 74)

The chapter is in five sections, dealing respectively with definitions of community care, the changing context of community care, its appeal, progress in its realisation, and future scenarios.

Community care: what is it?

Controversy has raged over the *meaning* of community care, the *motives* for its adoption by successive governments and its *implications* for the allocation of

responsibilities between different public agencies, non-statutory organisations and family—particularly female—carers. None of these features of community care has remained constant: for example, the motives for particular initiatives have at various times included different blends of social concern, public outrage and financial economy. This and subsequent sections of the chapter take up and develop these issues.

Community care is not easily defined. It has been described as a 'portmanteau' term conveying the point that it can mean all things to all people. Its very slipperiness and imprecision can be attractive to policy-makers who do not wish to be held to very tight definitions or to precise goals and objectives. It is nevertheless puzzling that so much confusion surrounds the term when a policy of care in the community has been a top priority of successive governments since the end of World War II.

In 1961 Richard Titmuss, a leading British sociologist and social historian, delivered a lecture on community care which has survived as an uncannily accurate comment on contemporary developments.

> Confusion has often been the mother of complacency. In the public mind, the aspirations of reformers are transmuted, by the touch of a phrase, into hard-won reality. What some hope will one day exist is suddenly thought by many to exist already. All kinds of wild and unlovely weeds are changed, by statutory magic and comforting appellation, into the most attractive flowers that bloom not just in the spring but all the year round. (Titmuss, 1961, p. 104)

Continuing with the botanical metaphor, Titmuss went on to pose the question

> And what of the everlasting cottage-garden trailer, 'Community Care'? Does it not conjure up a sense of warmth and human kindness, essentially personal and comforting, as loving as the wild flowers so enchantingly described by Lawrence in *Lady Chatterley's Lover*? (Titmuss, 1961, p. 104)

Titmuss, like others, failed to discover in any precise form the social origins of the term 'community care'.

It is important to try and unravel the various strands that go to make up the term **community care**. Policies for community care in the United Kingdom have varied in their emphasis over time. At their root, however, have been two basic themes:

- That policies should be directed at meeting individual needs rather than producing services.

- That this objective can best be met by replacing *inherited* services dominated by large institutions (especially long-stay hospitals) with a more balanced and flexible range of *alternative* services.

A statement published by the Department of Health and Social Security (DHSS) in 1985, and endorsed by the 1989 White Paper on community care, *Caring for People,* captures the essence of the policy and is as good a definition as any:

...community care is a matter of marshalling resources, sharing responsibilities and combining skills to achieve good quality modern services to meet the actual needs of real people, in ways those people find acceptable and in places which encourage rather than prevent normal living. (DHSS, 1985, p. 1, paragraph 3)

Later in the chapter we will return to the issue of 'normal living' and what is meant by this.

The policies of successive governments in the area of community care are directed at the so-called 'dependency groups' such as elderly, mentally

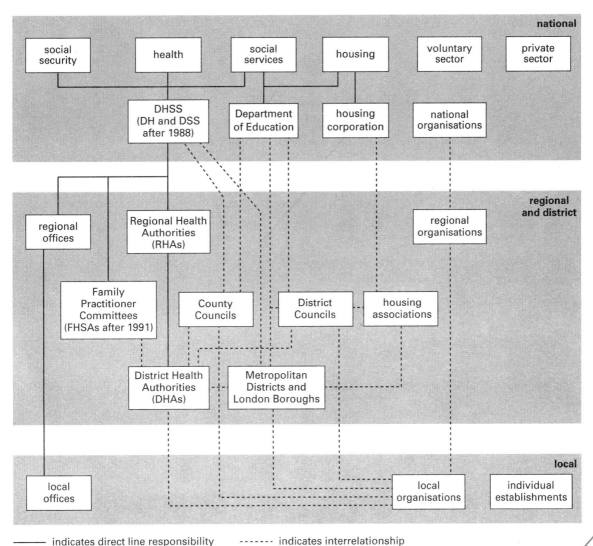

— indicates direct line responsibility   ------ indicates interrelationship

Figure 8.1 (referred to on p. 124) *The principal agencies involved in community care. (Adapted from Audit Commission for England and Wales, 1986,* Making a Reality of Community Care, *HMSO, London, p. 50)*

handicapped[2] and mentally ill people and it has increasingly been appreciated that an extensive range of government functions has a role in meeting their needs, including health services, social services, housing, education, social security, transport, employment and physical planning. Figure 8.1 (*previous page*) shows the principal agencies involved in providing community care services. Since 1986, when this diagram was first produced, no equivalent audit of community care has taken place. But, although a little dated (e.g. the DHSS was split into the Department of Health (DH) and the Department of Social Security (DSS) in 1988), the diagram remains essentially accurate. Voluntary organisations, the private sector and the informal caring networks of family and neighbourhood have also been given increasingly prominent positions in the provision of community care.

☐ On the basis of Figure 8.1, what do you consider to be the principal obstacles to achieving more effective collaboration between agencies?

■ Coordinating so many different agencies and functions is very difficult; the priorities of (say) government agencies and the voluntary sector are likely to be very different.

The obstacles to collaboration are multiple and complex and no single diagram can adequately convey them. Some of the obstacles are *structural* in origin, that is they arise from different organisational structures in the agencies involved. For example, there is an absence of common geographical boundaries between health and local authorities, different systems of accountability operate in these agencies (e.g. the members of health authorities are appointed, whereas members of local authorities are elected), there are different financing mechanisms in operation and different priorities (e.g. local authorities might give education or roads a higher priority than social services).

The implementation of community care policy as conceived by successive governments depends upon the fulfilment of three fundamental conditions:

• A shift in the balance of responsibilities and resources from the NHS to local authorities and voluntary organisations.

• A shift in the balance of care from institutions to community facilities.

• An increase in the ability of health and social services to coordinate their activities at all levels in policy and the service delivery processes.

As you will see later in this chapter, the thrust of recent policy reviews and changes is aimed at achieving effective implementation of these conditions. Important issues are at stake, including the boundary between what is a *health care* 'problem' and a *social care* 'problem'. For example, for many old people it is not possible to make a clear distinction since health and social care needs may be inextricably bound up together. Consider the following fairly typical situation.

Mrs A is aged 75 and has had a stroke, leaving her paralysed down the right side. She has severe speech difficulties. Saying 'yes' or 'no' is a major effort. Her son, aged 45, lives with her. He is working shifts, but is able to contribute to her care at weekends.

Mrs A gets support from the NHS, social services and voluntary sector for the following services (the service provider is shown in brackets):

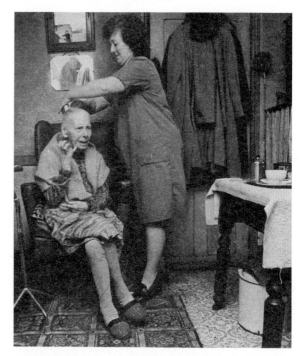

A home help caring for an elderly person in Battersea, London. The role of the home help is carefully defined by their social services employer, but many tasks have overlapping social care and health care functions. (Photo: Gina Glover/Photo Co-op)

[2]Although the term 'mentally handicapped' is still in widespread use in the health and social services, it is gradually being replaced by 'people with learning disabilities' in sources arising from this client group.

- personal care scheme—one hour each morning, Monday–Friday (Social Services)

- physiotherapy—twice a week (NHS)

- speech therapy—once a week (NHS)

- home help—two hours each week to relieve son (Social Services)

- day care centre + transport—once a week (Social Services or voluntary or private agencies)

- respite care—occasionally (Social Services or voluntary or private agencies or NHS)

□ Why do you think the boundary between health needs and social needs is difficult to draw?

■ The health and social care needs of many people, like Mrs A, are multiple and difficult to separate out in a straightforward fashion. Complex assessments would be required which tried to distinguish between health needs and social care needs.

The meaning of community care has become confused in recent years in part because of the perverse effects of social security policies. The ready availability of income support for *residential provision* in the private sector but not for community care was such that, as the Audit Commission put it in its critical report on community care policy in 1986:

> …social security policies appear to be working in a way directly opposing community care policies. (Audit Commission, 1986, p. 44, paragraph 90)

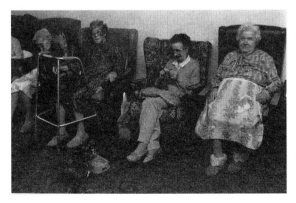

Financial incentives in the 1980s encouraged the growth of private residential care for elderly people at the expense of home-based community care. (Photo: Mike Levers)

The need to control the growth in social security spending on private-sector residential and nursing homes was a principal target of the 1993 reforms which are discussed later in the chapter. Spending on residential provision from this source of funds grew from £10 million in 1979 to £1 300 million in 1991. By the end of 1992 the figure was expected to be in the region of £1.9 billion. Because of the ready availability of such funds from a central government source that is not cash-limited, health and local authorities were encouraged to develop community care programmes which were biased towards traditional forms of residential care, since they did not have to pay for such provision from their own budgets. The Conservative government acknowledged in the 1989 White Paper on community care, *Caring for People,* that existing funding structures had worked against the development of home-based services. Moreover, income support was only available for *private*-sector residential care, which had the effect of sharply reducing the amount of *public*-sector provision available. The unintended effect was to dilute the government's definition of community care—a subject to which we now turn.

The changing context of community care

Government policy

During the late 1970s and early 1980s the policy of care *in* the community became care *by* the community, thereby reflecting the government's ideological stance in favour of self-reliance and the family as the bulwark of support in the community.[3] This was the result of various influences but chief among them was a desire on the part of the government to 'roll back the frontiers of the welfare state' and encourage a new and expanded role for *voluntary* and *informal* care. Under Norman Fowler, Secretary of State for Social Services from 1981 to 1987, the previous emphasis placed on voluntary and informal care was moderated by the government and replaced by a new emphasis on the *shared responsibility* of public agencies and informal carers for providing care.

[3]The history of this development is described in more detail in *Caring for Health: History and Diversity* (revised edition 1993), Chapter 7.

Demographic changes

The situation is also complicated by demographic changes leading to increases in the numbers of very old people (defined as over 85 years, see Figure 8.2), many of them suffering from dementia, together with changes in family structure and the declining number of potential informal carers—partly through age, but also because many women are seeking employment. Changes in family patterns brought about by divorce and the growth of co-habitation have added further elements of uncertainty. The Conservative government elected in 1992 acknowledged that demographic trends will have implications for the future availability of informal carers.

☐ What does Figure 8.2 show about the age distribution of elderly people?

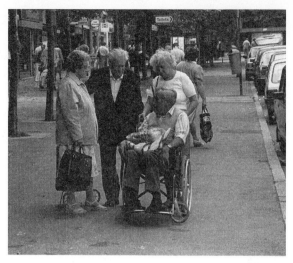

The care of elderly people in the community depends mostly on carers who are themselves often elderly. (Photo: Mike Levers)

■ The figure shows three main trends: (a) a decline between 1986 and 2001 in the 'young old', i.e. those aged 65–74; (b) a slight increase in the numbers of those aged 75–84; and (c) a sharp rise in the very old, i.e. those aged 85 and over.

Most people in need of community care are elderly. The numbers aged 85 and over are projected to rise from 695 000 in 1986 to 1 146 000 in 2001. Figure 8.2 provides a graphic illustration of the rapidly increasing trend towards an older population in Britain. Most older people lead fulfilled and independent lives. But inevitably there will, as a result of these demographic changes, be more people in the population with physical disabilities (which accounted for 73 per cent of those being cared for in 1985) and with both physical and mental disabilities associated with old age (16 per cent). Carers look after people of all ages, but principally those aged between 75 and 85. Carers, too, are growing older with the result that much of the care of older people will be carried out by people who are themselves in their 60s and 70s. Table 8.1 shows the relationship between the carer and person cared for in a study of the support given by family and friends to people who later die.

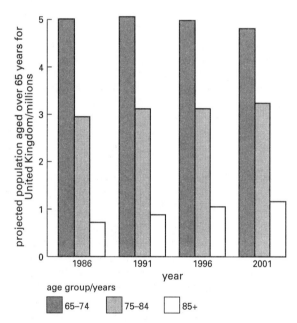

Figure 8.2 *Projected population of the United Kingdom aged 65 years and over, from 1986 to 2001. (Source: Dennis, G. (ed.), 1993,* Annual Abstract of Statistics 1993: no. 129, *HMSO, London, p. 10, Table 2.5)*

Table 8.1 Who bore the brunt of caring for a person who later died

The person who died was cared for by their:	When they died, they were living:				
	alone (%)	with spouse only (%)	with spouse and others (%)	with others only (%)	all (%)
wife	0	56	53	0	28
husband	1	29	31	2	16
daughter	23	3	11	29	15
son	6	1	0	16	5
other relative	11	1	0	33	9
friend or neighbour	20	1	0	5	7
official	38	7	0	11	16
more than one person	2	2	5	4	3
average number of relatives and friends who helped	1.7	1.9	3.1	2.0	2.0

Data from Seale, C. (1990) Caring for people who die: the experience of family and friends, *Ageing and Society*, **10**, p. 419, Table 3.

Taking account of carers

The position of informal carers is increasingly recognised by policy-makers. As the Minister for Health told the House of Commons Social Services Committee in 1990:

> Five or ten years ago it (i.e. carer) was a word that people would scarcely recognise in common parlance, whereas now I think the carers are very much a force, quite rightly and properly, to be reckoned with, and I think the priority they get in the White Paper and in all our guidance will ensure that there is actually practical assistance for them built in to the provision that local authorities undertake. (House of Commons Social Services Committee, 1990, p. v, paragraph 2)

The White Paper, *Caring for People*, makes clear that:

> ...the reality is that most care is provided by family, friends and neighbours. The majority of carers take on these responsibilities willingly, but the Government recognises that many need help to be able to manage what can become a heavy burden. Their lives can be made much easier if the right support is there at the right time, and a key responsibility of statutory service providers should be to do all they can to assist and support carers. Helping carers to maintain their valuable contribution to the spectrum of care is both right and a sound investment. Help may take the form of providing advice and support as well as practical services such as day, domiciliary and respite care. (Department of Health, 1989c, p. 9)

The most recent national survey of informal carers was carried out as part of the General Household Survey (GHS) in 1985. The study, called *Informal Carers*, was published in 1988 and revealed the nature and extent of care by people who were looking after, or providing some regular service for, a sick, handicapped or elderly person living in the carers' home or another private household (see Box 8.1, *overleaf*).

Only recently have the pressures and strains on carers been openly acknowledged and discussed. There are many first-hand accounts available of the experience of caring.[4] One witness questioned by the House of Commons Social Services Committee described some of the strains on carers (which are also reflected in the quotations we included earlier):

> ...many carers also live under a tremendous strain of guilt that is imposed on them—something which we do not impose upon any of the rest of us in society. Your children grow up, they become adults, they become independent. We are looking here at groups of people and we are saying, 'No! You must continue caring, you must continue doing this'. And the amount of guilt that so many parents feel is dreadful and I think it should be addressed. (House of Commons Social Services Committee, 1990, p. vi, paragraph 10)

[4]You will find it useful to refer to the article 'Caring for the spouse who died' by Ann Bowling and Ann Cartwright in *Health and Disease: A Reader* (1984 and revised edition 1994).

Another witness said:

> ...caring, of itself, isolates you. I think that one of the things that we, as a society, have to remember is that caring, because it isolates you, locks you into this relationship. It does not enable you, yourself, to build up the kind of relationships which, in turn, will give rise to you being cared for. (House of Commons Social Services Committee, 1990, p. vii, paragraph 10)

The government acknowledged in the 1989 community care White Paper that:

> ...(carers') total input was greater than the combined inputs financed from central and local government. (House of Commons Social Services Committee, 1990, p. 63, paragraph 8.11)

Box 8.1   Who are the carers?

- In Great Britain in 1985 (the most recent year for which census data are available), 6 million people over the age of 16 years—that is, one adult in seven, or 14 per cent of the population—was an informal carer for a mentally or physically disabled or elderly person.

- Of these carers, 3.5 million were women (15 per cent of the adult female population) and 2.5 million were men (12 per cent of the adult male population).

- The peak age for caring is 45 to 64 years, and in this age group 24 per cent of women and 16 per cent of men looked after a disabled or elderly person.

How much time does it take?

- 45 per cent of carers looking after someone in the same household devote at least 50 hours a week to informal care.

- 57 per cent of carers who spend more than 20 hours a week looking after a dependent person in the same house cannot take a break of two days, and 8 per cent cannot take a break of two hours.

- 25 per cent have been caring for a dependent person for over 10 years.

What are their responsibilities?

- 53 per cent of carers whose dependent person lives in the same household provide 'personal' care, e.g. bathing, toileting.

- 20 per cent of carers look after more than one disabled or elderly person.

- 29 per cent of carers spending more than 20 hours a week devoted to informal care also have reponsibility for looking after children.

What help do they get?

- 69 per cent of carers whose dependent person lives in the same household do not receive regular visits from health and social services (including voluntary agencies).

- Friends and relatives help to some degree (see Table 8.1).

What are the consequences for the carer's health?

- 44 per cent of carers spending at least 20 hours a week looking after a dependent person have a longstanding illness themselves.

Data from Green. H. (1988) Informal Carers, *OPCS Social Survey Division, Series GH5, No.15, Supplement A, HMSO, London; and Haffenden, S., 1991,* Getting it Right for Carers, *Department of Health, Social Services Inspectorate, HMSO, London.*

Changing attitudes to care in the community are also apparent on the part of potential users of services. It is not just government which has sought to redefine the balance between statutory provision and other forms of support. A new assertiveness on the part of service users is most apparent among disabled people who believe passionately in 'ordinary life' principles and cherish their independence. The Director of the British Council of Organisations of Disabled People told the Social Services Committee:

> …it worries me…when I hear this word 'care'. The fact that the Government paper *Caring for People* has 'caring' in the title worries me intensely, because many, many disabled people do not need caring for, but they are people who are entitled to benefits and they are people who need basic services in order to lead full and independent lives. (House of Commons Social Services Committee, 1990, p. vi, paragraph 7)

As part of its community care reforms, the government has insisted that, in the drawing up of community care plans, users of services (including carers) must be involved. Health and local authorities

> …should also consult with, and take account of, the views of …representatives of service users and carers in drawing up their plans. (House of Commons Social Services Committee, 1990, p. 42, paragraph 5.7)

Demographic trends in the younger age groups are likely to affect not only the availability of informal carers, but also the supply of *formal* carers. If the need for community care grows, as it will, then the need for sufficient numbers of suitably trained staff will also grow. Much of the work involved is unattractive to many, because it is low status and low paid. There are also issues of appropriate skills on the part of carers. Some searching questions need to be asked about whether those providing care in the community are over-professionalised or receive too much training for the tasks they go on to do. Sir Roy Griffiths in his 1988 review of community care (discussed later) raised the issue by suggesting that there might be a place for a *generic* community care worker who would combine many skills currently spread over a number of separate individuals.

Implications for service provision

With the expansion of the need for care and the implications this will have for new and enlarged services, the cost of care is inevitably a crucial issue. At the time of going to press early in 1993, the government had not taken a position on this issue. Griffiths was less equivocal in his report, echoing views expressed by the government in its White Paper, *Growing Older,* published in 1981, which stated that there would not be sufficient public finance to meet the growing needs of increasing numbers of older people.

> This will be a task for the whole community, demanding the closest partnership between public and voluntary bodies, families and individuals. (DHSS, Scottish Office, Welsh Office and Northern Ireland Office, 1981, paragraph 9.6)

Finally, in this brief review of the changing context of community care we should not omit to mention the impact on community services of developments in *medical technology* and health care *policy* and *practice* (discussed in the previous chapter) which are creating additional pressures on home-based provision. In particular, developments in hospital-at-home schemes,[5] outreach services, more rapid discharges from hospital (an issue raised by the report into day surgery which you read earlier),[6] less invasive medical interventions which can be carried out on a day-case or out-patient basis or by GPs, will demand effective and often intensive community care support. These innovations have also brought new categories of patients into the community care arena, who previously would have been treated as acute admissions in hospitals, requiring little or no community support upon discharge. Shorter hospital stays and more rapid throughput of patients have changed all that. Increasingly in future, community care will not be confined to the so-called priority groups.

[5] A television programme for Open University students entitled 'Who calls the shots?' is associated with this chapter, and highlights the decision to expand a hospital-at-home scheme for the care of very sick children.

[6] The extracts from the 1990 Audit Commission Report, 'A Short Cut to Better Services' in *Health and Disease: A Reader* (revised edition 1994).

Community care: why?

As we pointed out earlier, successive governments have supported policies on community care since the 1950s. For much of this time, and at least since the mid-1970s, community care has been a top policy priority. Most policy statements on the subject have followed the reasoning contained in a DHSS document published in 1981. It stated that

> ...most people who need long-term care can and should be looked after in the community. This is what most of them want for themselves and what those responsible for their care believe to be best. (DHSS, 1981a, p. 2)

It has to be said that no evidence was produced to support these assertions. Although it is probably true that most people in need of support would prefer to be cared for at home, this can only be achieved if appropriate services exist. It should be noted that not everyone will wish to remain in their own home. Given a choice, they may prefer to go into a residential care home.

The push for community care on the part of governments has been the result of a complex and shifting mix of humanitarian and economic factors. As long ago as 1956 a committee looking at the cost of the health service (the Guillebaud Committee) argued the case for promoting community care on both 'humanitarian and economic grounds'. The humanitarian reasons centred on the **normalisation philosophy** based on 'ordinary life' principles. This philosophy seeks to ensure for dependent individuals, especially those with a mental illness or with learning disabilities, the right to live a life as near to the normal as possible. The approach was initially most

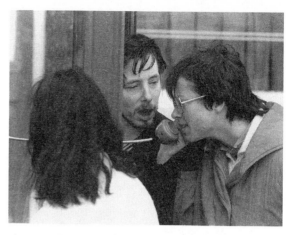

The 'normalisation philosophy' in the care of people with learning disabilities encourages the development of skills required in the community, rather than in residential homes. (Photo: Mike Levers)

influential in the development of thinking about care for people with learning disabilities but has since spread to developments in respect of other client groups. Perhaps the most important elements of this approach are its emphasis on services responding to individuals' needs in ways that respect their dignity and promote their growth and development. The need for services to be provided in the least restrictive settings possible is also a central feature of normalisation.

In practice, the normalisation philosophy has had two particularly important consequences for community care to date. It has:

- Focused attention on the values and principles that underpin community care policies and underlined the need for them to be made explicit and consistent.

- Led to an increasing appreciation of the role and importance of ordinary housing, as opposed to traditional residential-home care, being located at the heart of community care.

Costing community care

As we said above, there have also been economic, or cost, factors behind the push for community care, and not only humanitarian ones. By the mid-1970s *resource scarcity* rather than *client welfare* began to be a primary determinant of community care policy. In the government's 1976 priorities document covering health and personal social services, community care took its place alongside the pursuit of other 'low-cost' alternatives such as reducing average lengths of hospital stay.

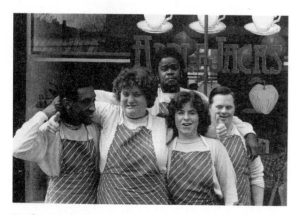

Employment in this restaurant in London enables people with learning disabilities to lead a life as near to normal as possible in their community. (Photo: Mike Levers)

Hard evidence that community care is cheaper care has been difficult to come by, as the DHSS was compelled to admit to Parliament in 1980. The following year, an in-house DHSS study concluded that:

> ...for some people community-based packages of care may not always be a less expensive or more effective alternative to residential or hospital provision, particularly for those living alone. In some cases, the community alternative might only appear cheap because its level of provision could be considered inadequate. (DHSS, 1981b, p. 29, paragraph 3.27)

The study also suggested that:

> ...the cost effectiveness of these packages often depends on not putting a financial value on the contribution of informal carers. (DHSS, 1981b, p. 3, paragraph 1.6)

More recent evidence from *reprovision* studies (that is, studies of people relocated in the community from long-stay hospitals) is less pessimistic and suggests that good community care need not be more expensive and may even be cheaper than other types of support.

Any discussion of the costs of community care compared with other forms of care is riven with difficulties. The issue is complex, in large measure because of the inconsistencies in the usage of the term 'community care' but also because of gaps in our knowledge. We lack the hard evidence to make robust claims one way or the other. In much of this area we simply do not know.

> Economic appraisal of alternative locations of care has often failed to provide conclusive evidence of the best form of care for people with a given set of characteristics because certain costs (e.g. of informal care) or measures of effectiveness have had to be omitted from the analysis. This applies to some key areas of resource allocation such as the substitutability of community for residential care of elderly people because it has not been possible in most studies to follow people over a sufficient period of time to ascertain whether it is better to keep people at home until they are very disabled and then admit to care or whether it is better to admit people to care before they become too disabled because they are able to adjust to new surroundings if they are in better health. (Wright, 1987, pp. 30–1)

There is also the problem of using *average* costs to determine the cost of community care. Most studies in this area rely on simple average costs. Concerns about such an approach have led some researchers to consider the usefulness of looking at the costs of a range of *individual* clients with varied needs. Their conclusion is that the variation in costs between clients would imply that average costs will not reflect the true costs for all patients/clients. A different group of individuals would produce a different average cost. Client needs change over time and costs vary in respect of peak times of need.

Much of the most recent costing of community-based services has been undertaken by the Personal Social Services Research Unit (PSSRU) at the University of Kent, focusing on three initiatives: the *Kent Community Care Project*, the DH's *Care in the Community Initiative* and the Darlington *Care in the Community Project*. These initiatives have spawned many similar service developments and have been influential in sharing a commitment to case (now commonly referred to as 'care') management, and to a rigorous evaluation of the model adopted. Case or care management aims to provide individuals with appropriate support based on a careful assessment of need and with an emphasis on coordinated services efficiently provided. These projects reflect the uncertainty we noted earlier in community care policy about what is *community* care and what is *residential* care.

The Kent project was concerned with the relative costs and outcomes of home-based compared with institutional care. The DH project, by contrast, was organised around a policy initiative designed to secure the transfer of patients from long-stay hospitals to community services, including other institutional settings. This distinction, as you will see in the next section, between community care as an alternative to *hospital*, or as an alternative to any form of *institutional* care, has been fundamental to the determination of national policy priorities and, as a consequence, to any evaluation of costs and outcomes.

The results of the PSSRU evaluation of the DH's Care in the Community Initiative (which ran from 1983 for about three years) provide evidence in relation to each of the following client groups:

- *Mental health:* Favourable outcomes were achieved at costs lower than the full costs of hospitalisation even after adjustment for the tendency of projects to take clients who were less dependent than the hospital average. This finding is supported by a further PSSRU study which predicted that the cost of community care for the full populations of two hospitals scheduled to close would be 'no larger and probably smaller than their present hospital residence costs', at least in the first years after discharge. (Knapp *et al.*, 1990a, p. 11)

- *Mental handicap:* In general, improved outcomes were found but at greater cost than hospital care, though 'the differences (were) not great' and were not statistically significant in the project 'where there was some budgetary delegation to care managers' (Knapp *et al.*, 1990b, p. 13)

- *Elderly people:* Better outcomes were reported at costs 'lower than the costs of hospital, particularly for those clients who moved from general hospitals'. (Knapp *et al.*, 1990b, p. 14)

An interim evaluation of the Darlington Care in the Community project (modelled on the Kent Community Care Project) and carried out by PSSRU on clients six months after hospital discharge, reported the existence of:

> ...lower levels of apathy and higher levels of morale, social activity and general quality of care, when compared to a controlled group of hospital residents. Informal carers experienced fewer difficulties than both the carers of elderly patients in hospital and the informal carers of another group of elderly clients receiving conventional packages of community care. Costs are likely to be no greater. (Knapp *et al.*, 1990a, p. 14)

The Darlington project appears to suggest that, compared with hospital provision, the consequences of home-based care were *neutral* in cost terms and *positive* in relation to outcomes. You should remember that the findings from a single study may not be reproduced in another study of a different scheme with its own unique features (a point raised in Chapter 4). Moreover, a *longitudinal* study (conducted over a long period of time to monitor changes in the object of the study) might produce different cost and outcome findings. Evaluations of costs and outcomes after, say, only a year must be treated with caution.[7] The PSSRU researchers are aware of this. As two of them have warned:

> ...as time passes, clients will become increasingly dependent and staff will tend to increase provision in response to need and jealously guard the elderly person's right to stay in their own home. Adequate monitoring built into service provision is necessary to detect such shifts. (Challis and Davies, 1986, p. 218)

[7]The interpretation of data generated by longitudinal and cross-sectional studies is discussed in *Studying Health and Disease* (1985 and revised edition 1994).

The few studies available on the costs of community care suggest that if there is effective targeting of resources on needs, and provided those groups for whom community care is likely to offer improvements are carefully identified, then there are grounds for concluding that community-based alternatives offer better value for a given volume of resources. But a key message to emerge also is the need for more longitudinal studies which seek to establish cost-effectiveness over time. In calculating costs in different settings, it is important to include the costs of care provided by informal or family carers where it is appropriate to do so. These costs will include income tax foregone as a result of people possibly not working in order to care for a spouse or relative, and the 'savings' to formal services as a result of a carer being present.

□ From the evidence available do you think we are in a position to say *for certain* whether community care is always cheaper than other forms of care?

■ Some study findings suggest that community care can be cheaper or no more expensive, but we lack studies over time which may show that as people become more dependent the cost of care increases. Few studies have dealt with the costs of community care. On available evidence it would be unwise to draw firm conclusions either way, although there is a view emerging that the costs of community care may be comparable with other forms of care.

Assessing progress

In the 1980s, the government's health adviser, Sir Roy Griffiths, was invited by the Secretary of State for Social Services to review the government's community care policy in respect of its management. He concluded that in few other fields could:

> ...the gap between political rhetoric and policy on the one hand, or between policy and reality in the field on the other hand, have been so great. (Griffiths, 1988a, p. iv, paragraph 9)

Not until the 1989 White Paper, *Caring for People*, and the subsequent *NHS and Community Care Act* of 1990 did the government take steps intended to close these gaps. As we show below, some observers believe that the gaps will not be closed and that community care has entered a period of considerable instability and uncertainty, the outcome of which is by no means clear.

Policy review in the 1980s

If we look back over the recent history of community-care policy, 1986 is something of a watershed. It marked the start of a lengthy period of policy activity. All that is happening at the time of writing early in 1993 and that is likely to happen over the next few years can be traced back to 1986 and to a series of events which began then.

At the close of 1986, the government-appointed (but independent) watchdog on efficiency, the Audit Commission, published a report, *Making a Reality of Community Care*, documenting the chief impediments to the development of a coherent policy. The report had a dramatic impact and proved influential in shaping subsequent events. Ministers felt compelled to act following a period of years when little attention was given to community care despite numerous studies, both academic and official, pointing to deficiencies and anomalies.

But the Audit Commission report (the main conclusions are set out in Box 8.2) spurred the Secretary of State for Social Services to take swift action. He asked Sir Roy Griffiths, the government's health adviser, to undertake a rapid review of the arrangements underpinning community care policy. The precise terms of reference were:

> To review the way in which public funds are used to support community care policy and to advise (the Secretary of State) on the options for action that would improve the use of these funds as a contribution to more effective community care. (Griffiths, 1988a, p. iii, paragraph 2)

Diagnosis and treatment: the Griffiths prescription

When he reported early in 1988, Griffiths made a number of detailed recommendations. The principal ones are listed in Box 8.3 (*overleaf*).

Three key policy assumptions underpinned Griffiths' analysis and recommendations:

- If community care means anything it is that responsibility is placed as near to the individual and his [sic] carers as possible. (Griffiths, 1988a, paragraph 30)

Box 8.2   The Audit Commission's diagnosis of the chief obstructions to developing a coherent community care policy

Mismatched resources

The separation of health and social services budgets had hampered the desired shift in resources from health to social services.

Lack of bridging finance

The lack of resources to support the transitional costs incurred by running down prior to closing long-stay hospitals while at the same time building up alternative services in the community had slowed down any shift from institutional to community care.

Perverse effects of social security policies

The ready availability of income support for residential provision but not for community care was such that it offered an incentive to develop residential rather than domiciliary-based care.

Organisational fragmentation

The division of responsibilities between different central government departments and different local agencies had resulted in conflicting and fragmented policy and practice.

Inadequate staffing and training arrangements

Staff planning and effective training were both 'conspicuous by their absence as far as community care is concerned'.

Source: derived from Audit Commission (1986) Making a Reality of Community Care, *HMSO, London, pp. 29–64.*

> **Box 8.3   The Griffiths agenda for improving the efficiency and effectiveness of community care policy**
>
> A clearer strategic role for central government including a Minister for Community Care
>
> A more facilitative and enabling role for social services departments as lead agencies
>
> The continuing need for collaboration at local level between different agencies including the development of care management
>
> New methods of financing community care including a specific community care grant
>
> A single gateway to publicly financed residential care
>
> Greater forms of encouragement for experiments to promote new forms of more pluralist provision
>
> Restricting housing involvement to a 'bricks and mortar' role
>
> Encouraging joint or shared training between different professions
>
> Exploring the introduction of community carers to carry out basic care tasks
>
> Establishing a better balance between policy aspirations and the availability of resources
>
> Facilitating more consumer choice
>
> Clarifying the respective responsibilities of health and social care

Source: derived from Hunter, D. J., Judge, K. and Price, S. (1988) Community Care: Reacting to Griffiths, *King's Fund Institute Briefing No. 1, King's Fund, London, p. 1*

• Nothing could be more radical in the public sector than to spell out responsibilities, insist on performance and accountability and to evidence that action is being taken; and even more radical, to match policy with appropriate resources and agreed timescales. (Griffiths, 1988a, paragraph 20)

• [There needs to be a Minister for Community Care who] would be responsible for ensuring that national policy objectives were consistent with the resources available to public authorities charged with meeting them. (Griffiths, 1988a, paragraph 6.21)

□ What does this (and Boxes 8.2 and 8.3) tell you about the relationship between the Audit Commission's diagnosis of the problems in community care and Griffiths' prescription for tackling them?

■ The Griffiths proposals for reform sought to confront head-on the principal criticisms put forward by the Audit Commission. They aimed to clarify the confusion in responsibility at national and local levels for community care policy, to sort out the funding problems in order to provide an incentive to develop home-based care services, to involve users in the development of services so that care provision would be more responsive to user preferences, and to extend opportunities for shared training between professional groups providing care.

As a result of his three key policy assumptions, Griffiths was convinced that local authorities were uniquely well placed to assume the major responsibility for ensuring that appropriate resources were brought to bear to meet individual needs. In advocating this, Griffiths was anxious to avoid major organisational restructuring. Success, in his view, lay in reshaping the managerial culture within *existing* organisations in order to deliver the necessary changes. Griffiths was also anxious to emphasise that his review was 'not about cost reduction' but about obtaining better value for money.

> What cannot be acceptable is to allow ambitious policies to be embarked upon without the appropriate funds.... If we try to pursue unrealistic policies the resources will be spread transparently thin. (Griffiths, 1988a, paragraph 38)

Griffiths' agenda for community care reform proved to be an explosive cocktail for a government which did not seek to conceal its dislike of local government and wanted to contain public spending and preferably reduce it. The Griffiths review caused the government some anxiety over how best to proceed and, in particular, over how to respond to his recommendations. The 15-month interval between publication of Sir Roy's report and the government's response provided evidence of the difficulties the report had created.

Government policy for the 1990s

When the government's response finally came it did so in two stages: a brief statement to Parliament in July 1989 which was then elaborated in a White Paper, *Caring for People,* published in November of that year. The White Paper was given legislative effect through the *NHS and Community Care Act* 1990. The reform proposals were largely based on Griffiths' recommendations. They sought to promote user choice and independence through improved assessment and care management, together with the *separation of purchase and provision,* so that local authorities became enablers, acting (in Griffiths' words) as the:

> ...designers, organisers and purchasers of non-health-care services and not primarily as direct providers. (Griffiths, 1988a, paragraph 1.3.4)

The intention was to develop a 'mixed market' of care in which maximum use would be made of the voluntary and private sectors in order to:

> ...widen consumer choice, stimulate innovation and encourage efficiency. (Griffiths, 1988a, paragraph 1.3.4)

You may well have spotted striking similarities between the emphasis in the government's proposals on user choice and independence, and the principles and values of 'ordinary living' which were discussed in the previous section. Under the *Caring for People* proposals, services were to be needs-led and not provider-led, with professionals determining what was in the best interests of users in a somewhat paternalistic fashion.

Financing community care

Despite much concordance between Griffiths' proposals and those contained in the White Paper, there were nevertheless key differences between them, notably in the fields of finance and the role of central government. Griffiths wanted to ensure that resources transferred to local government were protected (or *ring-fenced,* to use the current economic jargon) for their intended purpose of developing community care services. However, the government did not initially accept the need for such protection (with the exception of a modest specific grant for mental illness services). This was for various reasons,

including the view that it was for local authorities (not central government) to determine their own priorities, and because central government did not want to be held responsible for decisions on priorities for spending. Only

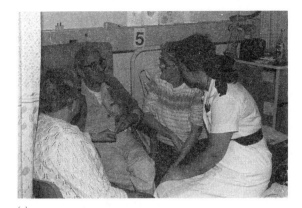

(a)

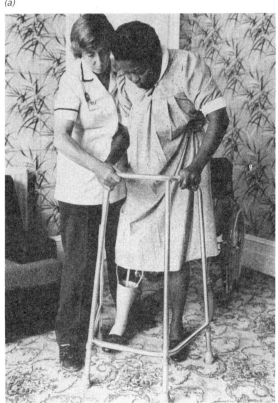

(b)

Many elderly or disabled people could be discharged sooner from acute hospital beds if community care services were in place to support them at home. (Photos: (a) Mike Levers; (b) Gina Glover/Photo Co-op)

under pressure from the Secretary of State for Health, Virginia Bottomley, did the government decide in June 1992 to ring-fence—for a period of four years only—the resources to be transferred to local authorities from income support.

Resources for expanding home-based care have become available by transferring to local authorities the care element of income support, which would have been claimed by people in residential care homes and nursing homes had the old system remained in place. The decision to ring-fence these resources to ensure that they reached their intended destination and were not diverted to other local government activities marked a major shift in government policy. Health service managers were especially worried because they feared that unless community care services were in place there would be a risk of acute hospital beds becoming occupied inappropriately (a practice known to insiders as 'bed blocking') by elderly people whose needs were primarily for social care and not health care.

However, the decision to ring-fence resources did not address the issue of whether the resources to be transferred would be *sufficient* for the purpose for which they were being transferred. Local authorities feared they would receive around half of the £800 million they believed was required to provide appropriate community care. The Conservative government elected in 1992 sought to reassure local authorities that 'adequate resources' would be made available to them. It announced in October 1992 that £539 million would be transferred; this was seen by many local authorities to represent a shortfall of some £200 million. But in the face of tight public-spending limits the settlement was seen as something of a political victory for the Secretary of State for Health. The amount to be transferred is important because (as Figure 8.3 shows) much of the increase in community care spending in the decade between 1980 and 1990 has come from the *care supplement* available through the social security system.

□ What does Figure 8.3 tell you about changes in social security sources of finance for community care in the decade between 1979–80 and 1989–90?

■ The data show that in 1979–80 the sources of finance did not include social security funds other than the care supplements, and then at a modest level. By 1989–90, these two sources of funding accounted for a substantial proportion of community provision.

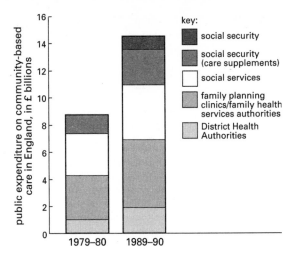

Figure 8.3 *Public expenditure on community care in England in 1979–80 and 1989–90, £ billions in 1989–90 prices. (Source: Audit Commission, 1992,* Community Care: Managing the Cascade of Change, *HMSO, London, p. 3)*

Obstacles to coordinated care

Although the reforms of the early 1990s are intended to end the practice whereby *public* resources were used to enable people to be looked after in *private* residential or nursing home care—regardless of whether it was appropriate or not—it is possible that a new set of unintended consequences for policy-makers may occur. The reforms seek to establish a clear dividing line between health care provided by the NHS, and social, or non-medical, care which is arranged and provided by local authorities or by the independent sector. It is notoriously difficult to make a clear distinction between the two.

For example, as you saw earlier in the case of Mrs A, an elderly person in need of support may have multiple needs which require inputs from health and social services simultaneously. There is in practice no clear divide between the two types of care. The problem, however, is one of resources and, in particular, one of who pays. In a climate of resource scarcity, there is a perverse incentive to identify need in terms of the *other* agency's responsibilities; indeed, it becomes a major preoccupation. It is also likely to make collaborative working and community care planning much more difficult to achieve. Joint planning in some form is critical to the success of community care because, as Figure 8.1 showed, many agencies are involved in providing community care services.

Most of the research evidence suggests that joint planning, as it has operated since the late 1970s, has been more generally marked by conflict or stand-off than by productive cooperation. Compared with the expectations and requirements of numerous government circulars, the experience of joint planning appears to be one of disappointment and failure in overall terms, with the occasional success being very much the exception. Some of the main obstacles to cooperation are listed in Box 8.4.

One policy analyst, Aaron Wildavsky, has written that:

> ...coordination is one of the golden words of our time. Offhand, I can think of no way in which the word is used that implies disapproval. But what does it mean? Policies should be mutually supportive rather than contradictory. People should not work at cross-purposes. Participants in any activity should contribute to a common purpose at the appropriate time and in the right amount to achieve coordination. (Wildavsky, 1979, pp. 131–2)

Griffiths, in his review of community care policy, made a clear distinction between a policy aimed at providing support to those who needed it to enable them to continue living in the community, and a policy that sought to run down and close long-stay hospitals. He was critical of a tendency on the part of governments to confuse the two instead of viewing them as quite separate. But confusion has reigned over the years with numerous initiatives expressly aimed at facilitating the speedy rundown and closure of long-stay hospitals for people with a mental illness or learning disabilities.

A limited success?

It will be clear by now that community care policy has had limited success in achieving the shift from institutional to non-institutional forms of provision. The Audit Commission in its 1986 report on community care concluded that progress had been 'slow and uneven'. The Commission's analysis suggested that progress in developing community home-based services had been generally slower than would be needed to offset the rundown in NHS provision. In a report published by the Commission in 1992, it argued that although steady progress was being made in implementing the reforms:

Box 8.4 Barriers to coordination of community care between health and social services agencies

Structural barriers

Fragmentation of service responsibilities across agency boundaries, within and between sectors
Inter-organisational complexity and a lack of common geographical boundaries

Procedural barriers

Differences in planning horizons and cycles
Differences in budgetary cycles and procedures

Financial barriers

Differences in funding mechanisms and bases
Differences in the availability of, and access to, financial resources

Professional barriers

Differences in ideologies and values
Professional self-interest and concern for threats to autonomy and domain
Threats to job security
Conflicting views about clients/consumers' interests and roles

Status and legitimacy barriers

Organisational self-interest and concern for threats to autonomy and domain
Differences in legitimacy between elected and appointed agencies

---

Source: Wistow, G. and Hardy, B. (1991) Joint management in community care, Journal of Management in Medicine, *5(4), p. 41.*

...big changes in policy and practice at all levels are still needed if the Government's objectives of a user-driven and cost-effective system of community health and care services are to be realised, and it is likely to take many years for this process to reach completion. (Audit Commission, 1992, p. 8, paragraph 15)

☐ From the evidence produced by the Audit Commission and others on the disappointing progress of community care, what do you consider to be the main explanations for this?

■ The reasons are complex, but include: lack of political will or real government priority; the difficulty in getting agreement from among so many agencies and professional groups; government concern about the cost of care; and suspicions about the competence of local government among national politicians.

Variations in policy in Britain

There is one final issue to be considered in this sobering review of progress. In all that we have said so far there has been an implicit assumption that the arguments and trends we have identified apply equally across the four countries making up the United Kingdom: England, Wales, Scotland and Northern Ireland. In fact, nothing could be further from the truth. Just as marked variations in service arrangements occur *within* each of the four countries, they also occur *between* them. Indeed, the differences go deeper because they reflect differences in the implementation of an agreed United Kingdom policy.

There is no such thing as a community care policy for the United Kingdom. Because Northern Ireland is so different from the rest of the United Kingdom for a variety of reasons, we shall restrict our comments to developments in England, Wales and Scotland. The major difference between Northern Ireland and the rest of the United Kingdom is the existence of integrated health and social services boards which should, in theory, overcome the organisational fragmentation evident elsewhere. Whether this has resulted in closer joint working between professional groups is less certain.

☐ The details of health and social service provision for hospital and community care in England, Scotland and Wales were given in another book in this series.[8] Briefly summarise the main differences.

[8]See *Caring for Health: History and Diversity* (revised edition 1993), Chapter 9.

■ A review of service patterns in each of the countries demonstrates a marked bias in expenditure on hospital services in Scotland, which is considerably greater per person than in England or Wales. Scotland provides a much higher ratio of hospital beds for the officially defined priority groups (elderly, mentally ill or mentally handicapped people) relative to its population size. Spending on community health services is marginally lower in Scotland than elsewhere in Britain, and considerably less is spent on day care and domiciliary services.

The development and implementation of community care in Britain has not followed a uniform pattern; it is marked by policy diversity rather than policy uniformity. Many influences appear to be at work to account for the differences in approach adopted by each country. The following are among the most important:

• Organisational structures, especially the fragmentation evident between health and social services at national and local levels in each of the three countries.

• Financial mechanisms which allow each country scope to adopt different policies.

• The strength of professional lobbies which have resulted in different pressures for change or for maintaining the status quo in the three countries.

• The effect of resource constraints which have been felt more acutely in England than in Wales or Scotland where resources (financial and personnel) have been more plentiful.

• The influence of political leadership which has resulted in different policy emphases in each of the three countries.

In Wales, for example, there is evidence of particularly imaginative policy development in the shape of the Welsh Office's All Wales Mental Health Strategy introduced in 1985. It was more radical in its conception and commitment to the tenets of the normalisation philosophy than anything adopted nationally in England and Scotland. A significant factor in this innovative approach was the leadership given by senior politicians in Wales. The emphasis of the All Wales Strategy is on building up services in the community to *prevent* hospital admissions. There was no equivalent of the push in England for patient transfers from hospital beds to community provision. Bed reductions and closures would gradually emerge from the process of building up community care.

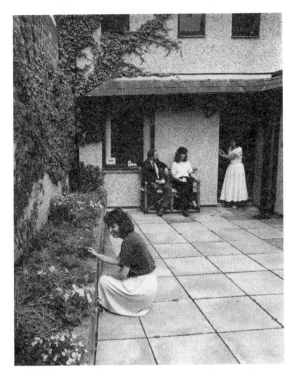

Community Mental Health teams developed as part of the All Wales Mental Health Strategy are multi-professional and based in ordinary buildings in the midst of the communities they serve. Services were formerly based in large psychiatric hospitals. (Source: Gwynedd Mental Health Services)

What is clear from the available evidence is that England, Wales and Scotland are set on rather different courses with regard to the balance between hospital and other provision. In England, health and social services interests are reasonably evenly balanced. In Wales, there is a clear bias in favour of social care. In Scotland, there remains an emphasis on a medical view of care for the priority care groups. Care continues to be largely based on traditional institutions for a variety of reasons including a continuing commitment by Scottish health ministers to such provision, the power of the medical lobby, and a less constrained resource position which provides fewer incentives for change.

Community care: future scenarios

You will be aware by now of how turbulent the policy environment of the early 1990s has become in the area of community care. There are no signs that the pace of change will slow down. Indeed, quite the opposite seems likely. Over the next decade or so, community care will be shaped by a number of pressures and developments. We cannot deal with all of these prospects here so the most important have been singled out for comment. Some of them have already been mentioned in previous sections.

Over the decade of the 1990s it is likely that:

- The average length of patient stay in acute hospitals will continue to fall, and there will be increased pressure on day care and other community-based facilities.

- Demographic trends will cause some changes in the balance between health and social care needs, with the likelihood of further pressure on the latter in line with the emphasis on home-based care for chronic conditions (although these will not be dramatic over such a short period).

- The demand for community health services and other community-based services will rise, in large part as a result of the two developments above.

In order to meet the growing demand for care and to finance it, a number of options are possible. These range from the introduction of long-term care insurance for elderly people, through greater scope for mixed public- and private-sector involvement in service delivery, to greater user involvement through self-help initiatives.

It is possible, too, that the organisational and managerial reforms in community care that are being implemented could be overturned by a new emphasis on primary health care and an enlargement of its scope to include social care. In this scenario, GPs would become key figures in coordinating and possibly purchasing community care from whatever source—health or social services (curiously, this coordinating role was envisioned for GPs but never implemented when the NHS was set up).[9]

Concern over local government's ability to cope with the responsibilities proposed for it have led to a reassessment of some of the thinking contained in the 1988 Griffiths report and picked up in the 1989 White Paper. In the words of the Audit Commission:

> ...if community care is to have any chance of success the change process itself will need to be managed with considerable skill...[Only in this way can] the potential chaos of the cascade of change...be turned into a more ordered agenda. (Audit Commission, 1992, p. 38, paragraph 100 and p. 39, paragraph 102)

[9] See *Caring for Health: History and Diversity* (revised edition 1993), Chapters 5 and 6.

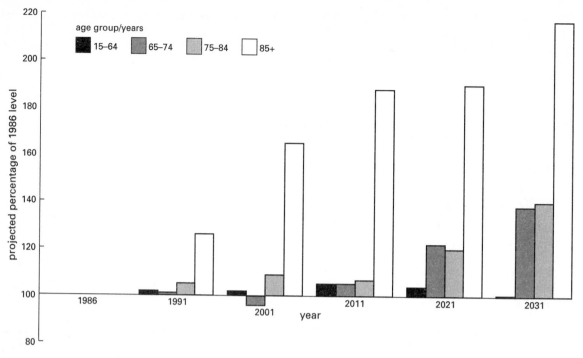

Figure 8.4 *Projected trends in the age-structure of the United Kingdom population aged over 15 years, 1990–2031, expressed as the percentage increase in each age group compared with the size of that age group in 1986. (Source: Dennis, G. (ed.), 1993, Annual Abstract of Statistics 1993: no. 129, HMSO, London, p. 10, Table 2.5)*

But the change agenda remains a massive one which, eventually, will change local and health authorities out of all recognition. As the Commission comments, they 'have every right to feel intimidated'.

A drawback in any major reassessment of community care which attempts to give a more prominent role to *health* services is that it will lead to an overly narrow conception of what constitutes community care. As we stressed earlier, community care goes beyond social care services and embraces housing, education and transport, together with other local authority services. There is therefore an important *corporate* dimension to local government's responsibilities for community care, which go well beyond the strict boundaries of social services.

By the year 2000, demand for community care services will rise as a result of policies to support people in need of care at home, to discharge mentally ill people and people with learning disabilities into the community from long-stay beds, to discharge patients more rapidly from acute hospital beds, and from an increase in the number of very elderly people. Changing patterns of health care,

including shorter stays in hospital, more day-case surgery and earlier discharge, will also result in additional pressures on community care services. At the same time, changes in employment patterns will reduce the potential number of informal carers and attention will need to be given to the capacity of the voluntary and private sectors to complement public-sector provision in order to cope with rising demand.

Demographic trends not only imply major new demands on community care services, but also major shifts in the composition of the work force. Figure 8.4 shows the forecast demographic trends in the United Kingdom to the year 2031. Whilst the number of people aged 15 to 64 remains fairly constant, the number of elderly people will increase well into the next century. As the population ages, the evidence suggests that the incidence of chronic illness, such as Alzheimer's disease, diabetes, coronary heart disease and cancers also rises, increasing the demand for long-term community care. These trends will have implications, too, for the recruitment of professional carers and the informal carers of the future.

The pace of social and economic change is so great that any proposals for reforming the provision of community care run the risk of dealing with yesterday's problems. A number of policy, practice and research questions for the future present themselves over the next decade. We have already mentioned the demographic issues, but other issues demand attention. Many of these concern the future funding of care. While there will always be a major role for the public sector, supplementary sources of finance may become more necessary. The rising level of owner occupation and the spread of occupational and private pension schemes may increasingly enable a section of the elderly population of the future to purchase the care and support they want for themselves. The converse of this growth in 'woopies' (well-off older people) is that a significant minority of elderly people are poor, and the gap between the most affluent and those in poverty is widening (a subject taken up in Chapter 11). The lack of financial resources is reflected in poor housing circumstances and scarce amenities.[10]

Sir Roy Griffiths, in his review of community care, was concerned about such issues although it was not part of his remit to dwell on them. But he did argue for more imaginative policy thinking, including the introduction of some form of social care insurance. He also suggested that corporate financial planning in future years may reflect growing concern about community care in the way that support for occupational pensions developed after World War II. Government may need to give a lead.

Conclusion

A theme running through this chapter is the confusion which pervades community care policy, the seeming lack of commitment to it (which is probably responsible for the confusion) and uncertainty about the future. There is a paradox in all this. Few of us are unaffected by community care in some way. Yet, despite its significance in shaping our lives, policy and practice in the field of community care continues to be muddled and haphazard. Good examples of practice are outweighed by the tales of inaction and insensitivity, of lives shattered by pressures on informal carers. Although the reforms announced in 1989 and launched in 1991 are intended to address these problems, at the time of writing it is not possible to assess their likely impact. Some difficult issues remain to be tackled, which inevitably gives rise to some scepticism about whether these reforms will be sufficient. Much more attention is needed from policy analysts and policy-makers if we are to succeed in turning rhetoric into reality in community care.

[10]The circumstances affecting the health and well-being of elderly people in the United Kingdom in recent times are discussed in *Birth to Old Age: Health in Transition* (1985 and revised edition 1995).

OBJECTIVES FOR CHAPTER 8

When you have studied this chapter, you should be able to:

8.1   Identify the dilemmas or critical issues that dominate discussion of community care.

8.2   Distinguish between the different meanings of the term 'community care' and how these have shifted over time in the policies pursued by successive governments.

8.3   Discuss the contribution made to community care by informal carers.

8.4   Comment on the social, economic, ideological and demographic forces that are shaping community care policy and practice, both in terms of those people being cared for and those doing the caring.

8.5   Describe community care policy and practice at the time of studying in the context of the reforms introduced in 1991, and comment on the major obstacles to progress.

8.6   Discuss the reasons underlying differences in community care policy in the countries of Great Britain.

QUESTIONS FOR CHAPTER 8

Question 1 (*Objective 8.1*)

Summarise the principal dilemmas in community care and say why they are difficult to resolve.

Question 2 (*Objectives 8.2 and 8.4*)

Describe (a) the underlying ideological position that has led to support for community care, (b) how this belief has changed over time under successive governments, and (c) the social, economic and demographic trends that policy-makers will have to confront over the next decade.

Question 3 (*Objective 8.3*)

What are the implications for community care policy of the indicators concerning informal carers listed in Box 8.1?

Question 4 (*Objective 8.5*)

What have been the main reasons for the community care reforms announced in the 1989 White Paper, *Caring for People,* and introduced in April 1991?

Question 5 (*Objective 8.6*)

Consider the data presented in Table 8.2. First describe the major patterns in the table. How would you account for the differences between the three countries? You will need to take into account the data on numbers of hospital beds and the extent of day-care and domiciliary services provided for priority groups in each of the countries, which were summarised earlier and are given in detail elsewhere.[11]

Table 8.2   Number of people in residential homes in Great Britain in 1985, per 100 000 population (*= number of places provided, whether occupied or not)

	Elderly	Mentally ill	Mentally handicapped
England	1 530	1 220	46
Wales	1 760	1 600	59
Scotland	2 100*	460*	36

(Sources: Department of Health and Social Security, Welsh Office and Scottish Office data)

[11]See *Caring for Health: History and Diversity,* (revised edition 1993), Chapter 9, Table 9.1.

9

Disease prevention and health promotion

This chapter refers back to the detailed description of patterns of health and disease in the United Kingdom which occurred in **World Health and Disease, Chapter 9**. *You will be expected to look back at the data presented there as you study the present chapter. During your study of this chapter you will be asked to read two articles: 'A health promotion primer for the 1990s', by Lester Breslow, and 'Assessment of screening for cancer', by Carlo La Vecchia and colleagues; both are in the Reader.[1]*

This chapter was jointly written by Helen Lambert, Lecturer in Medical Anthropology, and Klim McPherson, Professor of Public Health Epidemiology, and Head of the Health Promotion Sciences Unit, both in the Department of Public Health and Policy at the London School of Hygiene and Tropical Medicine. The Department is primarily concerned with health policy evaluation, human nutrition, environmental epidemiology, health promotion and health services research.

Is prevention better than cure?

Attempts to move the emphasis in health care away from a curative approach and toward disease prevention and health promotion are occurring worldwide. In 1986 the World Health Organisation (WHO) convened an international conference which issued the *Ottawa Charter for Health Promotion* and has encouraged its members—including the United Kingdom—to develop national strategic plans for improving health. In its campaign for *Health For All by the Year 2000,* the WHO has formulated a European strategy that identifies a number of targets in health promotion to be achieved by that year. Some

[1] *Health and Disease: A Reader* (revised edition 1994).

attempts have been made to move toward a preventive health strategy in the United Kingdom, and a government White Paper, *The Health of The Nation,* was published in the summer of 1992.

Most people would agree in principle that 'prevention is better than cure', and few would argue against the notion that actively *promoting* health is better than simply preventing disease. But these commonsense ideas conceal some important dilemmas in contemporary health care, which have surfaced several times in this book in other contexts. We begin this chapter by skimming briefly across this territory before looking in more detail at examples of disease prevention and health promotion strategies as diverse as price barriers to alcohol consumption, anti-smoking campaigns and hormone replacement therapy for women distressed by symptoms of the menopause.

The first dilemma lies in deciding the desirable balance between promotion, prevention and cure. Where resources are finite, expenditure on disease prevention and health promotion—within the formal health-care system at least—would probably divert funds from curative services. Given the choice, should we abandon help for some of those who are already sick in order to preserve or increase the future health of those who remain well?

The second dilemma arises from the difficulties involved in developing *appropriate* and *acceptable* strategies to prevent disease or promote health, and then in demonstrating their *effectiveness*. These difficulties do not apply to all prevention or promotion strategies.

☐ Can you name one such strategy where evaluation of effectiveness is reasonably straightforward?

■ Immunisations to prevent infectious diseases are given routinely under similar conditions to very large numbers of people, and the outcome can be readily assessed in terms of the incidence of infection.

But many strategies to prevent disease or promote health do pose serious problems of evaluation. This may be because they entail very long-term social, behavioural or environmental changes, or because the 'outcomes' involved cannot easily be defined and measured, or because it is difficult to control for influences external to the strategies themselves. For example, if reductions in morbidity and mortality for certain specified health problems are found to have occurred in an area following the introduction of a community health programme, this does not prove that the programme 'caused' the improvements, since other factors may have been at work. Nor does it necessarily imply that a similar programme would have the same effectiveness in another community elsewhere. The dilemma is whether we should allocate resources to interventions if their benefits to health cannot be accurately evaluated. Evaluation is discussed in more detail later.

A particular dimension of this dilemma in the medical sphere arises as a result of advances in medical technologies. How can we judge whether drugs developed by commercial interests and vigorously promoted to a mass market as preventing disease are really effective, safe and affordable innovations for use over long periods of time? For example, cholesterol-lowering drugs and hormone replacement therapy have been clinically demonstrated to be effective for the short-term reductions in disease risk or discomfort for which they were developed, but their long-term effects remain unknown (a subject we return to later). Moreover, the results of clinical trials may be used as a reason to allow or even promote the widespread use of such drugs, although the presence of substantial vested interests may entail a danger of general 'medicalisation' of life and health against which the public might need to be protected.

The problems inherent in evaluation lead us to a third dilemma. Since strategies for disease prevention and health promotion outside the medical sphere (such as health education, community action or government legislation) are rarely evaluated systematically, decisions about whether to adopt such strategies tend ultimately to be based more strongly on political or ideological grounds than on demonstration of their beneficial effects on health. Should the interests or preferences of citizens who might benefit from such interventions be considered, or can the best use of resources only be determined as part of a national strategy by central government, despite the likelihood of politically-expedient or ideologically-driven policies?

A fourth dilemma leads on from this, arising from the tension between individual freedom and social control. To what extent is health promotion and disease prevention socially or morally justified? Strategies to prevent disease or promote health can restrict individual freedoms (as in the banning of smoking in public places or the wearing of seat belts), or exert coercive pressure which arouses guilt over 'unhealthy' behaviour. Such strategies can reach into every aspect of people's daily lives—in their homes, workplaces and communities—and inevitably they focus yet more attention on health and disease. This may be beneficial in prompting people to become more aware of their health, but it may also have negative effects, such as the anxiety caused when screening is imposed on fit and healthy people. This dilemma is especially acute where health promotion or disease prevention strategies lack clear scientific evidence to justify their implementation.

Defining disease prevention and health promotion

Three levels of prevention

The central dilemma of 'prevention versus cure' can be ameliorated by redefining *all* health-care activities as entailing prevention in some sense. They can then be loosely classified into three levels according to the type of preventive activity they involve:

1   **Primary prevention**: strategies that aim to prevent the onset of disease.

2   **Secondary prevention**: strategies that aim to detect and cure a disease at an early stage before it causes serious irreversible problems.

3   **Tertiary prevention**: strategies that aim to minimise the effects or reduce the progression of an already established irreversible disease.

Strategies at all three levels can be readily identified from within the health-care system.

> ☐ Can you suggest an example of a strategy available in the formal health-care sector at each of these levels of prevention?

> ■ Many examples are possible, for instance: *primary prevention* includes immunisation against infectious diseases, and screening to detect and reduce possible risk factors for disease (e.g. high blood pressure); *secondary prevention* includes screening for early signs of disease (e.g. microscopic cancers in breast tissue); *tertiary prevention* includes such interventions as hip-replacement surgery, which may reduce immobility from osteoarthritis.

This medical focus is the context in which the terms primary, secondary and tertiary prevention are conventionally used. But it is possible to take a broader view.

Table 9.1 Examples of activities aimed at preventing disease

Type of prevention	Intervention	Responsibility for implementation
Statutory		
reduction in cigarette smoking	higher taxation	government
prevention of waterborne disease	safe water supply	water companies
reduction of road traffic accidents	breathalyser	police
reduction of childhood infections	housing the homeless	local authority
prevention of foodborne disease	inspection of food premises	environmental health officers
Voluntary		
reduction in cigarette smoking	education in schools	health promotion officers, school teachers
reduction in coronary heart disease	advice on reducing fat in diet	doctors, health promotion officers, school teachers
prevention of measles	immunisation	doctors
reduction of invasive cervical cancer	screening	doctors

Source: Royal College of Physicians (1991) *Preventive Medicine*: *A Report of a Working Party of the Royal College of Physicians*, RCP, London, Table 1.1, p. 6)

□ Can you suggest examples of disease prevention strategies at each of these levels arising from social welfare, education or environmental change?

■ Primary prevention might include health education advice (e.g. on dental care, or sexually transmitted diseases) broadcast in the media, in schools, etc.; secondary prevention might include community outreach schemes to persuade women to attend for breast-cancer screening; tertiary prevention might include legislation to enforce wheelchair access to all public buildings and transport.

Of these three levels, this chapter is concerned with primary and secondary prevention, some examples of which appear in Table 9.1. Notice the wide range of agencies involved (you may be able to think of others).

Secondary prevention mainly relies on specific technologies to detect disease early and so usually involves the public or private health-care system. These technological approaches to prevention will be discussed later in the chapter.

Primary prevention, on the other hand, must inevitably also promote health since it aims to stop the *onset* of disease. Many such strategies can be adopted by individuals to promote their own health.

□ Can you think of examples of ways in which you promote your own or your family's health?

■ Brushing teeth, taking exercise, preparing nutritious food, etc.

Health promotion and the concept of optimal health

The overlapping activities involved in disease prevention and health promotion at the community level are illustrated in the Reader article[2] by Lester Breslow, a leading public-health physician in the USA. In 'A health promotion primer for the 1990s', he discusses alternative definitions of **health promotion** which flow from ambiguities in what we mean by 'health'. You should read this article now.

□ What definition of health does Breslow favour and how does this influence his concept of health promotion?

■ He emphasises **optimal health**, which is more than the absence of disease, and more even than the WHO's definition of 'physical, mental and social well-being'. It encompasses a dynamic balance between the human organism and its environment, with reserves of capacity such that the person does not collapse or deteriorate under adverse pressure from the environment. Health promotion becomes action that enables the person to 'lead a buoyant life, full of zest, competent to meet challenges'.

The promotion of optimal health clearly requires more than medical intervention. Public-health policies focus increasingly on the role of individuals and groups outside

[2]See *Health and Disease: A Reader* (revised edition 1994).

145

the medical sphere, in addition to government-funded professionals such as environmental-health officers, health-education officers, doctors, health visitors and dieticians. Numerous non-governmental organisations, both professional and voluntary, are active in the health field at both local and national levels, ranging from pressure groups and charities such as Action for Smoking and Health (ASH), the Coronary Prevention Group and Help the Aged, to consumer watchdogs, trades unions, housing associations, environmental groups, community and self-help groups and other informal associations of activists.

Many such groups and agencies focus on specific health issues or the prevention of particular causes of ill-health, rather than the promotion of optimal health in a more general sense. They are often opposed by those with vested interests. For example, trades unions have an interest in workers' health, but their monitoring of accidents and diseases arising from workplace hazards or attempts to introduce safer working environments may be opposed by management. A tenants' association campaigning for better housing conditions might encounter opposition from local landlords. A consortium of industrial concerns might lobby Members of Parliament to oppose a legislative measure to introduce rigorous emission controls from factories, because this would necessitate the installation of expensive new equipment. The concept of optimal health and its promotion has been vigorously pursued by the alternative health-care sector, which is itself generally opposed by orthodox medicine.

Strategies for disease prevention and health promotion

Targeting individuals, communities or governments?

Conventional approaches to improving health in recent decades have tended to assume that as rational individuals people will make sensible choices about their health if they are given sufficient information. This assumption underlies most forms of **health education**, such as the leaflets in dentists' waiting rooms containing information about prevention of tooth decay, doctors' advice to individual patients on giving up smoking, and mass media campaigns intended to inform individuals how to protect themselves from HIV, the virus that causes AIDS. Medical action is most frequently directed at the individual, as the case study on the menopause in the next section illustrates.

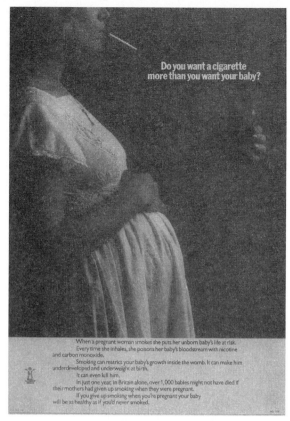

Do you want a cigarette more than you want your baby?

When a pregnant woman smokes she puts her unborn baby's life at risk.
Every time she inhales, she poisons her baby's bloodstream with nicotine and carbon monoxide.
Smoking can restrict your baby's growth inside the womb. It can make him underdeveloped and underweight at birth.
It can even kill him.
In just one year, in Britain alone, over 1,000 babies might not have died if their mothers had given up smoking when they were pregnant.
If you give up smoking when you're pregnant your baby will be as healthy as if you'd never smoked.

An example of health education that aims to change behaviour by targeting the individual. (Source: Health Education Council)

☐ According to Lester Breslow, what is the main drawback of a strategy that emphasises individual action and personal choice?

■ It ignores the social context in which individual choices are made and so cannot tackle the wider influences on health. It runs the risk of 'blaming the victim' for the disease (a subject to which we return at the end of the chapter).

☐ Breslow describes a *community* approach to health promotion. How does this differ from strategies aimed at individuals?

■ It seeks to protect and enhance the health of *all* members of a community or population, by creating social and environmental conditions that are more conducive to health.

The community approach is gaining ground in the 1990s. It requires the involvement of many sectors of a society (for example, the agencies in Table 9.1, and interest groups in the general population). Breslow uses the term 'community' to refer in a general sense to all members of a society, but it can also mean the members of any group inhabiting a particular geographical area and/or sharing some common interests. Interacting with, and in some cases directing, strategies aimed at individuals and local communities are the policies of central government, which have an impact on the health of the whole population. We can explore the strengths and limitations of strategies for disease prevention and health promotion aimed at each of these targets by considering three case studies: alleviating the symptoms of the menopause; local community action schemes; and government legislation concerning alcohol.

Medical action: reducing the harmful effects of the menopause

The menopause is associated with two significant changes in women's health status. First, women have lower levels of coronary heart disease (CHD) than men until after the menopause[3] (a subject we return to in Chapter 10), when the ovaries stop releasing eggs and the levels of female hormones in the body decline greatly. These circulating hormones may have a protective effect against CHD, since after the menopause the incidence among women begins to approach (but never matches) that among men. Second, after the age of about 50 years, bones begin to lose density and strength, but this process is much more apparent in women than in men and can lead to a condition known as *osteoporosis* (or holes in the bones). Osteoporotic bones are weaker and so more likely to fracture, which is a major cause of morbidity among older people, especially elderly women.

A treatment that may reduce the incidence of both CHD and osteoporosis has been available from doctors since the early 1970s, in the form of **hormone replacement therapy** (**HRT**), originally prescribed as an effective treatment for distressing menopausal symptoms such as hot flushes. HRT consists of taking a regular monthly 'cycle' of synthetic versions of those hormones— *oestrogen* and *progesterone*—whose levels are depleted during and after the menopause. HRT has attracted great attention not only because it has obvious short-term benefits in relieving discomfort but also because, if demonstrated to be effective at preventing disease, its manufacturers can expect an enormous and highly profitable market.

The question to be answered, however, is the extent to which the costs of such an intervention can be justified by its benefits. Does taking hormones during (and possibly before) the menopause and afterwards, perhaps for decades, do important harm as well as good? After all, the history of medicine is littered with 'attractive' interventions that turned out to have unsuspected harmful effects.[4]

Evidence from epidemiological studies in the mid-1970s indicated that taking oestrogen *alone* (oestrogen replacement therapy) increased the risk of cancer of the lining of the womb (endometrium) by a factor of about six. It was quickly found that if a synthetic progesterone was combined with oestrogen for part of a 'cycle' (combined replacement therapy), the increased risk of endometrial cancer was eliminated.

The effect of these hormones on subsequent risk of breast cancer also raises a dilemma. The epidemiological study of oestrogen-only therapy suggested that HRT does decrease the risk of heart disease, but also increases the risk of breast cancer after around 10 to 15 years of use. Thus while the risk of endometrial cancer was discovered quite quickly after HRT became available, the risk of breast cancer only emerged several years later. At the time of writing (1992) the effect of combined oestrogen-with-progesterone therapy on the risk of breast cancer is poorly understood because as yet it is too new to be able to evaluate the effects of long-term use. It is also unclear whether combined HRT is as protective against heart disease as oestrogen alone, and there are some strong epidemiological reasons for supposing it is not.

In these circumstances the possible effect of combined HRT on breast-cancer risk in the future can be down-played as hypothetical and much less important than its actual beneficial effects on menopausal symptoms and osteoporosis. But the question of whether the benefits outweigh the potential risks remains and this poses a dilemma for women faced with possible treatment now. The market could be exploited much more than it is; in 1992 around eight per cent of menopausal and post-menopausal women in the United Kingdom took HRT, but some (not least the manufacturers and many gynaecologists) feel that it should be taken as a *preventive* drug by many more (if not all) menopausal women. Indeed some of the promotional material indicates that no woman can be complete without HRT: one advertisement in a medical journal shows a woman who appears to be below menopausal age sitting alone on a sofa surrounded by party-goers, with the slogan 'By taking [brand name] she could be taking part.'

---

[3]The biological, sociological and personal dimensions of the menopause are explored in detail in *Birth to Old Age: Health in Transition* (1985 and revised edition 1995).

[4]See *Medical Knowledge: Doubt and Certainty* (1985 and revised edition 1994), which discusses iatrogenic illness (i.e. illness caused by medical treatment).

HRT illustrates a type of preventive intervention that is medical in nature, directed at the individual and only available within the health-care system; indeed, it derives much of its perceived credibility as a 'medicine'. The costs and effectiveness of HRT are gradually being evaluated, and compared with those of alternative therapeutic interventions for menopausal and post-menopausal health problems. Such systematic evaluation is difficult to undertake, as you will see later in the chapter.

Community action: participation in social change

Many health-promotion campaigns are targeted not on individuals but on specific groups or communities, such as the labour force in a particular workplace, elderly people in an urban neighbourhood, residents of a village, or a school population. Programmes at this middle level between the individual and the national population are large enough to consider some of the wider social and economic issues outside the control of the individual, while being small enough to address the specific needs and circumstances of the group. *Community participation*, or the active involvement of community members, is an essential part of these community-oriented strategies for health promotion, which echo the consumer participation campaigns described in Chapter 5 for health-service users.

> ☐ According to Breslow, what important process is community participation intended to encourage?

> ■ It is intended to enable individuals, through social action, to 'take control' of their own health.

This process is also sometimes referred to as *empowerment* because, through social action, individuals may gain the power to change their life circumstances and improve not only their own but also their community's health. For example, a health-promotion programme for parents on a housing estate might include conventional health-education classes on child care and nutrition, but the participants might also meet together informally and discuss other issues affecting their health. As a result they might begin to act jointly, for example by initiating meetings with council representatives to demand improvements in housing conditions, or advocating a change in the ante-natal clinic's opening hours to make attendance easier.

> ☐ What does social action at this local level of the community leave out?

> ■ Action aimed at business interests and central government, which make a powerful contribution to social and environmental conditions.

Some threats to health, such as air pollution or excessive consumption of alcohol, cannot usually be tackled by local community participation alone. Action at government level is an essential element in effective strategies to prevent alcohol-related disease and injury, as the following case study illustrates.

Government action: reducing alcohol consumption

In all industrialised countries, excessive alcohol consumption presents a serious health problem. Figure 9.1 shows the relationship between alcohol consumption and deaths from cirrhosis of the liver (progressive damage and death of liver cells) in Europe.

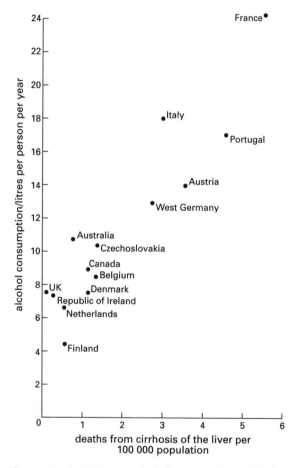

Figure 9.1 *Comparison of alcohol consumption and deaths from cirrhosis of the liver in 14 European countries in 1975. (Source: Popham, R. E. et al., 1975, cited in Royal College of Physicians, 1991, A Report of a Working Party of the Royal College of Physicians, RCP, London, Figure 3.1, p. 34)*

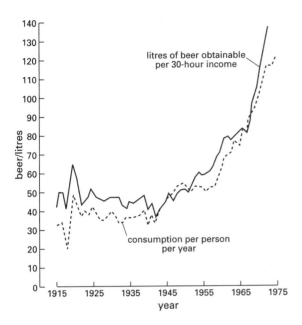

Figure 9.2 *Relationship between the price of beer and consumer purchasing in Denmark, 1915–75. (Source: Neilson, D. D. and Sorenson, D. D., 1979, cited in Royal College of Physicians, 1991, A Report of a Working Party of the Royal College of Physicians, RCP, London, Figure 3.2, p. 36)*

The 1991 report on *Preventive Medicine* published by the Royal College of Physicians of London suggested that in the United Kingdom, a fall in the relative price of alcohol between 1950 and 1980 was associated with a rise in consumption and an increase in deaths from cirrhosis of the liver during the same period. High rates of alcohol consumption are also associated with other public health and social problems including coronary heart disease, alcohol dependence and road accidents from drunk driving. According to Acquire (Alcohol Concern's Quarterly Information and Research Bulletin, 1992), in the early 1990s, one road death in six in the United Kingdom was drink-related and deaths caused by drink-driving were costing society about £530 million per year. The government's 1992 White Paper, *The Health of the Nation*, noted that alcohol-related absenteeism accounted for an estimated eight million lost working days annually.

Figure 9.2 shows the strongly positive relationship between the price of beer and levels of beer consumption in Denmark over a 60-year period.

One obvious strategy for preventing disease and death resulting from excessive alcohol consumption would be to reduce sales by raising prices significantly. But would the consequent health benefits outweigh the costs? The drinks industry in the United Kingdom generates considerable revenue for the government from duty and exports, and is also a major employer; in 1983 it had a 'turnover' of £6 000 million and employed 250 000 people. Damage to the drinks industry might *reduce* government resources for health and social care, and increase unemployment with its attendant health risks.

Another strategy would be to restrict or ban advertising, on which the industry spends over £150 million per year. However, as with cigarette advertising, there is only

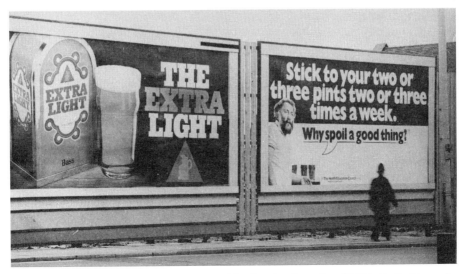

Contrasting messages on alcohol. (Source: Health Education Council and British Medical Journal)

indirect evidence that advertising really encourages *greater* consumption rather than merely encouraging consumers to switch or remain loyal to particular brands. Calls for legislation to ban all advertising of alcohol or cigarettes have not succeeded in convincing government to take such action, which could variously be seen as paternalistic interference with personal freedom or enlightened protection of the health of the whole community. Moreover, it now seems that people who drink alcohol in moderation have lower rates of some common fatal diseases than those who never drink alcohol. This finding further complicates policy formation.

Evaluating effectiveness

One important technical problem that may frustrate the adoption of strategies for disease prevention and health promotion is that the evaluation of their effectiveness is often much more difficult than it is for a *therapeutic* intervention (i.e. one aimed at treating existing disease).

□ What is the ideal way to evaluate the effectiveness of a health-care intervention?

■ Chapter 4 described the randomised controlled trial (RCT) in which morbidity, mortality or some other outcome measure among individuals who have received the intervention is compared with that of similar individuals who have not.

Evaluation is never easy because ensuring strict comparability between intervention and control groups is always a problem. However, RCTs of interventions aimed at *preventing* disease take longer and need more people in the two groups than RCTs of medical treatments for *existing* disease. To assess the effectiveness of any primary preventive intervention, we have to compare the rates at which initially-healthy people *become* ill or die in the intervention and control groups. Only in this way can all the other possible influences on subsequent disease be allowed for completely. Since not everyone *will* become ill, a much larger population sample is required to make a valid comparison, and they must be followed up for longer than when a medical treatment is subjected to an RCT in an already-ill population.

For example, for an RCT of a *preventive* intervention to have a reasonable chance of detecting a ten per cent reduction in mortality which could be attributed to it, the trial might well require *30 000* people, each of them followed for *ten* years. A 10 per cent reduction in mortality for a *therapeutic* intervention might be as reliably detected with *3 000* patients followed for *two* years, because the outcome to be compared will usually be both

more common and more immediate. In the preventive comparison an 'outcome' event rate (such as death) of five per *thousand* per year would be considered high, whereas in the treatment comparison an event rate of five per *hundred* per year would be low.

However, many health-promotion and disease-prevention strategies cannot be assessed by RCTs at all, especially where they are non-medical in nature.

□ Why would it *not* be feasible to assess the health outcomes of banning the advertising of alcohol through an RCT?

■ It would be impossible to obtain comparable groups (with and without alcohol banning) or eliminate all possible influences on the outcome in the intervention group other than the banning order.

Finally, because prevention strategies are largely matters of public policy, concerning healthy individuals who are not seeking care, and often requiring large amounts of public money, the evidence required to justify a preventive intervention must be especially accurate and compelling. By comparison, the standards of evidence required to justify new medical interventions are less rigorous, except in the case of new drugs (as Chapter 7 described).

But, despite the problems of evaluation, the health-care system, including the NHS, is a major provider of disease-prevention and health-promotion activities. We turn now to consider the financial costs of these services and whether we are getting value for money.

Balancing the costs of prevention and cure

The balance between prevention and cure may have begun to shift slightly in recent years. Since 1991, GPs have been required as part of their contracts with the NHS to fulfil target quotas for numbers of immunisations, cervical smears for cancer screening, and other preventive activities such as health education and 'well-woman' clinics offering check-ups and advice to the healthy. Nonetheless, the NHS is mainly devoted to curative services—indeed, an old joke states that it is really a 'National Illness Service'.

It is extremely difficult to calculate how much is spent on health promotion and disease prevention. One attempt to produce a rough estimate (see Table 9.2) put total United Kingdom expenditure on disease prevention in 1980–1 at almost £1 billion,[5] of which almost £550

[5]thousand million.

Table 9.2 Estimated expenditure on disease prevention (£thousands) in the United Kingdom, 1980–1

Source of funding	£ thousands on prevention	Percentage of total expenditure by that service
NHS		
community services	312 652	40
general medical services	75 978	10
general dental services	101 533	20
hospital services	59 385	0.8
Non-NHS		
Public sector		
Ministry of Agriculture, Fisheries and food	34	
Health and Safety Executive	72 167	
Department of the Environment	268	
Department of Health and Social Security (including health education, public health laboratories)	19 882	
Home Office	45	
Northern Ireland Office	109	
Scottish Office	1	
Department of Trade	30	
Central Office of Information	100	
Private and voluntary bodies	15 500	
Total of NHS and non-NHS expenditure on disease prevention	**966 648**	

Source: Cohen, D. and Henderson, J. 1983, A Minister for Prevention: An Initiative in Health Policy, *HERU Discussion Paper 2/83*, University of Aberdeen, Tables 1, 4 and 5

million was spent within the NHS. However, this represented less than 5 per cent of NHS expenditure on *curative* services in the same financial year; there is no reason to believe that this proportion has changed greatly since then.

Two important questions arise from this observation: 'Why is spending so low?' and 'Would greater investment in disease prevention actually improve health?'

Resources for health services are finite, so using them for disease prevention may mean foregoing other services or facilities. Policy decisions concerning the implementation of any preventive programme *should* depend on the careful assessment of costs and benefits, including possible alternative uses for the resources involved (recall Chapter 3 on rationing of health care), but—as we pointed out earlier—evaluation is often difficult and decisions tend to be made more on political and ideological grounds.

There are many reasons why the health-care sector is biased towards curative rather than preventive approaches to disease.

☐ Can you suggest why?[6]

■ Illness is often frightening and painful to patients and carers alike, so every possible effort is usually made to alleviate individual suffering—failure to provide immediate medical help would generally be considered unethical. It might also lead to public protest and accusations of malpractice, which could undermine the prestige of the medical profession. That prestige is itself indicative of the dominance of curative medicine in our culture; preventive medicine has a much lower status.

[6]See *Medical Knowledge: Doubt and Certainty* (1985 and revised edition 1994) for a discussion of the prestige of medicine in Western culture; the dominance of specialist hospital medicine over public health or community medicine has a long history, which is discussed in *Caring for Health: History and Diversity* (revised edition 1993).

☐ What reasons can you suggest for re-examining the emphasis on curative medicine in the 1990s?

■ As earlier chapters in this book have pointed out, increasing demand from an ageing population, coupled with advances in medical technologies and expertise in the provision of effective care, have led to escalating costs for curative health services both in absolute terms and as a proportion of GNP. Since funds are limited, there is *de facto* rationing in both acute and chronic health-care sectors.

A major argument for adopting general preventive strategies is that they may be more cost-effective than treating (or attempting unsuccessfully to treat) people who are already ill. If successful, disease-prevention strategies would reduce the dependency associated with illness and hence produce other benefits to society as a whole beyond the reduction in the cost of health and social services. On the other hand, preventing *one* disease may increase the likelihood that *another* will occur, which may turn out to be more costly than the disease that was prevented. Total costs per person over a *lifetime* may thus increase as a consequence of preventing one disease. Another possible drawback arises from the fact that most preventive services can only be offered, not enforced. Thus they may not reduce the *overall* incidence of disease in the population, but instead simply (and possibly expensively) be taken up only by the 'worried well'.

These uncertainties create dilemmas for those who must balance the costs and benefits of disease-prevention and health-promotion strategies. The pressure inherent in such uncomfortable choices is illustrated below by considering two specific diseases and the intervention strategies currently available to reduce their incidence. Since we cannot hope to prevent all diseases, particularly where funds are limited, suitable targets for prevention programmes must be selected.

☐ What criteria do you think a disease should satisfy if a prevention programme is to have a significant impact?

■ It should be (a) relatively common in the population, (b) result in relatively high levels of morbidity and mortality, (c) the main underlying causes should be sufficiently well understood to enable (d) some effective preventive response to be taken.

In the first half of the twentieth century, attention was focused primarily on infectious diseases such as polio, diphtheria and tuberculosis, for which effective immunisation now exists.

☐ Can you suggest some diseases that fit criteria (a) to (d) above in the United Kingdom in the 1990s?[7]

■ Chronic conditions such as coronary heart disease (the subject of Chapter 10), strokes and certain cancers, particularly lung cancer because of its known association with smoking. You may also be aware of the resurgence of tuberculosis.

Primary prevention of lung cancer: a comparison with breast cancer

The profound effect of lung cancer on individual and population health is undisputed. It is more common among older people and, despite a falling incidence among men since the 1970s, it has been increasing among women (see Figure 9.3). Lung cancer can rarely be cured and treatment largely consists in attempting to prolong life while reducing the suffering produced by symptoms. Even with the best efforts of therapeutic medicine, the average survival time is currently less than two years from diagnosis and the prospects for a medical breakthrough in treatment are not encouraging.

The epidemiology of lung cancer has been intensively studied since World War II and it is well understood that the principal cause of this disease is the amount and duration of cigarette smoking, with environmental and occupational exposures to carcinogens (agents that cause cancer) contributing only a small proportion of the incidence. The changing mortality rates over time are largely explained by changing smoking habits among men and women, and hardly at all by changes in medical treatment. A reduction in tobacco smoking would have a dramatic effect on this disease, because 80–95 per cent of cases of lung cancer are a direct consequence of cigarette smoking or passive smoking. Rarely is evidence about disease prevention so uncomplicated.

For lung cancer, then, there is no doubt that prevention is better than cure because abandoning smoking would largely prevent the disease. In contrast, consider another common cancer—cancer of the breast among women—until recently the commonest fatal cancer among women, but overtaken by lung cancer in several parts of the United Kingdom in the 1990s. Each year there are about 13 000 deaths each from breast cancer and lung cancer among British women. In recent decades, the incidence of breast cancer in the United Kingdom has been increasing by about 2 per cent per year and the mortality by about 1 per cent per year (most of this increase occurring among women aged over 55). Time trends in mortality are shown in Figure 9.4.

---

[7]Mortality and morbidity rates from major diseases and disabilities in the United Kingdom in the 1990s were described in *World Health and Disease.*

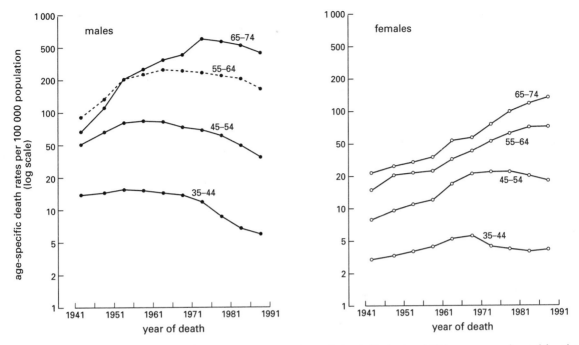

Figure 9.3 *Time trends in mortality from lung cancer per 100 000 population in England and Wales, among males and females aged 35–74 years at death between 1941 and 1991. Note that a logarithmic scale has been used for the vertical axis.[8]*
(Source: Cancer Research Campaign, 1992, Lung Cancer and Smoking, Factsheet 11.1, CRC, London, Figure 3)

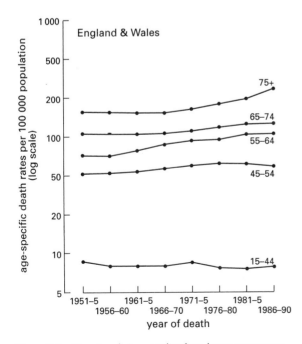

Figure 9.4 *Time trends in mortality from breast cancer per 100 000 population in England and Wales, for women aged over 15 years at death between 1950 and 1990. (Data derived from Cancer Research Campaign, 1991, Breast Cancer, Factsheet 6.2, CRC, London, Table 1)*

In order to consider the problems inherent in devising prevention strategies for breast cancer you need to appreciate the complexity of its underlying causes. Breast cancer is in part a *hormonal* disease; the transformation of breast cells from a normal to a malignant state is influenced by their sensitivity to the female hormones involved in pregnancy and the menstrual cycle.[9] This is evident from some of the major **risk factors** for breast cancer (i.e. factors that have been found to be associated with an increased risk of the disease, see Table 9.3, *overleaf*).

In Table 9.3 the apparent **relative risks**[10] quoted are for the extreme values of the variable in question. Thus 'young menarche' is taken to be the age by which about 5 per cent of girls will have started periods and 'late menarche' is defined as the age by which about 95 per cent will have done so.

[8]Logarithmic scales are often used in graphs in which one variable is changing very rapidly; this is fully explained in *Studying Health and Disease* (1985 and revised edition 1994).

[9]The biological changes (as well as the sociological and personal ones) associated with the female reproductive cycle are discussed in *Birth to Old Age: Health in Transition* (1985 and revised edition 1995).

[10]The interpretation of relative risks is discussed in *Studying Health and Disease* (revised edition 1994).

Table 9.3 Factors associated with an increased risk of breast cancer, in a review of epidemiological research in a variety of populations

Risk factor	Higher risk	Lower risk	Approximate relative risk
age at first menstruation	young	late	3
age at first full-term birth	late	young	3
family history of breast cancer	mother/sister affected	none	2
weight	high	low	2
age at menopause	late	young	2
diet	high fat	low fat	2

Terms such as 'high' or 'late' refer to extreme values in the country under investigation; thus the actual age at which (say) the menopause would be classified as 'young' will vary slightly from country to country. (Data derived from Kalache, A. and Vessey, M. P., 1982, Risk factors for breast cancer, *Clinics in Oncology*, **1**(3), pp. 661–78, various Tables)

□ What does a relative risk of 3 for young age at first menstruation (menarche) mean in this table?

■ The annual risk of breast cancer among women who had an early menarche is on average, over all ages and countries, three times as high as the risk among women who had a late menarche.

Some of the relative risks listed in Table 9.3 can be taken as roughly multiplicative; for example, a woman with both early menarche and late first full-term birth might have a relative risk of breast cancer of around nine times higher than a woman who experienced both a late menarche and early first birth. (But note that these combinations of risk factors will only arise in a very small proportion of the female population.)

□ What differences would you expect to see between Table 9.3 and a similar one for lung cancer?

■ Two important differences. First, there are many risk factors for breast cancer but only one major risk factor (smoking) for lung cancer. Second, each one of the risk factors for breast cancer has a relatively weak influence on the overall risk, unlike smoking which has a very strong influence on the risk of lung cancer.

Smoking bestows at least a tenfold increase in risk of lung cancer (depending on how many cigarettes are smoked per day and for how long), but it has hardly any effect on breast-cancer risk. Moreover, even being in a higher risk group for *all* of the breast-cancer risk factors gives rise to an overall relative risk, compared to being in the lower risk column, of not much more than ten. With such a

relatively small and complicated effect, behaviour changes that could shift a woman into a low risk category for breast cancer are of less relevance than in the case of lung cancer.

□ Can you foresee the difficulties of attempting to prevent breast cancer by advocating behavioural changes?

■ To maximise the reduction in her risk of breast cancer a woman would have to start menstruating late, carry a full-term pregnancy while young and undergo menopause early, watch her weight and her diet, and not be closely related to someone with the disease. These are not easily 'chosen'.

Such preventive strategies are not comparable to giving up smoking to reduce the risk of lung cancer, nor is there evidence that they would be effective even if they could be achieved. By contrast, British doctors gave up smoking in large numbers during the 1950s and 1960s and their lung cancer rates went down in a predictable fashion.

□ Taking a great deal of exercise before puberty is known to delay menarche. What kind of evidence would be the minimum required to justify persuading girls to do this in order to reduce their risk of getting breast cancer?

■ You would have to prove that:

1   Late menarche is strongly associated with a reduction in breast-cancer risk;

2   A delayed menarche induced by exercise is associated with the same reduction in breast-cancer risk as a natural delay;

3   This much effort preceding puberty, and the possible costs in terms of (say) exercise-induced injuries or loss of social life, is worth the benefit of reduced breast-cancer risk much later in life.

For breast cancer no practical and effective means of primary prevention has been found and this is unlikely to change unless more is understood about the biology of its underlying causes. Even when the cause is well understood, as is the case with lung cancer, primary prevention is not easy, as anyone who has tried to give up smoking will testify. Primary prevention of lung cancer is gradually capturing the imagination of many different groups, partly because stopping smoking (or better still, not starting) also reduces the risk of a large number of other diseases, especially CHD. One in six deaths—around 300 per day—are caused by cigarettes in the United Kingdom and this is by far the largest single preventable cause of death. Reducing the burden of breast cancer, on the other hand, must for the present rely on *secondary* prevention by screening to detect and treat the disease early, a subject to which we now turn.

The case for and against screening

Screening is a medically-driven strategy for disease prevention: it relies on a test involving medical technology and expertise, and acting on the test results is a medical responsibility. Screening tests may be designed to detect physiological changes that commonly happen before the onset of a particular disease (a *primary* prevention strategy if the disease can thus be prevented), or to detect an early stage of the disease itself (*secondary* prevention if the disease can be treated more effectively than if detected later). For example, screening to detect and reduce a risk factor such as raised blood cholesterol may result in the primary prevention of coronary heart disease (the subject of the next chapter), whereas screening to detect and treat microscopic breast cancers is secondary prevention. Cervical screening for so-called 'precancerous cells' falls somewhere between the two, since it is not known what proportion of these cells would revert to normal or progress to cancer if left untreated.

There are two main approaches to disease prevention through screening.

1   **Population screening** (or **mass screening**): the whole or a cross-section of the population is investigated for the presence of early disease or a risk factor.

2   **High-risk screening** (or individual screening): individuals who are thought to be at higher than average risk are screened, often during routine consultation with

health professionals, to establish whether early disease or a risk factor is indeed present.

The choice of approach depends partly on the disease but can be strongly influenced by the prevailing medical, economic and political climate. For example, as you will see in Chapter 10, screening to prevent CHD in the United Kingdom has been targeted on high-risk individuals, whereas the USA has adopted a mass screening programme.

Screening is often considered to be intrinsically 'in the public interest', but this view ignores several important difficulties. For example, the increasing number of screening tests being developed to detect *genetic* abnormalities may produce major ethical dilemmas. Although conditions such as cystic fibrosis, sickle-cell disease and Tay-Sachs disease can be identified and genetic counselling offered, no fully effective treatment is available.[11] Where carriers of abnormal genes are identified, the only form of 'prevention' possible is to avoid reproduction, and where screening consists in pre-natal testing, termination of an affected pregnancy is the only 'preventive' option available.

Moreover, the value of screening is entirely dependent upon the effectiveness of subsequent measures for curing the disease, or preventing its development or transmission. Without such measures, individuals could be identified as prone (or certain) to develop an untreatable disease long before it becomes manifest, casting a blight over otherwise healthy life-years (for example, screening for HIV or Huntington's disease (also known as Huntington's chorea) may have this outcome).[12]

Also, in contrast to most *non-medical* prevention strategies (such as taking more exercise), which usually involve individuals making up their own minds, screening is offered to, or may be imposed upon, perfectly fit people, the majority of whom may not benefit from it. Thus the acceptance of a screening policy requires rather careful justification.

The article in the Reader[13] by Carlo La Vecchia and his colleagues on 'Assessment of screening for cancer' discusses the issues involved in evaluating the usefulness

[11]Genetic screening and its consequences are discussed in more detail in *The Biology of Health and Disease* (1985) revised as *Human Biology and Health: An Evolutionary Approach* (1994).

[12]HIV testing is discussed in a special supplement for Open University students only, prior to the publication of the revised edition of another book in this series, *Experiencing and Explaining Disease* (Open University Press, 1995).

[13]*Health and Disease: A Reader* (revised edition 1994).

of cancer-screening programmes. You should read this now.

☐ According to La Vecchia *et al.,*, what is the most basic criterion necessary to justify adopting a screening programme to detect early disease?

■ Early diagnosis as a result of screening must increase the duration and/or quality of life compared with the outcome of clinical diagnosis at the 'usual' time by the best standards of medical practice.

Difficulties inherent in deciding whether this criterion is met can be illustrated most effectively by means of a specific example.

Screening for breast cancer: a case study

There are several possible ways of detecting breast cancer at an early stage. The disease is normally diagnosed by a woman (or her partner) feeling a solid lump in the breast. This can also be accomplished by regular and systematic monthly breast self-examination. However, the greatest chance of successful secondary prevention lies in detecting a tumour before it can be felt as a lump and this is most effectively achieved by **mammography**, the detection of changes in the structure of breast tissue revealed by a *mammogram*, a low-dose X-ray film of the breast. In 1988 a national breast-cancer screening programme was implemented in the United Kingdom offering a mammogram to all women aged 50–64 every three years. On what grounds has the considerable expenditure involved been justified?

Breast cancer is a common disease, as we mentioned earlier, and primary prevention strategies are generally inappropriate. Doctors have devised a system for classifying four *stages* of the disease (measured by tumour size and the degree of infiltration of cancer cells in neighbouring tissue), each of which can be thought of as a progression from the previous stage. At each stage, predictions can be made concerning—on average—the likely outcome of the disease (see Figure 9.5).

☐ From Figure 9.5, what might you conclude about the value of screening to detect early breast cancer?

■ The earlier the stage of disease progression at diagnosis, the better the survival after five years, so you might conclude that earlier detection through screening will increase relative survival rates.

Such a conclusion requires careful evaluation. The article by La Vecchia *et al.* pointed out that screening programmes can be evaluated by comparing the distribution

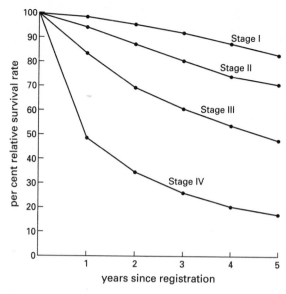

Figure 9.5 *Percentage relative survival rates for women with breast cancer at different stages of disease progression when reported to the Cancer Registry, England and Wales, 1975–80. Note that cancer is a 'notifiable' disease and cases must be registered soon after the diagnosis is made. Stage I cancers are small tumours confined to the breast, Stage IV cancers have already spread to distant organs, and Stages II and III are intermediate. (Source: Cancer Research Campaign, 1991, Breast Cancer, Factsheet 6.2, CRC, London, Figure 5)*

of stages and survival rates from cancers detected through screening with those detected by other means. However, they warned that three different types of bias could enhance the *apparent* effectiveness of screening.

☐ What were they?

■ *Length-time bias* occurs because screening is likely to pick up a disproportionate number of slowly-growing cancers with a good prognosis, creating the false impression that screening-detected patients have a better outcome; *selection bias* arises because people who attend voluntarily for screening tend to have youth and education on their side, which may also improve their chance of survival; and *lead-time bias* results from moving the date of diagnosis earlier without altering the date of death.

Lead-time bias is the most important of the three and may need further explanation. Follow-up studies of survival such as the one shown in Figure 9.5 do not necessarily mean that earlier diagnosis and treatment *cause* longer survival. For example it is known that earlier (pre-symptomatic) diagnosis of lung cancer through detection of cancer cells in sputum or X-rays does not alter the inexorable progression of the disease or the patient's prognosis. Earlier diagnosis from screening would merely label people as ill earlier, without bestowing any benefit on their actual survival, but it creates the illusion that screening-detected cancers have a better prognosis because the period between diagnosis and death is increased. It is essential to exclude this bias when evaluating a screening programme, including one for breast cancer.

All screening tests, mammography included, are evaluated to assess the extent to which they actually detect the disease or risk factor which they claim to measure. Two questions are important:

1   Is the test **sensitive** (that is, does mammography detect *all* breast cancers reliably)?

2   Is the test **specific** (that is, does mammography *only* detect actual breast cancers)?

A screening test that is insufficiently *sensitive* would result in **false negatives** (in this case, failure to detect actual breast cancers), with obvious consequences for treatment delay. The consequences of a test that is inadequately *specific*—the detection of changes in the breast which are falsely attributed to breast cancer, or **false positives**—are quite as serious, since the usual treatment for a condition labelled as breast cancer is surgical removal of all or part of the breast (mastectomy or lumpectomy). Sensitivity and specificity are not truly independent of one another; usually improving the sensitivity automatically makes a test less specific, and vice versa. There is thus a 'trade off' between the two.

The sensitivity of mammography is about 95 per cent on average (in 1992) for women screened for the first time—that is about 5 per cent of results are false negatives. Thus, if 10 000 women were screened and 100 of them actually had breast cancer, you would expect the test on average to miss five of these cancers.

The specificity of mammography is currently also about 95 per cent, that is about 5 per cent of results among women without breast cancer are false positives.

□ If 10 000 women were screened and 100 actually had breast cancer, how many false positives would you expect?

■ 9 900 women don't have breast cancer, but 5 per cent of them will *appear* to have breast cancer, falsely detected by mammography. This produces 495 false positive results.

In practice, mammography is not used on its own, otherwise there would be too many (in this case nearly 500) unnecessary mastectomies. Positive mammographic findings give rise to further tests, in which small samples (biopsy) of the detected lump undergo microscopic investigation in order to distinguish between false and real positives. However, a biopsy often causes serious anxiety for women, who receive notification of a possible positive result, a request for a repeat visit, and a small operation. Repeating the test at fixed intervals can increase the specificity of mammography, often to as high as 99 per cent. But sensitivity and specificity are not the only criteria by which a screening test should be judged.

□ From the article by La Vecchia *et al.*, can you remember other important criteria?

■ It must be acceptable, convenient, safe and painless, affordable by society, and the benefits must outweigh the costs.

The uptake rate for most breast-screening programmes is between about 60–90 per cent, depending on age (older women are less likely to accept an invitation to be screened), social class, publicity and other factors, for example, the extent to which the programme is seen as an essential part of healthy living. Mammography can be inconvenient because women have to travel to the screening centre, take their clothes off and undergo an uncomfortable and somewhat undignified procedure, but it is acceptable to most women. What remains is to establish whether mammography actually prolongs survival.

The article by La Vecchia *et al.* reviews non-randomised methods of evaluating the effectiveness of a screening programme but points out that, despite their cost in time and money, randomised controlled trials (RCTs) have the greatest potential to settle the question. By the early 1990s, four RCTs of breast-cancer screening programmes had taken place, involving about 300 000 women who were followed for ten years or more. In all these trials there were around 30 per cent fewer deaths from breast cancer among the screened groups in women over age 50, with most of this difference being observed after the programme had been operating for five years. However, the true effect on mortality of the programme outside experimental settings has yet to be fully assessed. The quantitative improvement in survival was not seen among younger women, probably because mammography cannot distinguish a possible tumour from their more dense breast tissue, and because ten years was not enough time for cancers to develop in these younger women.

Table 9.4 Cost per quality-adjusted life year (QALY) for different health interventions, updated to 1993 prices using NHS price index

Health intervention	Cost per QALY (£)
10 years oestrogen replacement therapy for hysterectomised women with severe menopausal symptoms	200
advice by GP to stop smoking	300
10 years oestrogen replacement therapy for hysterectomised women with mild menopausal symptoms	500
10 years combined replacement therapy (oestrogen with progesterone) for women with mild menopausal symptoms	900
coronary artery bypass graft for severe angina with left main coronary artery disease	1 750
action by GP to control hypertension (high blood pressure)	2 850
prophylactic treatment of hysterectomised women (no menopausal symptoms) for 15 years with oestrogen replacement therapy	3 450
coronary artery bypass graft for moderate angina with disease in three coronary arteries	3 800
breast-cancer screening programme	5 550
heart transplantation	8 350

Source: Daly, E. *et al.* (1993) Hormone replacement therapy in a risk-benefit perspective, paper delivered at the 7th International Congress on the Menopause, Stockholm, June.

Effectiveness at saving lives among women aged over 50 does not, in itself, ensure that such a screening programme will be adopted. Analysis of the financial costs coupled with the benefits in quality and quantity of life, give rise to a rough estimate of around £5 550 per quality adjusted life year (QALY) gained through breast-cancer screening.[14] This method of reducing the toll of disease is towards the expensive end of the spectrum of interventions for which similar data exist, as Table 9.4 shows.

Screening represents the current 'best hope' for the prevention of *advanced* breast cancer, but it cannot prevent women from *getting* breast cancer. This short case study serves as a reminder that screening has costs as well as benefits, which must be carefully weighed against each other before the decision to start a new screening programme is taken.

The ideology of sickness, disease prevention and health promotion

In the final part of this chapter, we take a step back from the detailed analysis of methods of prevention and promotion to ask 'Who is responsible for protecting the nation's health?' and 'Can interference with individual freedoms be justified in preventing disease?'

These questions flow from divergent assumptions about the origins of ill-health that can currently be distinguished in society. One type of approach assumes that the *individual* is responsible for his or her own health: it follows that the prevention of disease and the promotion of health are a consequence of individual behaviour, *voluntarily* chosen, but stimulated and encouraged by relevant health education. In this version, people are left essentially free to choose their *lifestyle* and hence their level of health. At the opposite extreme, the agencies of the *state* are held to be responsible for the nation's health: they can enforce healthier choices upon the population by *statutory* means (such as legislation enforcing the wearing of seat-belts, or banning smoking in public buildings), and sustain a health-promoting social, physical and economic *environment* through a network of public-health, fiscal and other policies. Somewhere between the two is an approach that incorporates elements of both individual and state action.

In practice, preventive measures directed at the individual and at the environment often blend into one another: a ban on smoking in public places not only compels individual smokers to change their behaviour, but also enforces a healthier environment for non-smokers. But an excessive emphasis on one or other ideology raises particular dilemmas for the individual and the state.

[14]QALYs are discussed in the article in *Health and Disease: A Reader* (revised edition 1994) by Alan Williams, 'Priority setting in the NHS', which was set reading for Chapter 3 of this book.

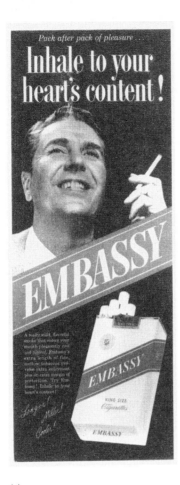

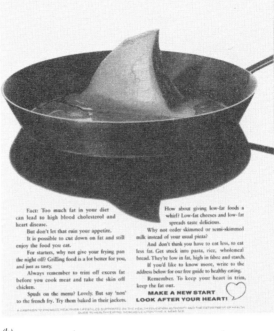

(a)

(b)

Changing messages about lifestyle and heart disease.
(a) 1949 Embassy cigarette advertisement; the small print made
an oblique reference to health risks by claiming that the brand
provided 'an extra margin of protection'. (b) 1990s poster
produced by the Health Education Authority as part of their
'Look after your heart' campaign. The complex relationship
between smoking, dietary fats and heart disease is analysed in
Chapter 10 of this book. (Photos: (a) Advertising Archives;
(b) Health Education Authority)

Individual behaviour

One reason that health is widely seen as dependent on individual behaviour is that many epidemiologists and doctors believe 'lifestyle' to be a major determinant of the chronic diseases which are now the most important causes of death in Western industrialised countries.[15] Accordingly, individual responsibility for health has been emphasised by health-education campaigns sponsored by government agencies such as the Health Education Authority. This is illustrated more fully in Chapter 10, which takes CHD as a case study and examines the contribution of lifestyle factors (such as smoking and high-fat diets) which have been prominently featured in health-education campaigns.

The 'messages' carried by health-education campaigns are determined partly by the statistical probability of a given risk (thus cigarette packets carry explicit warnings about the risks of smoking), partly by the cost-effectiveness of a preventive measure (distributing leaflets and free hypodermic needles to injecting-drug users is cheaper than treating them for AIDS), and partly by public perceptions of what constitutes a serious health problem (action to educate children about the dangers of solvent abuse has popular support).

The success of these campaigns in changing individual behaviour is subject to complex influences. These include lay beliefs about the causes of illness and lay perceptions of the level of health risk associated with a given behaviour.

---

[15]An analysis of the extent to which differences in individual lifestyle factors such as smoking, alcohol consumption, exercise, etc. can explain differences in patterns of chronic disease can be found in *World Health and Disease,* Chapter 10.

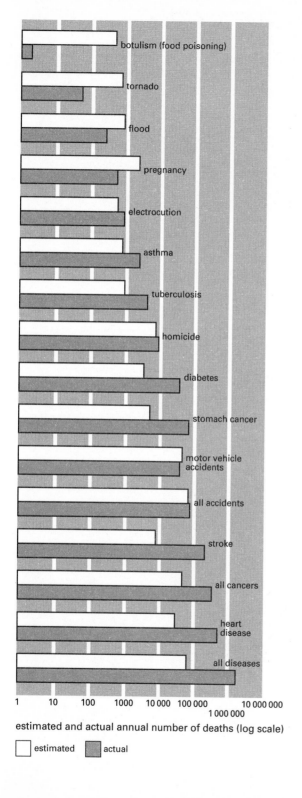

estimated and actual annual number of deaths (log scale)

☐ estimated ▨ actual

□ What does Figure 9.6 suggest might be a barrier to convincing people to change health-damaging behaviour?

■ People tend to *under*estimate the health risks of common everyday activities such as smoking or crossing a road, while *over*estimating the likelihood of major disasters such as plane crashes or mass food poisoning. This has implications for disease-prevention and health-promotion measures that depend on individual behaviour change, since if people perceive the risk of a particular health problem to be remote, they are unlikely to be motivated to avoid it.

For example, a perception among women that breast cancer is not a significant health risk might mean that uptake of screening would be low (as it is among older women). In a lay person's guide to living with risk, the British Medical Association has suggested that the extent of information available about a particular event influences people's perceptions of the likelihood of such an event occurring. Thus, more media attention to common health risks and less frequent reporting of unusual disasters and accidents, might lead to a shift in public perceptions about the major causes of disease and disability and hence improve the effectiveness of health-education messages.

However, focusing on individual behaviour *alone* is unlikely to be sufficient to abolish gross inequalities in health, even if lay beliefs about health and lifestyle could be radically changed by education. There exist powerful social influences on behaviour which can over-ride belief: for example, most smokers believe that tobacco is damaging to health, but persist in the behaviour. Should we 'blame the victim' if they fall sick, or is there a wider social responsibility?

Socio-economic dimensions

Individuals do not live in isolation: 'individual' behaviour is in reality influenced by the distinctive characteristics of the social group to which each person belongs. Sociologists such as Mildred Blaxter suggest that lay people have sophisticated views of disease causation that are related to their social group, and which in turn influence

Figure 9.6 *Relationship between estimated and actual number of deaths per year in the USA from selected causes. (Data from Lichtenstein et al., 1978, adapted from British Medical Association, 1990,* The BMA Guide to Living with Risk, *Penguin, London, p. 232)*

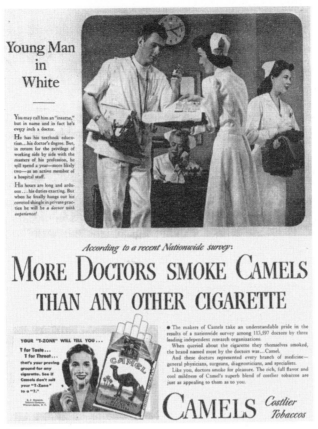

(a)

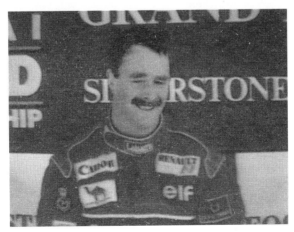

(b)

Figure 9.7 (referred to on p. 162) *The influence of commercial pressures. (a) The prestige of the medical profession was used to promote Camels in the USA in the 1950s. (b) Sports personalities carry similar prestige in the 1990s. BBC television shows Nigel Mansell wearing the Camel and Labatts lager logos at the end of the Silverstone British Grand Prix, 1991. (Photos: (a) Advertising Archives; (b) Health Education Authority, 1992,* Tobacco and the BBC, *photo 15, p. 11)*

their health and illness behaviour.[16] For example, according to the results of a national survey she published in 1990, people from working-class backgrounds are less likely to attribute illness to the state of their local environment, housing, workplace and income than are middle-class people, despite the fact that they are more at risk from adverse social conditions. Major differences exist not only in health status, but in the uptake of preventive services between different socio-economic groups. In addition, the influence of low income and other sources of stress arising from poor social circumstances, may conspire to make 'healthier' lifestyles (e.g. stopping smoking, eating more vegetables and fruit) difficult to sustain or afford.[17]

The social climate in which individuals make health choices can also be influenced by powerful commercial interests, which (for example) promote products such as tobacco and alcohol as socially desirable even though they are detrimental to health (see Figure 9.7 on p.161).

Some public-health activists, pointing to the clear association between poverty and ill-health, argue that only income redistribution and major legislative measures to alleviate social deprivation and improve environmental conditions will significantly improve the population's health. Such a strategy could have unforeseen consequences for economic growth (see Chapter 11 of this book).

Environmental dimensions

Environmental hazards can pose major threats to health. The area of most obvious state involvement in protecting and promoting the nation's health is in environmental-health legislation.

□ Can you suggest examples of environmental-health measures requiring statutory enforcement?

■ The range of possibilities is enormous: e.g. legislation to regulate levels of pollution in drinking water, or to add fluoride; inspection of catering establishments, poultry flocks and abattoirs; regulation of levels of pollutants in vehicle and factory exhaust gases; banning stubble-burning after grain harvests; regulations on the disposal or storage of

[16]Mildred Blaxter discusses her research in a television programme for Open University students, 'Why me? Why now?', associated with *Medical Knowledge: Doubt and Certainty* (revised edition 1994).

[17]This is discussed further in *World Health and Disease*, Chapter 10, and in an audiotape for Open University students entitled 'Smoking and women's health'.

toxic waste; safety standards enforced in workplaces, public buildings and utilities, and local-authority housing. You may have thought of many others.

Such legislation covers hazards that have already been identified, but environmental changes can have unforeseen consequences for health which come to light only after some time, as a report commissioned by the King's Fund highlighted:

> …new methods of food production, aimed at increasing efficiency and profitability, have not only increased the risks of contamination with such well-recognised micro-organisms as salmonellae but may also have exposed us to new hazards such as the agent of bovine spongiform encephalopathy [BSE, or 'mad cow' disease]. (Jacobson, Smith and Whitehead, 1991, p. 3)

Another example is the predicted increase in the incidence of skin cancers as the ozone layer in the atmosphere is progressively damaged and gives less protection from ultraviolet radiation. Measures to reduce the incidence of morbidity and mortality from skin cancers could entail action at the levels of both the state and the individual.

□ Can you suggest what these might entail?

■ Statutory measures to stop emission of gases (for example, from refrigerators and aerosol sprays) that damage the ozone layer; and voluntary reduction in sunbathing and the increased use of effective sunscreens.

These examples raise the dilemma of how far we are prepared to go to develop effective prevention strategies for threats to health that we are unable fully to evaluate. Can we foresee a time when there would be a public consensus to ban sunbathing, as there is currently for the ban on smoking in underground trains? Where would you draw the line between health promotion and infringement of civil liberty?

Conclusion

Providing health care is expensive and as each decade passes it absorbs increasing amounts of human and financial resource. Moreover, avoidable illness causes avoidable suffering. We know enough about the causes of some common diseases and disabilities to reduce these burdens by devising strategies for their prevention (or at least their reduction), but this requires a considerable shift in emphasis in government and local-authority policies directed at social and environmental change, as well as supporting changes in individual behaviour.

Since the late nineteenth century, enormous advances have been made in preventing infectious diseases and promoting greater health, largely through public-health legislation, immunisation programmes and improved standards of living.[18] The next century faces us with the challenge of reducing the incidence of those avoidable or deferrable diseases and disabilities that are at least in part a consequence of industrialisation and patterns of employment and income, as well as individual behaviour. Should we continue to expect advances in medical technology to provide cures, or redirect our efforts into disease prevention and health promotion? That choice returns us to the dilemma with which we began this chapter: where resources are finite and insufficient to meet present demands from those who are already sick, should we divert funds to pursue the goal of optimal health for those who are well?

[18]See *World Health and Disease,* Chapter 6 and the associated articles by Thomas McKeown and Simon Szreter in *Health and Disease: A Reader,* (McKeown's article is included in both the 1984 and 1994 editions; Szreter's only in 1994).

OBJECTIVES FOR CHAPTER 9

When you have studied this chapter you should be able to:

9.1   Distinguish between primary, secondary and tertiary levels of disease prevention and give examples of each.

9.2   Compare and contrast strategies for disease prevention and health promotion that focus either on individual behavioural change or on the wider social, economic and physical environment.

9.3   Discuss the difficulties inherent in evaluating the effectiveness of preventive interventions, including screening.

9.4   Identify and discuss the criteria for a cost-effective screening programme.

9.5   Illustrate the principal economic, social and ethical dilemmas raised by shifting the balance of health care away from curative medicine, towards disease prevention and health promotion.

QUESTIONS FOR CHAPTER 9

Question 1 (*Objective 9.1*)

Categorise the following interventions into primary, secondary or tertiary levels of disease prevention:

(a)   A kidney transplant for someone with kidney failure

(b)   Protective clothing for workers handling asbestos

(c)   Vitamin supplements for pregnant women

(d)   Rubella (german measles) immunisations for schoolgirls

(e)   Free eye-testing for pensioners

Question 2 (*Objective 9.2*)

The 1992 White Paper *The Health of the Nation* sets out the government's strategy for improving the standard of nutrition in the British population:

> • continue and enhance research into the links between diet and health, and into influences on consumer choice;

• continue to secure expert advice on nutrition and health;

• continue national surveillance of diet, nutrition and health of the population;

• seek ways of improving and targeting information and advice on healthy eating and weight control;

• seek ways of improving information on the nutritional content of food;

• produce and disseminate voluntary nutritional guidelines for catering outlets.

(Department of Health, 1992, p. 53)

What does this strategy reveal about the government's view of the causes of diet-related illness and where the principal responsibility lies for promoting nutritional health?

Question 3 (*Objective 9.3*)

Lead pollution has been implicated in a reduction in children's performance in intelligence tests. Describe the most reliable method available *in theory* for evaluating the effect on IQ (intelligence quotient) of reducing lead pollution by providing a price incentive to buy lead-free petrol, and explain the problems inherent in using such a method *in practice*.

Question 4 (*Objective 9.4*)

At the time of writing in 1992, free NHS screening for breast cancer in the United Kingdom is offered only to women between the ages of 50 and 65, at intervals of three years. Which criteria for screening programmes have been involved in determining this pattern of service provision?

Question 5 (*Objective 9.5*)

John Stuart Mill, the English nineteenth-century philosopher and social reformer, wrote:

> The only purpose for which power can rightfully be exercised over any member of a civilised society is to prevent harm to others. His own good, either physical or moral, is not a sufficient warrant. (Mill, 1859, cited in Gray, 1979, p. 157)

What dilemma does Mill's philosophy raise in relation to the banning of smoking in all public places?

10 Coronary heart disease: a cautionary tale

Coronary heart disease (CHD) is discussed in different contexts in other books in this series.[1] Here CHD is used as a case study exemplifying a number of the dilemmas raised in earlier chapters of this book. We assume a familiarity with the incidence of CHD in the British population in the 1980s, and with conflicting explanations for its unequal distribution across different social groups, as discussed in World Health and Disease, Chapters 9 and 10. You should also be aware of the difficulties in demonstrating an association between Western diets and heart disease from Chapter 11 of that book.

This chapter was written by Richard Holmes, a Senior Lecturer in the Biology Department of The Open University, who has a long-term interest in potential links between diet and health.

Why 'a cautionary tale'?

Up to now in this book we have considered the dilemmas inherent in many different aspects of health care, including evaluation of interventions and outcomes, the adoption of medical innovations, screening, and disease prevention. Faced with limited resources, choices have to be made between these various options: money spent on surgery is not available for health education and so on. Sometimes such choices may be relatively easy to make. For example, as you learnt in the previous chapter, the medical treatment of lung cancer is largely ineffective, but epidemiological studies have shown that around 90 per cent of cases are associated with smoking tobacco; in this case the rational approach is to reduce tobacco consumption rather than invest more resources in treatment.

However, for other diseases, the most appropriate forms of intervention are not so clear-cut. This is true of several of the conditions responsible for much of the mortality, morbidity and disability in industrialised countries. How do we make rational choices when treatments have not been adequately evaluated, and the causes of the condition are not fully known? How should doctors, health-service managers, health educators, central government and the public proceed in such circumstances? To illustrate the dilemmas arising from these questions, we shall take coronary heart disease (CHD) as a case study.

Since World War II, coronary heart disease has occupied a high public profile. In 1990 in the United Kingdom, it accounted for about 94 000 deaths among men and 76 000 among women. Six thousand hospital beds are in constant use by sufferers of this condition, while the lives of tens of thousands are restricted by its disabling symptoms.

A disease which is so important, both as a cause of premature death and as the major killer of the over-75s, has inevitably engendered calls for effective action, as well as a great deal of anxiety among the 'worried well'. Indeed, so great are people's fears of a heart attack that some are prepared to make radical changes in their lifestyle in the hope of avoiding a disease whose impact has been likened to plague. Innovations in surgery, screening for early diagnosis, and preventive strategies all have had their advocates, many of whom are highly committed to their own particular approach and dismissive of all others—the debate is quite acrimonious at times,

[1]Medical understanding of the heart from ancient times to the present day is described in *Medical Knowledge: Doubt and Certainty* (revised edition, 1994). *World Health and Disease* also contains relevant information (see above). The interaction of multiple contributory factors in heart disease is discussed in *The Biology of Health and Disease* (1985), and also in the revised edition of that book, *Human Biology and Health: An Evolutionary Approach* (1994).

despite, or perhaps because of, the considerable uncertainty that surrounds many aspects of CHD. Thus, although CHD has been declining in the United Kingdom since 1978, any new development in treatment, or new outcome of a research trial, has for many years been newsworthy and vigorously promoted in the media.[2]

The by-pass road to recovery

Coronary artery by-pass grafts are the sort of operation doctors would like to see more people with heart disease undergo. A meeting organised last week recommended that an extra 10,000 sufferers a year should be offered the operation. (Olivia Timbs and Lorraine Fraser, 1984, *The Times,* November 27)

Eat less salt to save 40,000 deaths a year

Eating half a teaspoonful of salt less a day would save one in six from heart disease, one in five from a stroke and one in two from needing blood pressure drugs. (Dr K. C. Hotchin and David Fletcher, 1991, *Daily Telegraph,* April 5)

Scanner may end heart deaths

Coronary artery disease, which claims 180,000 lives a year, may be practically eliminated by new screening techniques and drug treatments, a leading heart specialist said yesterday. Mobile scanning trailers similar to those used by mass X-ray screening for tuberculosis could be introduced to provide early diagnosis, he suggested. (Nicholas Timmins, 1984, *The Times,* September 21)

Cholesterol Risks 'Underestimated'

The risk of death in middle age from high blood cholesterol was being dangerously underestimated because results of trials were misleading, Dr Rory Collins of Oxford University claimed yesterday. Some scientists believed this to be 'one of the most damaging false negative results in the history of medical statistics', he said. (Christine McGourty, 1992, *Daily Telegraph,* 30 May)

The persistent chorus of 'certain' voices has often drowned out discussion of the uncertainties about CHD. The discussion here may convince you that it is indeed 'a cautionary tale'.

The background to the CHD dilemma

Up to the mid-1960s, CHD presented a frightening and rapidly growing problem for the population of the West, but it did not really pose a health care *dilemma* (i.e. an uncomfortable choice between problematic alternatives). There was almost no active treatment other than bedrest, and therefore no difficult choices to make. The only controversy was whether people should exercise after recovery from a heart attack, or lead the quietest possible life. Intervention—primary, secondary or tertiary—was not an issue, although even in the late 1930s a few medical physiologists were suggesting that people with a family history of CHD should eat a low-salt, low-fat diet and exercise every day. However, trials were not conducted to evaluate whether this strategy was in reality effective, and there was no medical consensus.

However, new treatments for those suffering from CHD were being vigorously pursued, and in the late 1950s the use of the anti-coagulant substance *dicoumerol* (previously marketed as the rat poison Warfarin), was prescribed to protect against repeat attacks. It was considered a breakthrough, and indeed is still used quite extensively, but research studies showed that it had little impact on CHD mortality, and after a major trial by the Medical Research Council in the 1960s, it was accepted that anti-coagulants were not the answer to the problem.

So while the pressure continued to find more effective *treatments*, there was a growing conviction that the only real answer would be found in *prevention*. Through the late 1960s and 1970s, medical and scientific opinion became increasingly convinced that CHD was primarily a disease of Western affluence caused by the Western diet and, in particular, the consumption of saturated fat. Proving this became a major focus of medical research.

Meanwhile, new and more effective treatments were being developed, notably surgery to by-pass blocked coronary arteries, probes manipulated within the arteries, drugs to dissolve blood clots, and the establishment of specialised coronary care units. Most of these were, and remain, expensive and in the United Kingdom, where government spending on health care is relatively low compared with that in most other Western economies,[3] this led to a dilemma about resource allocation by the early 1980s. Clearly, if the link between CHD and diet was as strong as many believed, resources focused on a large primary prevention campaign could have a significant effect on both health and health-care spending. If it were not, then such a campaign would not only be a huge

---

[2] See also the news report of 'clot-busting drugs' in Chapter 1 of this book.

[3] See *Caring for Health: History and Diversity* (revised edition, 1993), Chapter 9.

waste of resources, but could also raise public scepticism about health education in general. What was needed was reliable information on the effectiveness of both the primary prevention approach, and the various treatments for existing disease.

Although considerable resources have been committed to both approaches in the West since the early 1980s, at the time of writing in 1993 there is still no consensus on the most effective strategy for reducing the burden of CHD. Hence the dilemma.

What is CHD?

Biomedical definitions

The term *coronary* heart disease or CHD (from the Latin for 'a crown', so named because the arteries encircle the heart) and *ischaemic* heart disease or IHD (from the Greek verb 'to restrict') are used in this chapter to describe the same phenomenon. Ischaemic heart disease is a condition in which the heart muscle, or part of it, receives an insufficient blood supply—and thus *oxygen* supply—to continue to function. This is most commonly due to obstruction or spasm of the coronary arteries, and in this case the condition may also be described as **coronary heart** (or artery) **disease**. Here, we use the term CHD except when citing research in which the authors referred to IHD.

An important cause of the insufficient blood supply is a narrowing of the coronary arteries by fatty deposits, known as *atheromas* (also sometimes called *plaques*). These may start to form in childhood, and are probably present in most adults, but only give rise to symptoms if the bore of the inside of the arteries become considerably narrowed—a condition known as *atherosclerosis*. The symptoms of CHD are also thought on occasion to result from *spasm* (sustained contraction) of the muscle in the arterial wall.

There are two main coronary arteries, the right and the left (see Figure 10.1), but the left divides into two major branches (the circumflex branch and the left anterior descending branch), so the blood supply to the heart muscle travels in *three* major blood vessels. As you will see later, the number of diseased vessels has a significant effect on treatment outcome.

CHD affects people in three different ways. First, it may cause sudden death if the blood supply to the heart muscle stops, often but not always, as a result of *thrombosis* (a blood clot or *thrombus* attached to an atheroma blocking an artery). Sudden coronary death sometimes

occurs without a clot being present, usually because irritation from an atheroma interferes with the coordinated rhythm of contraction of the heart muscle, causing the heart to stop pumping altogether. Second, it may

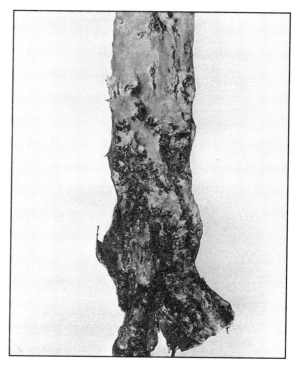

Atherosclerosis in a major artery. (Photo: Department of Pathology, Edinburgh University)

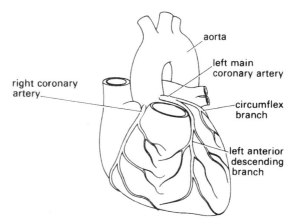

Figure 10.1 *Anatomy of the heart showing the two main coronary arteries (right and left) and the two branches of the left main coronary artery.*

cause a *myocardial infarction* in which a portion of heart muscle (myocardium) is permanently damaged by lack of oxygen. This may lead to death, though in most cases the person recovers. These first two consequences of CHD are often referred to as **heart attacks.** Third, it may cause *angina* (chest pain) which, if severe and frequent, can lead to considerable disability. This appears to be caused by partial spasm of the coronary artery walls, resulting from damage and irritation by local atheromas.

Epidemiological distribution

CHD began to be described in the medical literature as a significant cause of death in 1925 and, while other diseases of the circulation gradually declined in fatality, the incidence of CHD rose strongly through the 1930s, 1940s and into the 1950s.

Although CHD is the commonest cause of death among males in most industrialised countries, there are marked international differences in mortality rates (see Figure 10.2). This phenomenon may partly be due to

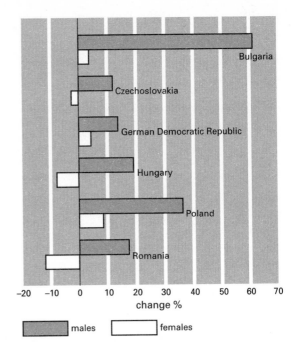

Figure 10.3 *Change in heart disease mortality, 1970–85. Age-standardised rates for people aged 30–69 years in selected Eastern European countries. (Source: Davey Smith, G. and Marmot, M., 1991, (Suppl) Trends in Mortality in* Britain, Annals of Nutrition and Metabolism, *pp. 61–2)*

variations in diagnostic criteria, but it is accepted that underlying differences in the national incidences of CHD exist.

Figure 10.2 raises some intriguing questions. What has accounted for the marked decline in the USA since the 1960s? Why did the decline in the United Kingdom not start until about 1978? And why are Japanese rates so low? We return to these questions later in the chapter when discussing strategies for prevention. The picture is very different in Eastern Europe, where CHD mortality is rapidly rising (see Figure 10.3).

In many ways the Eastern European pattern resembles that of the United Kingdom between 1920 and 1940. It may be that Eastern Europe is now going through a similar *epidemiologic transition* to that seen earlier in the United Kingdom, and more markedly in the USA and Australia. Whether the Western experience can be used to speed this transition remains to be seen.

The treatment of CHD

The treatment of CHD has three main objectives. The first is prevention of death immediately after a heart attack. This involves giving drugs that strengthen and regulate

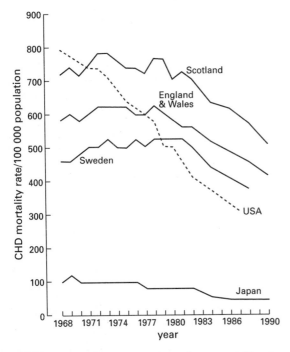

Figure 10.2 *Trends in coronary heart disease mortality rates for men aged 35–74 years (age-standardised rates per 100 000 population), in selected industrialised countries, 1968–90. (Sources:1968–82, U205 Course Team (1985)* Caring for Health: Dilemmas and Prospects, The Open University Press, Milton Keynes, Figure 10.2, p. 167. 1983, *personal communication, and for 1983–90 from World* Health Organisation, annual publications, 1984–91, World Health Statistics, WHO, Geneva)

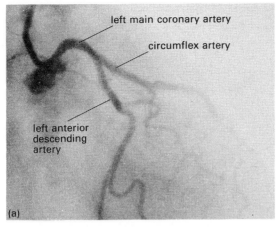 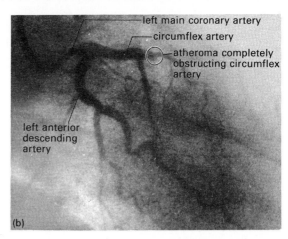

(a)

(b)

Figure 10.4 *Coronary angiograms showing (a) a normal left coronary artery and (b) one in which the circumflex branch is completely obstructed by atheromas.*

the heartbeat, or that inhibit further clotting and (in recent years) 'digest' clots, and life-support procedures such as intravenous fluids and oxygen. However, intensive treatment helps only a minority of patients to survive. It has been estimated that, until the late 1980s, and the arrival of more effective drugs, less than 5 per cent of people benefitted from being admitted to an intensive care unit rather than simply being nursed in their own home. This is primarily because most deaths occur in the first two hours after a heart attack—before it is usually possible to get someone into intensive care—and, if a person has already survived that long, they usually stand a good chance of recovery wherever they are subsequently treated.

The second objective is the prevention of further heart attacks, thus prolonging the lives of people who are already suffering from CHD. This can involve drugs or surgery.

The third objective is to alleviate the disabling symptoms of severe angina. For most people this is attempted with drug treatment, but for the most seriously disabled, surgery is becoming increasingly popular.

It is not possible, or appropriate, to discuss all the available treatments in detail in this chapter, so we will consider one well-established surgical treatment in some detail to illustrate the difficulties of evaluating effectiveness, and then briefly consider two other approaches.

Coronary artery by-pass grafting

The use of surgery to relieve angina is not new, but was not very effective until about 1965, when it became technically possible to produce accurate images of the coronary arteries and pin-point the exact location of obstructions in the blood supply to the heart. The

technique is called *coronary angiography:* a dye that is relatively opaque to X-rays is injected into the coronary arteries so that the vessels show up on an X-ray film (or angiogram, see Figure 10.4).

This newly-acquired imaging technique enabled American surgeons to develop **coronary artery by-pass grafting (CABG**, often referred to by doctors as 'cabbage') in the late 1960s and early 1970s. The aim of CABG is to relieve angina and reduce the risk of a heart attack in people with severely blocked coronary arteries. Obstructions in the coronary arteries are by-passed by grafting on a piece of blood vessel obtained from elsewhere in the patient's body, usually a vein from the leg (see Figure 10.5). CABG is a major operation, in which the chest wall is opened and the heart is temporarily stopped from beating.

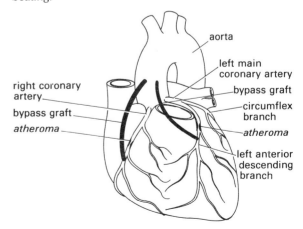

Figure 10.5 *Heart and coronary arteries showing the position of atheromas and two by-pass grafts in position.*

The new operation proved to be highly effective in relieving the disabling symptoms of angina. About 90 per cent of angina sufferers gain immediate relief from the operation, although some relapse each year. Ten years after surgery, 50 per cent of patients are still free of pain. Given the high prevalence of CHD, it is perhaps not surprising that CABG became the biggest 'growth industry' in surgery in the USA between 1970 and 1990, by which date more than 250 000 by-pass operations were performed each year.

CABG also *appeared* to increase life expectancy, but how effective is it? There is still considerable debate about its effect on survival. The issue was studied in three major *randomised controlled trials* (RCTs) between 1977 and 1983, two in the USA and one in Europe, in which CABG was compared with medical (drug) treatment. The results were conflicting, but suggested that the effectiveness of surgery depends on the exact location, extent and number of obstructions in the coronary arteries. For example, there was agreement that surgery improves survival if there is an obstruction only in the left main coronary artery, before it branches into two (see Figure 10.6).

However, only about six per cent of CABG patients have an obstruction in the left main coronary artery. In most patients the obstructions are further down, in the anterior descending and circumflex branches of the left main artery, and in the right main artery (see Figures 10.1 and 10.4). In these patients the results of the RCTs were

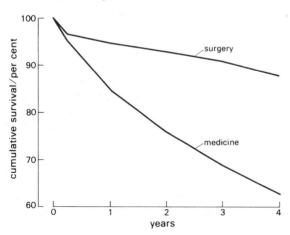

Figure 10.6 *Cumulative survival with CABG and with medical treatment in people with disease of the left main coronary artery. Based on 1 492 patients. The difference between the two treatments is highly statistically significant. (Source: Chaitman, B. R. et al., 1981, Effect of coronary bypass surgery on survival patterns,* American Journal of Cardiology, **48***, p. 767)*

less clear-cut, and the most recent (CASS, 1983, which cost $24 million) showed no improvement in survival after CABG compared with drug treatment.

Difficulties in evaluating the effectiveness of CABG are similar to those found in evaluating other complex surgical procedures.

☐ Why do you think evaluation is so difficult?

■ It is difficult to ensure that patients in the surgical groups are actually receiving the same treatment. There are inevitable variations in the skill and technique of surgical teams supposedly doing the same operation; differences in other interventions performed in parallel (e.g. drug treatments); and differences in post-operative care. (Indeed, in the USA the early evaluations of CABG showed that the mortality from the operation itself varied between hospitals from 1.5 to 29 per cent!)

Henry Aaron and William Schwartz (whose research, published in 1984, was discussed in Chapter 3) estimated that about 5 per cent of people given CABG operations in the USA in 1979 would have died without the surgery. About 250 000 CABG operations were performed annually in the USA in the 1980s, so even a critical assessment such as this suggests a more than negligible saving of lives, plus thousands of people relieved of severe angina. However, when viewed in the context of about 1.25 million deaths a year from CHD in the USA, the contribution of CABG to overall survival is slight.

In the United Kingdom, where the CABG rate in 1990 was about one-fifth of that in the USA (1 400 operations per million population in the USA; 286 per million in the United Kingdom, see Figure 10.7), the contribution of CABG in reducing mortality has been even less significant. For example, in England and Wales in 1991, the rate of CABG was approximately 28 operations per 100 000 population, but the crude mortality from CHD was 450 per 100 000. Furthermore, it does not follow that all those operated on were in immediate danger of losing their lives; many will have had the operation to relieve angina.

Why is the rate of CABG so much higher in the USA than in the United Kingdom? There are two possible reasons. The first concerns the difference in the method of payment for health care between the two countries. As one American cardiologist put it:

> The entrepreneurial aspect of surgery in this country makes it imperative for surgeons to pursue the recruitment of patients aggressively. (Cited in Aaron and Schwartz, 1984, p. 67)

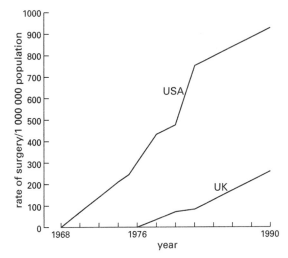

Figure 10.7 *Rate of coronary artery by-pass surgery in the United Kingdom and USA, per million population, 1968–1990. (Source: 1968–82 data from U205 Course Team (1985)* Caring for Health: Dilemmas and Prospects, *The Open University Press, Milton Keynes, Figure 11.6, p. 169. 1990 from British Heart Foundation)*

In contrast, most surgeons in the United Kingdom derive most of their income as salaried employees of the NHS. The second reason is related to the first. The United Kingdom spends a much smaller proportion of its Gross Domestic Product (GDP) on health care (6 per cent in 1990) compared with the USA (around 12 per cent).[4] Costly procedures such as CABG are mainly performed in cash-limited NHS hospitals where the number of operations is restricted (though some occur in the private sector).

Angioplasty and 'clot-busters'

Two product innovations in the treatment of CHD in the 1990s are worth a brief mention, because their adoption and diffusion into medical practice may follow the same pattern seen 20 years earlier for CABG, which they could overtake in popularity.

Angioplasty is a surgical technique for clearing coronary artery obstruction, which does not involve opening the chest wall. A fine tube, with a small inflatable balloon at its top, is inserted into an artery in the groin and then steered into the blocked coronary artery. Manipulation of the tube and inflation of the balloon can dislodge a clot, break up an atheroma or stretch the artery.

[4]International variations in spending on health care are discussed in *Caring for Health: History and Diversity* (revised edition, 1993), Chapter 9.

□ What are the advantages of angioplasty compared with CABG?

■ Much less trauma for the patient (because the chest wall is not opened, and grafts are not taken from other arteries). As a result, the procedure takes less time, and less hospital after-care, so overall costs are lower.

Angioplasty carries some risk, but it seems to prolong survival and reduce angina in a proportion of patients. However, the long-term success rate compared with CABG is not yet clear, and the comparison may be hard to establish because a different type of patient may be selected for each procedure. Despite this uncertainty, the number of operations rose in the USA from a few dozen in 1978 to 150 000 per year in 1988.

The other major development in the treatment of CHD is the **'clot-buster' drugs**, which 'digest' thrombi in the coronary arteries, breaking up the protein *fibrin* which binds the thrombus into a mechanically strong clot. One of these drugs, *streptokinase*, is an enzyme derived quite cheaply from the bacterium *streptococcus*, and given with aspirin, is as effective as more expensive drugs (ISIS, 1992).

Clot-busters are, by definition, only useful when the heart attack involves a blood clot. Such attacks are often very serious, but if the clot can be dissolved within a few hours, the chances of survival are greatly improved. Advocates of 'clot-busters' claim that many lives could be saved if the drug is given to patients very quickly (for example, see the news report in Chapter 1).

The dilemmas of treatment

In a civilised society, should everyone suffering from a potentially fatal disease have access to any effective treatment available? It may seem unacceptable that funds should not be available and that the necessary research to extend and improve such treatments should not be vigorously pursued. Indeed there are regular public calls from both doctors' and patients' organisations for more funds to be made available for treatment, especially CABG and angioplasty, and large sums of charitable money are raised from the public for research into heart disease. Yet both treatment and research are expensive and, as you have seen, have so far had only a very modest effect on the premature mortality caused by CHD. CABG is very costly and is rationed, in part, by waiting lists, which may unfortunately be self-limiting. Angioplasty is less expensive, but only appropriate in certain cases.

Although some of the clot-buster drugs are very expensive, and have been aggressively marketed by drug companies, they seem to be no more effective than cheaper equivalents. But the cost of the drugs is insignificant compared with the potential cost of administering them quickly enough. Ideally, a person trained to make an initial diagnosis and with the necessary resuscitation equipment and drugs to hand, should attend someone whose heart has stopped beating within a few minutes. Costly procedures would be required to achieve this, involving the emergency services, perhaps like those being piloted in some American cities, where paramedical resuscitation teams are deployed by the fire service. In the United Kingdom there have been limited moves in this direction with the installation of resuscitation equipment in some ambulances, and 'fast-track' admissions procedures for suspected coronary thrombosis patients in some hospitals, which have halved the time between the attack and initial treatment.

Thus, active treatment of CHD, whether to save a life or to improve the quality of life, is expensive. In a fee-for-service system where undertaking more medical intervention generates more cash for staff and hospitals, the major limit on treatment is the ability of the population to pay the insurance premiums. In a cash-limited public health system, painful decisions about how much it can afford to develop and administer innovative treatments have to be taken as a matter of strategic policy. It is in this context that a vigorous debate is taking place within the medical profession about the ethics of performing heart surgery on patients who can't or won't stop smoking. The success rate of CABG is lower and the recurrence of problems is higher among smokers, and—given the scarcity of resources—this has led some surgeons to question whether they should treat continuing cigarette-smokers. Other doctors have challenged the ethics of withholding treatment in these circumstances.

Prevention of CHD

From the foregoing discussion you will appreciate why efforts at primary *prevention* of CHD have assumed such importance. The rational way forward seems to be to adopt prevention strategies, if any can be found that actually work. Effective prevention requires a clear understanding of the *causes* of a disease. However, the exact causes of CHD are still far from clear, in spite of the truly enormous sums which have been spent on research since the 1960s. The dilemma here is whether we can justify prevention campaigns despite uncertainty about the causes of CHD. Is action, even if shown subsequently to be misguided in some respects, nonetheless preferable to inaction in the face of such high levels of mortality?

The best epidemiological evidence we can offer at present points to certain major **risk factors for heart disease**—factors which are statisically associated in the population as a whole with a higher incidence of CHD. The six most important risk factors are:

- a family history of CHD;
- being male;
- low social class;
- smoking cigarettes;
- high blood pressure;
- high levels in the blood of some fats, particularly cholesterol.

These factors cannot be seen in isolation from each other; they almost certainly interact in complex ways.

Although it is difficult to change the first three factors in the list, their contribution might be offset if information could be gained about how they cause an increase in risk. But the last three risk factors, sometimes irreverently known as 'the holy trinity of CHD prevention', could in theory be reduced by changes in individual 'lifestyles'. They are also implicated in several other major degenerative diseases, such as strokes and certain cancers. Chapter 9 will have alerted you to the dilemmas inherent in preventing disease by persuading or enabling people to alter their lifestyles.

Lifestyle and CHD

In reviewing the association between smoking, high blood pressure, blood cholesterol and the incidence of CHD, the discussion that follows highlights the nature and extent of the risk posed by each of these factors, and the controversies associated with them.

Smoking

By the 1970s, a strong association between cigarette smoking and CHD had been established (see Figure 10.8). The fact that stopping smoking reduces the risk of CHD strengthened the evidence that the relationship is causal, and further justified an anti-smoking campaign previously directed at preventing lung cancer.

However, the *size* of the CHD risk from smoking may have been overestimated. Research by epidemiologist George Davey Smith and M. J. Shipley, published in 1991, suggested that earlier studies had not made enough allowance for the fact that smokers tend to be in lower social classes—itself a risk factor for CHD (we return to this later in the chapter). On the face of it, the strength of the evidence for a causal connection between smoking

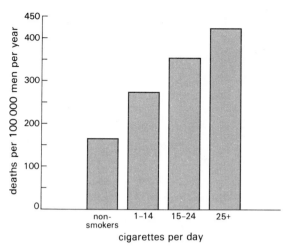

Figure 10.8 *Mortality from CHD in non-smokers and cigarette smokers by level of consumption for men under 65 years. (Source: based on data from Doll, R. and Peto, R., 1976, Mortality in relation to smoking: 20 years' observation on male British doctors,* British Medical Journal, *2, Table III, p. 1527)*

and several serious diseases seems to justify disease prevention campaigns targetted at smokers. In practice, however, radical changes in social and economic structures would be required to support such initiatives.[5]

High blood pressure

The statistical association between high blood pressure (hypertension) and CHD is now well established (see Figure 10.9).

From this association it has been assumed that reduction of blood pressure (whether by drugs, increased exercise, weight loss, reduction in salt or alcohol intake) will lead to a reduction in the incidence of CHD. However, establishing that there is a causal connection has proved to be controversial. Reduction of elevated blood pressure by exercise and by the use of some drugs may lead to a reduction in CHD mortality, but some of the most commonly used drugs do not seem to increase survival. This could in part account for the variable results of several large trials: in general, lowering the above-average blood pressure of whole sections of a community has not led to a significant reduction in CHD mortality. For example, results of a trial lasting almost seven years of drug treatment for hypertension in 4 400 older adults, were published by the Medical Research Council in

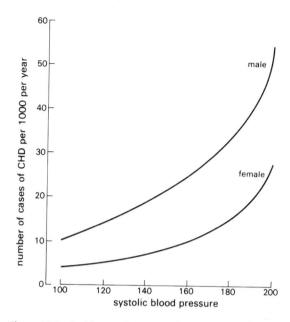

Figure 10.9 *Incidence of CHD in relation to systolic[6] blood pressure, for men and women aged 55–64 years. Annual incidence based on average over a 16-year period following blood pressure measurement being made. (Source: Ball, K.P., 1979,* The Heart Patient I, Epidemiology, *Update Publications, Guildford, Surrey, Figure 9, p. 7)*

1992. As Figure 10.10 (*overleaf*) shows, when blood pressure was reduced to normal levels by *diuretic* drugs (which reduce blood volume and thus blood pressure) there was a significant reduction in 'coronary events', but when it was controlled by two widely used *β-blockers* (which act by slowing the heart and dilating some of the blood vessels), there was no reduction at all. (Indeed, total mortality from all causes rose slightly.)

☐ What purpose was served in the MRC trial by giving one group a placebo for nearly seven years?

■ Administering a sham treatment generally produces some effect not seen in a comparable group of completely untreated people (the *placebo effect*). This may be due to the patient's expectation of benefit and/or to unconscious behavioural changes. Results in the placebo group are an essential 'baseline' against which to evaluate the genuine treatment groups.

---

[5]See Chapter 11 of this book, and the audiotape band 'Smoking and women's health' associated with *World Health and Disease.*

[6]Systolic blood pressure is measured in a main artery (e.g. in the upper arm) when the heart *contracts* and forces blood out; diastolic pressure is measured when the heart relaxes and refills with blood.

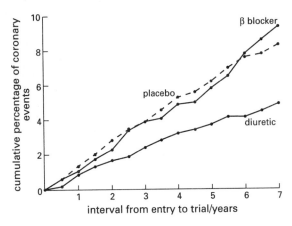

Figure 10.10 *Effects of anti-hypertensive drugs on CHD incidents: cumulative percentage of patients experiencing coronary events by randomised treatment. (Source: Medical Research Council working party, 1992, Medical Research Council Trial of treatment of hypertension in older adults: principal results,* British Medical Journal, ***304**, p. 408)*

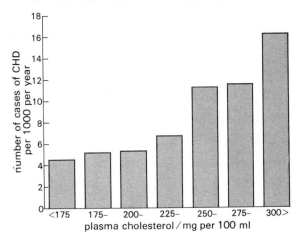

Figure 10.11 *Incidence of CHD in relation to plasma cholesterol level in men aged 30–59 years at entry to study. Incidence based on first major events (myocardial infarctions, sudden deaths) over a 10-year period. 'Plasma cholesterol' refers to initial level. (Source: based on data from Stamler, J. and Epstein, F., 1972, CHD risk factors as guides to preventive action,* Preventive Medicine, ***1**, p. 27)*

R. S. Paffenbarger *et al.* showed in 1986 that men gain some protection against the risk of CHD from taking regular exercise, which also reduces blood pressure. It is not clear, however, whether the reduction in blood pressure is important, as distinct from other possible gains in 'fitness' such as improved circulation and increased strength of the heart. The value of exercise as protection against CHD in women is not yet established, and may be hard to demonstrate because the association between elevated blood pressure and CHD mortality is weaker in women than in men.

There are at least three possible reasons for the very mixed success of programmes to lower blood pressure in reducing CHD mortality. One is that the association is not causal, or only when blood pressure is very high (but this suggestion is undermined by the results of the MRC trial mentioned above). A second reason might be that the damage done by high blood pressure is not usually reversible by treatment. Third, the effect of reducing blood pressure might be small and require larger trials to demonstrate it.

However, reducing hypertension seems to decrease the incidence of stroke[7] in both sexes, more or less independently of the means used to achieve the reduction. So despite some uncertainty about high blood pressure and CHD, there is good reason for GPs to screen their patients for hypertension and attempt to reduce it, whether by

medical treatment or counselling behavioural change. Once again, enabling such changes in lifestyle to be maintained requires more than willpower.

Cholesterol

The most controversial of the 'trinity' of risk factors is high blood cholesterol. Cholesterol is a fat which is, among other things, an important component of most cell membranes and a precursor of certain hormones. It is continuously taken up from the blood and used by the tissues of the body. Normally about 80 per cent of the supply is manufactured by the liver and released into the circulation, and about 20 per cent is obtained directly from the diet.

The association between high blood cholesterol and CHD was established in the early 1970s (see Figure 10.11). At that time and for at least the next decade, the levels of cholesterol in the blood were widely believed to be determined primarily by the amount and type of fat consumed in the diet. In particular, the consumption of fat which is biochemically described as 'saturated'[8] was thought *generally* to lead to higher levels of blood cholesterol. Most animal fats are saturated, many plant oils (e.g.

---

[7]In a stroke, damage to brain tissue results from blockage or rupture of a blood vessel in the brain.

[8]Saturated fats are those in which the chain of carbon atoms that forms the 'backbone' of the molecule cannot accept additional hydrogen atoms; mono-unsaturated fats can accept one hydrogen per carbon atom, and poly-unsaturated fats can accept more than one hydrogens per carbon atom.

sunflower oil) are 'poly-unsaturated' and some (e.g. olive oil) are 'mono-unsaturated'.

In the United Kingdom, the definitive statement is probably that of the (then) Health Education Council's National Advisory Committee on Nutritional Education (NACNE). In 1983, NACNE called for the fat content of the national diet to be reduced from 40 to 30 per cent of total energy intake, of which saturated fats should provide no more than 10 per cent. Caroline Walker and Geoffrey Cannon (the former was the secretary to NACNE) reflect the certainties of the time:

> A high level of cholesterol in the blood is an established cause of heart disease…high blood cholesterol itself is caused by high levels of saturated fat in food. (Walker and Cannon, 1984, p. 6)

As a consequence of this widespread view, strong dietary advice to 'look after your heart' by reducing fat intake has been issued by many official bodies and informal groups (see, for example, the Health Education Authority's 'Kitchen Killer' poster in Chapter 9). Health education campaigns against fats have had a profound effect throughout the Western world on people's perception of what constitutes a 'healthy diet', and have altered the commercial production, processing and marketing of food.

However, there is some doubt about the value of such dietary advice aimed at the whole population. There are very wide variations in the blood cholesterol of individuals, and only those with the highest levels experience higher risks of CHD (see Figure 10.11) and, as you will learn later in the chapter, the risk is far lower for women than for men. Moreover, only a minority of people can alter their blood cholesterol levels significantly by changing their diet, because a feedback system exists in the body which 'tops up' the level of cholesterol in the blood as it gets used—if less is available from the diet, then more will be manufactured in the body.

Recently it has emerged that the association of CHD with blood cholesterol may in fact be with one form of the molecule, cholesterol combined with *low-density lipoprotein* (LDL-cholesterol). LDL-cholesterol in the blood is taken up by macrophages (scavenger white cells) and some smooth muscle cells in the artery walls. The macrophages swell up, taking on a foamy appearance and appear to set up local inflammation, which may give rise to atheromas. Conversely, high levels of cholesterol combined with *high-density lipoproteins* (HDLs) may actually have a *protective* effect against CHD.

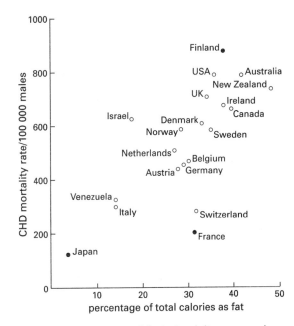

Figure 10.12 *Percentage of the national diet consumed as fat compared to CHD mortality in 20 countries. (Source: Brisson, G., 1982,* Lipids in Human Nutrition, *MTP Press, Toronto, p. 81)*

International comparisons of fat consumption and CHD mortality (see Figure 10.12) do not resolve the issue: the relationship is inconsistent and depends very much on which countries you select.[9]

☐ If you look at those countries in Figure 10.12 in whose national diet 30–40 per cent of calories are obtained from fat, what can you conclude about the association of dietary fat and CHD?

■ That there is no very consistent association—countries with similar intakes of fat may vary in their CHD rates by a factor of four—compare Finland and France for example.

The inconsistency does not, of itself, undermine a possible causal connection between dietary fat and CHD, because the risks posed by a fatty diet could vary depending on other differences between countries (e.g. the extent to which different rates of exercise, alcohol consumption, smoking, etc. interact with diet).

[9]For example, compare Figure 10.12 with Figure 11.3 in *World Health and Disease.*

The trends over time between countries offer little more help. It is argued (though not proven) that the downturn in CHD in the USA and the United Kingdom may have started *after* the eating of saturated fats became an issue. However, the downturn in CHD rates in Finland, Canada and Australia certainly *preceded* any change in the national consumption of fats. And in Japan, fat consumption has *risen* over the last 35 years, almost to Western levels, but CHD mortality has *fallen* and remains lower than in any other developed country (recall Figure 10.2).

Moreover, there have now been numerous intervention trials with high risk groups in the population of several countries (people with two or more risk factors above normal), some of them extensive and enormously expensive, some setting out to reduce multiple risks (smoking, cholesterol, blood pressure), others focusing on cholesterol alone. The results have been variable, and generally inconclusive. In 1992, George Davey Smith and J. Pekkannen surveyed the major primary prevention trials in which blood cholesterol was lowered either by dieting or by drug treatment (see Table 10.1).

☐ From the data in Table 10.1, what were the effects of cholesterol reduction on CHD deaths?

■ Compared with the controls, the intervention group suffered fewer CHD deaths in two out of three diet trials and four out of five drug trials, although the reduction was sometimes very small.

☐ What were the effects of cholesterol reduction on deaths from causes *other than* CHD?

■ In all trials except one (Minnesota Coronary Survey), there were *more* non-CHD deaths in the intervention group.

☐ Taking all causes of death (CHD and non-CHD) what were the overall effects on mortality of reducing cholesterol?

■ In most trials there were only small differences between the intervention group and the controls; in two trials (Finnish Mental Hospital and Colestipol–Upjohn) there were many *fewer* deaths in the intervention group, but in another two trials (WHO and EXCEL) there were many *more* deaths in the intervention group.

In a number of large trials where there was intervention for multiple risks (e.g. smoking and blood pressure as well as cholesterol level), a similar pattern emerges: lowering cholesterol across the board saves some lives from CHD, but raises mortality from other causes, notably cancers and accidental death. A further problem for mass dietary intervention is that a very vigorous, supervised dietary regime is required to produce a significant reduction in CHD. Such a regime may be possible in a trial, but is probably impractical for the population at large.

Table 10.1 Summary of effects on mortality of eight large-scale trials of cholesterol reduction by diet or drug treatment

	No. of participants		Deaths						Years of follow-up
			CHD		Non-CHD		All causes		
	I[1]	C[2]	I	C	I	C	I	C	
Diet trials									
1 VA Diet Study	424	422	41	50	133	127	174	177	8
2 Minnesota Coronary Survey	2 197	2 196	39	34	119	119	158	153	1
3 Finnish Mental Hospital	902	928	34	76	154	141	186	217	6
Drugs trials									
4 WHO Study	5 331	5 296	36	34	92	53	128	87	5
5 Colestipol–Upjohn Study	546	546	9	22	8	5	17	27	2
6 Lipid Research Clinics	1 906	1 900	32	44	36	27	68	71	7
7 Helsinki Heart Study	2 051	2 030	14	19	31	23	45	42	5
extended follow-up			16	28	43	27	59	55	6.5
8 EXCEL	1 663	6 582	n.a.	n.a.	n.a.	n.a.	33	3	1

[1]I = Intervention Group; [2]C = Control Group; n.a. = data not available. (Source: Davey Smith, G. and Pekkannen, J., 1992, Should there be a moratorium on the use of cholesterol lowering drugs?, *British Medical Journal*, **304**, p. 432, Table 1)

The dilemmas arising from all these data are clear enough. In the absence of precise information about each individual's cholesterol levels, and their ability to reduce blood cholesterol by dietary change, should health educators condemn high fat diets 'across the board', or remain silent and be accused of neglecting the nation's health? Should doctors intervene with cholesterol-lowering drugs which might reduce their patient's risk of death from CHD, but increase their risk of death from other causes?

There is certainly a case for advising a large reduction in the dietary intake of cholesterol and saturated fats in those individuals who have abnormally high levels of blood cholesterol (some of whom are suffering from a genetic condition called *hypercholesterol-aemia*)—but what about everyone else? Only a small number of people have highly elevated blood cholesterol levels, from whatever cause, and therefore most CHD deaths occur in people with *normal* or only *moderately elevated* blood cholesterol. But if the sceptics have got it wrong (as one of the news reports we quoted earlier claims), then lives are being needlessly lost because the threat from cholesterol has been underestimated.

At the end of this chapter, we return to the debate about cholesterol to illustrate what happens when the prevailing view of the causes of a major disease begins to be undermined by evidence.

Preventing CHD in women

One aspect of the prevention/treatment dilemma that we have not yet explored arises from the fact that while we have been viewing CHD as a 'scourge of the population', it is really only a scourge of *men*. In women, death rates from CHD are 30–50 per cent of those in men (see Figure 10.13), and even this is misleading as the female rate only rises significantly after the menopause. The female advantage holds across all social classes and is particularly marked if mortality is calculated in terms of years of potential life lost:[10] on average, men under the age of retirement lose at least ten times as many years of potential life from heart disease, compared with women below pensionable age.

Differences in lifestyle between British women and men do not supply an explanation—their smoking habits, blood cholesterol and blood pressure levels are now similar—but obesity (which may not in fact be an independent risk factor) and lack of exercise are more common in women. However, although these factors carry

[10]See *World Health and Disease*, Chapter 3, which discusses years of potential life lost as a method of calculating mortality.

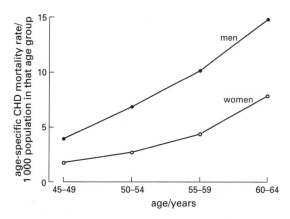

Figure 10.13 *Age-specific CHD mortality adjusted for all other risk markers. (Source: Isles, C. G . et al., 1992, Relation between coronary risk and coronary mortality in women of the Renfrew and Paisley Survey, compared with men, Lancet, 339, p. 703)*

the same *relative* risk (i.e. a woman who smokes, or who has high blood cholesterol, has a higher risk of CHD than a woman who does not), they result in a far lower *absolute* risk. In one study, for example, the 20 per cent of women with the *highest* levels of cholesterol still had a lower incidence of CHD than the 20 per cent of men with the *lowest* cholesterol levels (Figure 10.14).

HDL-cholesterol levels tend to be higher in women than men, which might account for some of their advantage, and it has often been surmised that oestrogen exerts

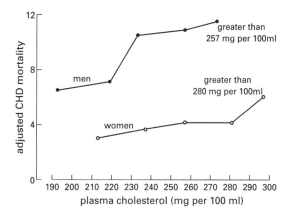

Figure 10.14 *CHD mortality, adjusted for all other risk markers, in deaths per 1 000 patient years for men and women by quintile (i.e. 20 per cent bands) of plasma cholesterol. (Source: Isles, C. G . et al., 1992, Relation between coronary risk and coronary mortality in women of the Renfrew and Paisley Survey, compared with men, Lancet, 339, p. 703)*

a protective effect—a view reinforced by the lower rates of CHD in post-menopausal women on oestrogen-only hormone replacement therapy (no longer prescribed because it promotes certain cancers, see Chapter 9). However, remarkably little research has been done on women and CHD, for reasons at which one can only guess, and it leaves open the question of whether it is justified to target women in anti-CHD campaigns just as if they were men.

Family history and the prevention of CHD

The strong emphasis on lifestyles and CHD has tended to obscure the heritable element of the disease. The neglect may also partly be due to the view that as you cannot change your genetic endowment, you might as well put the issue to one side. Many official reports and sources of advice do not mention inherited risks.

As yet little is understood about the ways in which genes may predispose a person to develop CHD, and few attempts have been made to quantify the level of heritable risk. In 1988, researchers at the Royal Free Hospital School of Medicine in London reported the results of a study on the risk of heart attack in a group of nearly 8 000 men aged between 40 and 59 years, grouped according to whether their parents were alive, had died of CHD or had died of other causes. They took the level of CHD incidence of men whose mother or father was still alive as 1.00, and calculated the relative risk of CHD of men

whose parents had died, after adjusting for the men's age and risk factors (blood pressure, smoking habits, cholesterol). Table 10.2 gives a summary of their findings after a follow-up of 6.2 years.

☐ What is the relative risk for men whose fathers died of heart trouble?

■ 2.11—more than twice the risk of men whose fathers were still alive, and substantially higher than the 1.37 risk of men whose fathers died of other causes.

In addition (not shown in Table 10.2), the effect of *both* parents dying of heart disease was to double the relative risk of their sons to 4.22. It is possible that the elevated risk is due to a familial tendency to high blood pressure.

☐ Does this study prove that the familial risk is genetic in origin?

■ No—despite the fact that differences in all the major risk factors were taken into account, other aspects of shared family environment or culture might be important. But the study strongly suggests a genetic component because the risk doubled if *both* parents had died of heart disease.

The complex interaction of genes and environment is illustrated by a study of 4 000 adults of both sexes in California, published in 1986 after a nine-year follow-up,

Table 10.2 Heart disease risks of men aged 40–59 years in England, Scotland and Wales, as defined by parental 'coronary status'. Those in all categories with (a) living fathers or (b) living mothers have been given a risk of 1.00

Parental status	No. of men	Relative risk of CHD standardised for age and risk factors[1]
(a) Father		
alive	1 738	**1.00**
died of heart trouble	1 429	2.11
died of other cause (known or unknown)	4 402	1.37
(b) Mother		
alive	3 318	**1.00**
died of heart trouble	850	1.32
died of other cause (known or unknown)	3 492	1.26

[1]Systolic blood pressure, total cholesterol, HDL-cholesterol and cigarette-smoking years. (Source: Phillips, A. N. *et al.*, 1988, Parental death from heart disease and the risk of heart attack, *European Heart Journal*, The European Society of Cardiology, **9**, p. 245)

by Kay-Tee Khaw and Elizabeth Barrett-Connor. A family history of heart disease increased the risk associated with *smoking* markedly in both sexes, but had no effect on the risks associated with high blood pressure or blood cholesterol. The authors estimated that 68 per cent of all the additional (excess) deaths occurring among those with a family history of heart disease were in fact brought about by the interaction of family history and smoking. Where there was *no* family history of CHD, the relative risks of CHD associated with smoking were quite small—1.1 in men and 1.7 in women, compared with 1.0 in non-smokers.

☐ What strategy for preventing CHD does the California study suggest?

■ Support for giving up (or not starting) smoking could be targeted more strongly at people with a family history of CHD.

Once again, the data from these trials increases the dilemma of everyone hoping to formulate a CHD prevention policy: are mass intervention strategies likely to be the most effective, or should precisely-defined 'high-risk' groups in the population be targeted? Could prevention policies of the future be based on genetic screening?[11]

Influence of the early environment

The influence of the *early environment* (defined as the time in the uterus and for a year after birth) on the risk of CHD in adult life has become the focus of considerable research in the 1980s and 1990s. There are, however, some formidable problems to overcome in undertaking retrospective investigations.

☐ What methodological problem would you encounter in such research?

■ CHD is predominantly a disease of middle age and beyond, so an investigator needs accurate data on the early environment of babies born more than 50 years ago, and these are scarce.

A further problem is that the environment encountered in the first year of life is likely to be very similar to the one experienced for many years subsequently, so the risk of CHD in an adult is hard to attribute to *early* environment alone.

[11]Genetic screening and the ethical issues it raises are discussed in *Human Biology and Health: An Evolutionary Approach.*

In spite of these problems, a succession of studies was published from the mid-1980s onwards which strongly suggested that factors such as birthweight and early feeding patterns may affect the incidence of CHD in middle age. However, you should note that these factors are themselves affected by social class and are difficult to disentangle from it.

In one study, a group at Southampton University led by epidemiologist David Barker obtained the birth, infant development and death records of 6 500 male babies born in Hertfordshire between 1911 and 1930, and compared their weight at one year of age and the subsequent incidence of fatal heart disease (see Table 10.3).

☐ Describe the pattern in Table 10.3, and suggest possible explanations for it.

■ The mortality from heart disease bears a strong inverse relationship to weight at one year. This might reflect a genetic predisposition to both CHD and slow infant growth, or perhaps indicate that the health and nutritional state of the infant and/or the mother during pregnancy and the first year thereafter has an influence on CHD in adulthood.

There is a similar, but less strong, relationship between weight at *birth* and CHD, which suggests that the environment inside the uterus might influence future development. For example, babies with higher birthweights tend to have lower blood pressure as adults. Another study, by Fall, Barker, Osmond, *et al.* (1992), showed that infant feeding and weaning routines may be important, with a sharply-rising relative risk of adult CHD in those babies who were breastfed for longer than one year.

Table 10.3   SMRs for ischaemic heart disease and all non-circulatory disease according to weight at one year of 6 500 men born in Hertfordshire, 1911–30. (Standardised for men of corresponding age and year of birth in England and Wales = 100)

Weight at one year (lb)	Ischaemic heart disease SMR	All non-circulatory disease SMR
less than 18	100	74
20	84	99
22	92	74
24	70	67
26	55	84
more than 27	34	72

Source: Barker, D. J. P. and Martyn, C. N. (1992) Maternal and fetal origins of cardiovascular disease, *Journal of Epidemiology and Community Health*, **46** (1), p. 10.

The Southampton group have concluded from their various studies that a significant degree of 'programming' of an individual's metabolism takes place within the uterus and during the first year of independent life, and that the effect of this programming may persist throughout life.[12] This view is controversial and has been challenged, especially on the difficulty of separating the effects of the earliest environment from the effects caused by the environment encountered *throughout* development and indeed in maturity. Men born over 60 years ago have had much to contend with during their lives, including one or even two World Wars. Furthermore, these are essentially *descriptive* data—the associations are merely observed, and are difficult to subject to trials that would test the strength or causality of the associations.

□ What are the implications of the 'programming' hypothesis for CHD prevention policy?

■ It suggests that less effort should go into bringing about 'lifestyle' changes in the behaviour of today's adults, and more into promoting higher birthweights and infant growth, perhaps by improving the health of women during pregnancy and breastfeeding.

Since this has, in fact, been happening since the 1940s as nutritional standards and antenatal care improved, perhaps we should do *nothing* in the expectation that CHD rates will fall as the better nourished post-war generation ages? It seems that every new line of research produces a different proposal for preventing CHD and increases the dilemma of those faced with formulating policy.

CHD and social class

We noted earlier that low social class was a major risk factor for CHD.[13] Table 10.4 shows the annual age-standardised rate of years of potential life lost as a result of CHD, per 1 000 population, distinguished by the Registrar-General's classification of social class.[14]

[12]The 'programming' hypothesis is also discussed in *Studying Health and Disease,* Chapter 10, and *World Health and Disease,* Chapters 10 and 11.

[13]See *World Health and Disease* , Chapters 9 and 10 for an analysis of the interaction between social class and ill-health, with particular reference to CHD.

[14]The Registrar-General's classification distinguishes social class on the basis of the occupation of the 'head of household'; see *Studying Health and Disease* (1985 and revised edition 1994).

Table 10.4   Annual age-standardised rate of years of potential life lost from ischaemic heart disease in England and Wales per 1 000 population in 1981

Social class	Potential years of life lost per 1 000 population from	
	All causes	Ischaemic heart disease
men aged 16–64		
I	37	12
II	42	14
III Non-manual	53	18
III Manual	58	20
IV	68	21
V	103	29
women aged 16–59		
I	13	1
II	15	1
III Non-manual	18	1
III Manual	18	2
IV	22	2
V	28	3

Source: Blane, D., Davey Smith, G. and Bartley, M. (1990) Social class differences in years of potential life lost: size, trends and principal causes, *British Medical Journal,* **301**, p. 430.

The gap between the highest and lowest social classes has been widening slowly in recent decades and is likely to increase further, given that the gap in incomes between those classes has also widened between 1981 and 1991. The reasons underlying this social-class gradient in CHD mortality have been investigated in a longitudinal study of over 17 000 civil servants working in Whitehall between 1968 and 1990.[15] The CHD mortality rates for people in the four main occupational grades is shown in Figure 10.15, which estimates the contribution made to those deaths by a wide range of risk factors.

Although some of this difference in CHD mortality between occupational grades can be explained in terms of known risk factors (for example, the prevalence of smoking is higher in unskilled workers than in professional staff), *most of it cannot.* George Davey Smith and M. J. Shipley (1991) concluded that many surveys have overestimated the effect of smoking on CHD by up to 25 per cent, and obscured some of the risk from low

[15]The Whitehall study is also discussed in *World Health and Disease,* Chapter 10.

social class. However, it must not be forgotten that smoking also greatly increases the risk of some other common, potentially fatal diseases.

◻ What are the possible underlying reasons for the large element in social-class variations in heart disease which cannot be explained by variations in known risk factors?

■ Differences exist between social classes in income, housing quality, nutrition (perhaps especially in early life), rates of childhood illness, and that most difficult aspect of human lives to define or quantify—*stress*.

If the contribution of social class to heart disease—separated from the risks associated with 'lifestyle factors'—has been underestimated, what aspects of prevention policy might need to be rethought? More attention might need to be given to social and economic factors that are largely beyond the control of the individual, and less to education about lifestyle. Health education is simpler and cheaper than major social and economic change (a subject we turn to in the next chapter), but is the evidence now good enough to conclude that to focus on lifestyles is to 'blame the victim' for the disease?

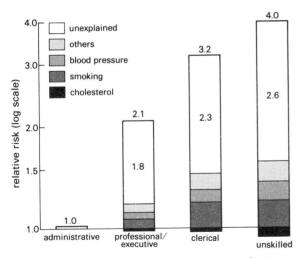

Figure 10.15 *Relative risks of death from CHD according to occupational grade in the civil service. Note that a logarithmic scale has been used. Proportions of the differences between grades that can be explained by differences in known risk factors are shown. 'Others' include age, height, over-weight, leisure-time activity, and glucose tolerance (a test for diabetes). (Source: Rose, G. and Marmot, M., 1981, Social class and CHD, British Heart Journal,* **45***, p. 17).*

Action or inaction? The case against cholesterol

People who are professionally (or otherwise) involved with CHD, and who encounter its disabling and tragic effects daily, are under great pressure to initiate or support *some* action which they believe, perhaps from their own research or practice, is likely to alleviate the problem—even if the action proposed is not fully supported by scientific evidence. Such action is often defended by saying that on any major issue there will always be controversy and argument, and somewhere there will always be sceptics. Therefore, (the argument runs), actions that might save lives should not be postponed pending the resolution of intellectual disagreements—which indeed may never be resolved!

Throughout the 1980s, the causal relationship between diet and CHD was the seldom-challenged paradigm within which research was evaluated and the policy of mass intervention to reduce the lifestyle factors was vigorously pursued. Yet there were numerous published investigations, some dating back to the mid-1960s, which suggested that the relationship was not straightforward, and that mass intervention might not work, or was not working. In warning of the flawed nature of the evidence, J. R. A. Mitchell, Professor of Cardiology at Nottingham University Medical School complained of:

…the harm to our credibility as scientists and as health advisers; if we go public on diet and CHD on the basis of poor evidence we are weakening our position in respect of measures for which there is clear evidence. (Mitchell, 1984, p. 297)

His was an isolated voice however, and largely ignored, as were the results of several trials which did not support the accepted view. In 1992, Uffe Ravnskov reviewed the scientific trials that had been published on the effects of reducing blood cholesterol on CHD mortality, and categorised them as either supportive, inconclusive or contradictory. He found that trials classified as supportive were cited six times more frequently in the scientific literature than unsupportive or contradictory research. After 1970, none of the unsupportive trials were cited, although there were almost as many of them as there were supportive ones.

Moreover, another survey of trials that failed to get published revealed that only 15 per cent of unpublished research showed statistically significant effects of intervention on the incidence of CHD, but 44 per cent of trials showing that intervention had no significant effect failed to find a publisher.

What can we conclude from all this? Is good evidence that undermines the prevailing view being ignored (as the quote below suggests), or is the case against cholesterol strong enough to withstand challenge?

> The strong implication which flows from the contemporary 'healthy lifestyles' movement is that, for example, all saturated fat is bad for everyone. The fact that this type of message is at best a distortion of the epidemiological evidence appears not to have diminished the zeal of its delivery. (Davison, Davey Smith and Frankel, 1991, pp. 16–7)

As evidence accumulates on both sides, we may be on the edge of a paradigm shift in the received wisdom about diet and CHD. But as with all paradigm shifts (and you may recall John McKinlay's analysis of the rise and fall of a standard medical procedure in Chapter 7), reputations have been built on the denunciation of saturated fats and advocates will not be easily persuaded to change their view.

A rational approach for the future?

The evidence suggests that, important though the improvements in treatment are, they are not likely to have a major impact in the near future on total CHD mortality. Even if CABG, angioplasty and the clot-busters between them save 20 000 lives a year in the United Kingdom (a generous estimate), this must be seen against a background of about 170 000 deaths annually from CHD.

The current orthodoxy is prevention, supported on the twin pillars of education about risk factors and the encouragement of lifestyle modification. Accepting this, and recognising that the pillars have been expensively constructed, one must ask if they have good foundations.

A large reduction in cigarette smoking might be expected to lead to a modest reduction in CHD in the population as a whole, primarily among men with a family history of heart disease. Hypertension is a reasonable predictor of CHD, but blood pressure reduction by drug treatment has a variable effect on CHD mortality.

Reduction in blood cholesterol levels by an intensive regime of diet and drugs among people who are at high risk of CHD seems justified, but in mass intervention trials the reduction in CHD mortality is partly or wholly offset by increased mortality from other causes.

Mass intervention to alter the major lifestyle factors is now open to serious question. This is the view of Michael Oliver, a leading cardiologist:

> As multiple intervention against risk factors for CHD in middle-aged men at only moderate risk seem to have failed to reduce both morbidity and mortality, such interventions become increasingly difficult to justify. (Oliver, 1992, p. 394)

Oliver suggests that given the results of the extended follow-up of the Helsinki heart study (see Table 10.1 earlier), it may be unethical for doctors to engage in mass intervention programmes to reduce CHD.

In the next century, the genetic background to CHD and the physiological events that link genes to visible signs such as atheromas may be understood. Such knowledge would create the possibility of screening to detect those at genetic risk and perhaps allow gene manipulation to reduce those risks. But the 'new biology' will face us with new dilemmas about the ethics of inspecting each person's DNA for imperfections.

The inadequacy of other approaches drives us to consider whether an attack on poor socio-economic circumstances might be the most effective strategy for reducing CHD. When individuals move from one social class to another (by marriage, or other selective processes), they tend to acquire the health patterns of their adoptive class. This, among other evidence, encourages the view that raising the standard of living of those in social classes IV and V would, over time, result in a shift to the lower rates of CHD that are currently experienced in higher social classes.

Socio-economic change of this kind is not likely to happen quickly in the United Kingdom, nor is it certain that it would have the desired effect on health if it did, without other unintended consequences. In the final chapter in this book, we evaluate the prospects for such change.

OBJECTIVES FOR CHAPTER 10

When you have studied this chapter, you should be able to:

10.1 Explain what is meant by coronary heart disease (CHD), coronary artery by-pass grafting (CABG), angioplasty, and clot-busters, and discuss the dilemmas and difficulties associated with the medical treatment of CHD.

10.2 Summarise the major risk factors associated with an elevated incidence of CHD, and evaluate the strength of the evidence that the association is causal.

10.3 Illustrate the dilemmas inherent in formulating a rational policy for the primary prevention of CHD, given the currently available evidence about its causation and the results of trials of mass intervention and 'high-risk group' strategies.

10.4 Use the case study of CHD to illustrate some of the dilemmas and issues raised in earlier chapters of this book about health care in the United Kingdom in the 1990s.

QUESTIONS FOR CHAPTER 10

Question 1 (*Objective 10.1*)

Suggest examples of *process innovations* (defined in Chapter 7) in CHD treatment and point out the difficulties that might block their introduction.

Question 2 (*Objective 10.2*)

What are the main criteria you should look for in deciding whether or not to intervene to lower the blood cholesterol levels of those considered most at risk of CHD?

Question 3 (*Objective 10.3*)

On what grounds would you defend launching a mass campaign to lower CHD mortality by reducing the prevalence of cigarette smoking in the population as a whole? What arguments could you construct against such a strategy?

Question 4 (*Objective 10.4*)

In what ways does CHD illustrate issues about primary prevention, rationing, evaluation, and innovation in health care?

11

Poverty, economic inequality and health

Beyond health care

While to specialists in public health the most attractive points of initial attack (on health inequalities) are health promotion initiatives to reduce risk factors such as smoking, poor diet, and physical inactivity there is a limit to the extent to which…improvements are likely to occur in the absence of a wider strategy to change the circumstances in which these risks arise, by reducing deprivation and improving the physical environment. (Sir Donald Acheson, *Guardian*, 1991, September 13, p. 4)

Thus spoke the retiring Chief Medical Officer at the Department of Health as he launched his last annual report on the state of the nation's health in 1991. He was highlighting one of the most profound dilemmas in health policy at the end of the twentieth century: that health care

has a very limited contribution to make to reducing the persistent and considerable inequalities in the experience of health and illness in this and other countries.

So far in this book we have explored some of the dilemmas inherent in the organisation and delivery of health-care systems. In this final chapter we move beyond the relatively narrow confines of the health service, beyond the middle ground where health and social services meet in policies for community care, disease prevention and health promotion, and focus on the potential for a wider strategy to reduce poverty and economic inequality as a means of preventing disease and promoting health. First, we briefly reconsider the main dimensions of inequalities in health and their possible explanations. We then discuss the meaning, scale and causes of poverty and economic inequality in contemporary Britain and the broad outlines of the strategic policy options available to address these inequalities. Finally, we examine the evidence for the likely effectiveness of these options both in terms of reducing poverty and economic inequality, and of reducing inequalities in health and disease.

Like the other issues discussed in this book, the pursuit of an effective strategy to reduce poverty and economic inequality is beset by difficulties, two of which run through the narrative presented here. First, there is the problem of definition. Poverty and economic inequality are complex and disputed terms which, as with community care, may fuel endless debates but constrain action. Second, there is the problem of public attitudes towards poverty and economic inequality. The introduction of an effective strategy to improve the standard of living of the poor, and to reduce the gap between the rich and the poor, would depend on widespread public support—yet public attitudes appear at best contradictory.

There is also an apparent dilemma. Since World War II there has been a general concern in the United Kingdom to ensure fairness and equality of opportunity. During the 1980s and 1990s this has been eroded by anxiety about the effects of welfare spending and taxation on economic prosperity. Will policies that reduce economic inequalities and (arguably) thereby improve the nation's health, end up by damaging economic incentives and reducing the nation's wealth?

Social inequalities in health revisited

The pattern of ill-health in the United Kingdom, as in many countries, does not display a random distribution in the population. Rather there is a distinct and persistent inequality in the distribution of premature death, disease, illness and disability.

> □ What are the major demographic and other characteristics by which inequalities in the distribution of health in the United Kingdom can be distinguished?[1]

> ■ The most frequently discussed are inequalities between groups with different socio-economic characteristics, such as social class, income, occupation, and housing. In addition, there are significant inequalities between groups distinguished by their gender, marital status, geographical area and ethnic background.

In the 1991 government White Paper, *The Health of The Nation*, one of the criteria set out for deciding whether an issue should be a public-health priority is that it should be a major cause of premature death or avoidable ill-health in the population as a whole, or among specific groups. The scale of the burden associated with social inequalities in health would appear to meet this criterion. Drawing on a number of different sources, for example, the deputy editor of the *British Medical Journal* argued that:

> If the whole population had experienced the same death rates as the non-manual classes, there would have been 700 fewer stillbirths, and 1 500 fewer deaths in the first year of life in England and Wales in 1988, 750 fewer deaths in children in 1981 and 17 000 fewer deaths in men aged 20–64 in Great Britain in 1981. (Delamothe, 1991, p. 1 047)

> □ Summarise four alternative explanations for these inequalities in the experience of health and illness.[2]

[1]Described in detail in *World Health and Disease,* Chapter 9.

[2]The evidence for and against each of these explanations is analysed in *World Health and Disease,* Chapter 10.

> ■ The four most prominent explanations are: that such patterns are *artifacts* of the way in which data are collected; that they result from processes of health-related *social selection*; that they arise from the *behaviour* of individuals; and finally, that they arise from inequalities in the *life circumstances* and *material conditions* of different groups in the population.

There is now growing evidence from research that, no matter how many risk factors or behavioural differences are taken into account, substantial inequalities in the health of different socio-economic groups remain. Less research has been conducted on the relative contribution of behaviour to inequalities in health between men and women, or between people from different ethnic groups, but a similar outcome is likely. Although genetic inheritance and aspects of individual lifestyle play their part, it appears that the material circumstances in which people live and work are dominant causes of inequalities in the distribution of health and illness. The case study of coronary heart disease in the previous chapter illustrates this point. Poverty and economic inequality—not smoking—could therefore be argued to be the most important health hazards in late-twentieth century Britain. But what exactly is meant by poverty and economic inequality? We begin with the problematic definition and measurement of poverty.

Defining and measuring poverty

Absolute and relative poverty

Adam Smith, the economic philosopher, is possibly best known outside economics (and perhaps within) for his theory of markets. In his famous book, first published in 1776, *The Wealth of Nations*, however, he also addresses a debate about the definition of poverty which continues to this day:

> By necessities I understand not just commodities which are indispensably necessary for the support of life, but whatever the custom of a country renders it indecent for creditable people, even of the lowest order, to be without. (Smith, 1812 edition, p. 693)

> □ What two approaches to the definition of poverty are inherent in this statement by Adam Smith?

> ■ Smith talks first about a level of commodities 'indispensably necessary to support life' and second he identifies a level necessary to support a decent life according to 'the custom of a country'. The former

would today be described as an *absolute* approach to the definition of poverty whilst the latter is a *relative* approach.

Arguments about the merits of absolute and relative definitions of poverty have characterised debates about poverty in Britain in the post-war years.[3] The concept of **absolute poverty** focuses attention on the minimum standards of food, shelter and clothing necessary to ensure physical survival. This approach has its twentieth-century advocates, as illustrated by the following quotation (Sir Keith Joseph was Secretary of State for Social Services at the time):

> A family is poor if it cannot afford to eat. A person who enjoys a standard of living equal to that of a medieval baron cannot be described as poor for the sole reason that he has chanced to be born into a society where the great majority can live like medieval kings. By any absolute standards, there is very little poverty in Britain today. (Joseph and Sumption, 1979, p. 27)

Opponents of this approach argue that, despite the apparent clarity, it is not possible to define an adequate standard of living in any absolute way. Rather they would agree with Adam Smith's relative definition of poverty, as this statement from the social policy analyst Peter Townsend (a prominent critic of the concept of absolute poverty) typifies:

> In fact, people's needs, even for food, are conditioned by the society in which they live and to which they belong and just as needs differ in different societies, so they differ in different periods of the evolution of single societies. Any conception of poverty as 'absolute' is therefore inappropriate and misleading. (Townsend, 1979, p. 38)

This approach to defining poverty—relative to the living standards of a society in general, or **relative poverty**—has been adopted by the European Commission. The European Commission also incorporates social as well as economic dimensions into the definition of poverty, with the Council of Ministers describing the poor as:

> ...persons whose resources (material, cultural and social) are so limited as to exclude them from the minimum acceptable way of life in the member state in which they live. (European Commission, 1991, p. 2)

[3]See *World Health and Disease*, Chapter 10.

The Commission has subsequently developed this approach even further and started to talk about 'social exclusion', rather than about poverty.

☐ What difficulties can you foresee with the relative approach to the definition of poverty?

■ There is still the problem of defining the standard of living, or level of resources, below which people can be said to be living in poverty. Using the relative approach, it is necessary to identify the standard of living which is generally considered to be 'necessary' or 'acceptable' within a society.

A number of researchers have sought to identify a **relative poverty line** in Britain. In a survey commissioned for the television series 'Breadline Britain 1990s', Joanna Mack, a journalist and Stewart Lansley, an economist, used *social consensus* as a basis for defining such a line. They asked a large representative sample of people across Britain, which items—out of a long list provided—they would regard as *necessities* and found a perhaps surprising degree of consensus. At least two-thirds of the people asked thought that the items shown in Box 11.1 were necessities.

Box 11.1 Items regarded as necessities by at least two-thirds of British adults surveyed for 'Breadline Britain 1990s'.

- Self-contained damp-free accommodation with an indoor toilet and bath.

- A weekly roast joint for the family and three daily meals for each child.

- Two pairs of all-weather shoes and a warm waterproof coat.

- Sufficient money for public transport.

- Adequate bedrooms and beds.

- Heating and carpeting.

- A refrigerator and washing machine.

- Enough money for special occasions like Christmas.

- Toys for the children.

Source: Frayman, H., 1991, Breadline Britain 1990s, *Domino Films/London Weekend Television, London, p. 4.*

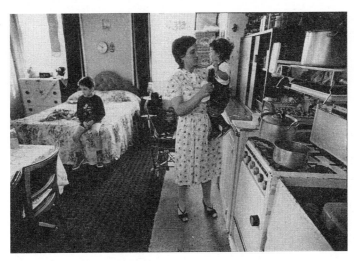

The threats to health and well-being are obvious for this family of four living in one room in Great Britain in 1987. In the 1990s, about 11 million people live without certain basic household items such as self-contained accommodation with adequate bedrooms and beds, which the majority of adults consider to be necessities. (Photo: Mike Abrahams/Network)

Numbering the poor

Without a working definition of poverty and therefore a way of measuring it, we cannot estimate how many people are experiencing poverty now, nor assess how changes in policy might affect the number of persons living below the poverty line. If we don't know the *scale* of the problem then it is difficult to begin to think about the *cost* of doing anything about it. Four different methods of estimating the total number of people experiencing poverty, and within that total the number of children affected, are shown in Table 11.1.

☐ How would you sum up the data presented in Table 11.1?

■ Different measures of poverty give broadly similar estimates of the number of people involved. There are, however, important differences at the extremes. The lowest estimate of the numbers of people experiencing poverty is two million below the highest estimate, and the number of children involved according to different measures differs by half a million.

☐ In addition to differences in the ways that poverty was measured, what other aspect of data collection might account for some of the variation in the numbers of people experiencing poverty shown in Table 11.1?

Table 11.1   Number of individuals living in poverty in Great Britain in the 1980s and 1990, using different definitions of poverty

People living on income at or below the level of:	No. of people (millions)	Percentage of the total population	Of which children (millions)	(%)
State Income Support (1987)[1]	10.0	19	2.5	20
Half national average income (1988–9)[2]	12.0	22	3.0	25
Half average income, European Commission estimates (1985)[3]	10.3	19	2.6	20
Households lacking basic necessities (1990)[4]	11.0	20	3.0	24

Sources: [1]Institute for Fiscal Studies, 1990, *Poverty in Official Statistics,* IFS Commentary No. 24, London, pp. 10–11. [2]Department of Social Security, 1992, *Households Below Average Income—A Statistical Analysis, 1979–1988/89,* HMSO, London, pp. 91–7. [3]European Commission, 1991, *Final Report on the Second European Poverty Programme, 1985–1989,* European Commission, Brussels, pp. 12 and 17 (data relate to the United Kingdom). [4]Frayman, H., 1991, *Breadline Britain 1990s,* Domino Films/London Weekend Television, London, p. 10.

■ The estimates relate to different years during the 1980s. Whilst differences of one or two years are unlikely to have a significant impact, differences of five years—for example between the European Commission estimates and the 'Breadline Britain' study—may affect the outcome.

All four of the approaches used in Table 11.1 to the measurement of poverty are in some sense relative, albeit to a greater or lesser extent. The level of income below which State Income Support is paid is often referred to as a *subsistence level* by groups actively trying to improve the circumstances of people living on benefits. In the 1940s, William Beveridge wished to set the level of state benefits (following the research by Seebohm Rowntree at the turn of the century) on the cost of a basket of goods considered necessary to provide for 'subsistence'. However, from the beginning of the welfare state the Treasury has exerted pressure to reduce benefit levels.[4] At the time of writing in 1993, benefits are increased annually, but the rate of increase over time is determined largely by political considerations. Using the state benefit level as a *poverty line* gives the lowest estimates of the numbers experiencing poverty,[5] whereas the highest estimate results from using the number of people living below half the national average income (see Table 11.1).

The causes of poverty

The development of effective anti-poverty strategies is not simply a matter of finding an agreed definition of poverty. Effectiveness will also depend on the extent to which the *causes* of poverty have been correctly identified. Some insights into the causes of poverty can be obtained from looking at who is at most risk of experiencing it.

□ According to Table 11.2, what factors are associated with an increased risk of poverty?

■ Poverty seems to be associated most strongly with the lack of a paid job, either through unemployment or retirement, having children (particularly if there is only one parent), and having a disability or sickness.

But the data in Table 11.2 do not tell the whole story. Although in 1987 only 8 per cent of those in full-time work were poor (using this definition of poverty), 26 per cent of the poor were in fact in *full-time work*. This raises the issue of low pay.

[4]The background to the setting up of the welfare state in Britain is given in *Caring for Health: History and Diversity*, Chapters 5 and 6.

[5]See *World Health and Disease*, Table 10.7.

Table 11.2 The risk of poverty in Britain, by economic and family status, 1987

	Percentage with incomes below 50% of average after deducting housing costs
Economic status	
pensioners	25
full-time workers	8
sick/disabled people	32
single parents not in paid work	58
unemployed people	59
Family status	
married couples with children	20
married couples (all)	10
all single parents	47
single people	15

Source: Oppenheim, C. (1990) *Poverty: The Facts,* Child Poverty Action Group, London, p. 30.

Another problem with the data in Table 11.2 (and more generally with traditional approaches to the definition and measurement of poverty) is that they ignore the possibility that people living in the *same* household may have *different* standards of living. Research in the 1980s has found that women are much more vulnerable to poverty than men, but the full extent of their poverty has been hidden by earlier research which focused on *household* living standards, rather than on the living standards of individuals in the household. Unless women are in receipt of earnings from paid employment, or head their own household as single parents, they are invisible in poverty statistics. It is assumed that they share the same living standard as others in the household. However it appears that this is often not the case.

Research by Holly Sutherland at the London School of Economics (quoted in Atkinson, 1991) has looked at the incomes of women and men in couples. She found that 9 per cent of *couples* had joint incomes below the state income support level. She then looked at women and men in these couples as *individuals* to see if income was equally shared (i.e. to see what proportion of each sex had incomes below *half* the state income support level). She found that 5 per cent of men had incomes below half the state income support level compared with 50 per cent of women.

Research has also documented how women frequently shield their partners and children from the full effects of low income and poverty by doing without themselves. The following quotation is typical of many others:

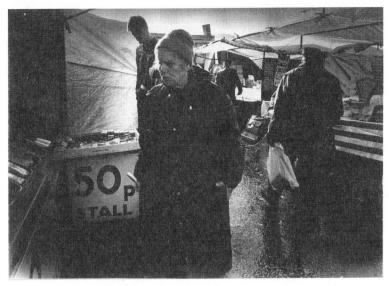

Women in low-income households frequently 'do without' to protect other family members and in old age they are over-represented amongst the poor. (Photo: Glaswegians Photo Archive/Cranhill)

I'll go to jumble sales for my clothes...but I'm not seeing me kids and me husband walk to town with secondhand clothes on. I'll make do myself, but I won't do for them. (Mother of three, partner unemployed, quoted in Oppenheim, 1990, p. 102)

Women's primary responsibility for the care of others—including children, but also other dependants—has profound implications for their relationship to the labour market. Characteristically, women are concentrated in low-paid work, are heavily reliant on part-time work, and have interrupted employment histories; consequently they have diminished social security, occupational benefits, and private provision (such as pensions or insurance policies). Their longer life expectancy also means that women form the majority among pensioners—a group with a relatively high risk of poverty (see Table 11.2).

A final neglected aspect of the experience of poverty that should be noted is its concentration amongst black and other minority ethnic groups. These groups are more likely than others to be in low-paid jobs (as Chapter 6 described for health-service employees) and to experience unemployment, partly at least as a result of discrimination. They are therefore at greater risk of experiencing poverty than white Britons.

Inequalities in income and wealth

So far we have been considering definitions of poverty *per se*. However, poverty—defined in absolute or relative terms—is entangled in some definitions with the wider issue of **economic inequality**. The European Commission, for example, considers poverty to be 'the extreme form of inequality'.

□ Can you suggest how the concept of economic inequality might differ from the concept of poverty?

■ Economic inequality is a broader concept than either absolute or relative poverty, which takes into account the distribution of income and personal wealth across the whole society; it includes the richest in society, as well as the average or 'norm', along with those who could be considered as living in poverty.

By all accounts, Britain is an economically unequal society, and in recent years has become more so. For example, data from the Department of Social Security (OPCS, *Social Trends 23*, 1993, Figure 5.17) reveal changes over time in the distribution of *household income* in the United Kingdom. Households are divided into five equal bands (20 per cent groups or quintiles), and the share of national income that each quintile takes is calculated.[6] In 1989, the richest 20 per cent of households took 40 per cent of the nation's total income after tax, compared with a 34.8 per cent share a decade earlier. In contrast, the poorest 20 per cent of households took only 7.9 per cent of total income in 1989, compared with a 9.9 per cent share a decade earlier.

The gap between the rich and poor, in terms of household income shares, had increased by almost 30 per cent in just ten years. The distribution of income, having become more equal in the years immediately following World War II—a trend that continued at a decreasing rate in the 1960s and 70s—then reversed earlier gains and by the 1990s had returned to the levels of inequality of the 1950s (Townsend, 1991, p. 29).

The biggest inequalities, however, are not those of income, but of **wealth**, which includes marketable assets such as property, land and shares. According to a special analysis carried out for the *Sunday Times* in 1991, just 400 people owned between them wealth which was equivalent to almost a tenth of the national income, and land equivalent in size to six average counties (Beresford, 1991, p. 2).

Government statistics show that one per cent of the population owns almost a fifth (18 per cent) of the nation's personal marketable wealth. This is three times the proportion owned by the poorer *half* of the population between them. This privileged but tiny group owned between a third and a half of all private land and nearly half of all company shares. The richest 10 per cent owned more than half of the total personal wealth, including three-quarters of all the privately-owned land and company shares (OPCS, *Social Trends 23*, 1993, p. 78).

Strategies for economic equality

The post-war perspective

Given the problems of definition discussed above, developing effective strategies to reduce poverty or economic inequality is far from simple. Should such policies be directed at the eradication of absolute or of relative poverty, or at the reduction of wider economic inequalities within society? It is not simply a question of choosing between the alternatives and then implementing the appropriate policies. If the issue is economic inequality rather than poverty *per se*, however defined, then policies aimed only at reducing or removing poverty while leaving the inequalities in society unchanged may

---

[6]This method of evaluating income distribution is also discussed in *World Health and Disease*, Chapter 10 (see Figure 10.8).

fail. Additionally, our particular concern here is not with the problems of poverty and economic inequality in their own right. Rather it is with the extent to which policies focused on these problems will make an effective contribution to improving the health of the nation. We need to ask what type of anti-poverty policies would be most effective in achieving this aim.

In their pursuit of a fairer society, governments since World War II, particularly but not exclusively Labour governments, have pursued a policy of **income redistribution** which can be described as being 'after the event'. The policy was to allow economic competition in a free market and social processes (such as discrimination against certain social groups) to determine the distribution of material resources among the population, and then intervene 'after the event' to reduce the inequalities in living standards and life chances that this created. Intervention was directed through the *tax and benefit systems* as well as through *public expenditure*, notably in the fields of health, education and housing. The expectation was that taxation on income would redistribute money from richest to poorest by financing both the benefit system and public expenditure on services directed at least in part at the poor.

Richard Tawney, an historian and social critic, in his book *Equality* (first published 1931, re-published 1964) described these post-war policies as part of a 'strategy of equality'. However, the strategy has not resulted in a major redistribution of resources to the poorer sections of British society: official figures show that even in 1979 five million people were still living in poverty (Institute for Fiscal Studies, 1990, pp. 10–11). Rather, the distribution of income and wealth in the early 1990s has seen a return to the situation in the immediate post-war years, reversing the moderate redistribution which occurred in the early 1950s and more slowly through the 1960s and 1970s. Moreover, the proportion of people in relative poverty is increasing, and social inequalities in health remain considerable.

It has been suggested that there are three main reasons why post-war policies met with such little success in terms of reducing economic inequalities or poverty. First, the post-war policies were superimposed onto an already unequal society. Inequalities in income and wealth reflect inequalities in power and access. After World War II, higher socio-economic groups were better placed than poorer sections of society to gain from the provision of universal welfare services in health care, housing and education. The same is true of the tax and benefit systems: to give one example, tax relief (for mortgages or pensions) are of no value to those who neither pay tax, nor have a mortgage nor private pension.

Second, William Beveridge, the architect of the present social security system, argued that if this system was to reduce the proportion of people living in poverty, it was essential that full employment and adequate levels of child benefit should be maintained. If these two conditions were fulfilled, then poverty, he suggested, would be confined to a very small number of people not currently participating fully in the labour market.

☐ Considering the discussion earlier on who is most at risk of experiencing poverty, and your general knowledge of the economic situation in the 1990s, have Beveridge's conditions been fulfilled?

■ We mentioned earlier that around a quarter of the poor in 1987 were in full-time paid work, and that people with children are at greater risk of experiencing poverty than those without (Table 11.2). This reflects the fact that salaries and wages can be below the poverty line, and that child benefit levels have not been sufficient to compensate for this. More generally, unemployment was high throughout the 1980s and much of the 1990s.

The 'rediscovery of poverty' in the late 1960s included a rediscovery of the 'working poor' and a growing realisation that a full-time job was not a guarantee against poverty, as indeed it never had been. New benefits have been introduced to compensate for low wages, but these have many problems associated with them, including low take-up, partly due to the complexity of the benefit system. Since the 1970s, the control of inflation has taken precedence over the maintenance of high employment levels and rates of unemployment have risen sharply. The third reason that the post-war 'strategy for equality' has failed is that it did not adapt to changing social and demographic circumstances.

☐ Drawing on material that you studied in earlier books in this series, can you identify some of the major aspects of demographic and social change since World War II that you would expect to have had an impact on the welfare system?[7]

[7]Demographic changes involving the age-structure of the British population were discussed in Chapter 8 of this book, and in *World Health and Disease* and *Birth to Old Age: Health in Transition*; the latter also comments on changes in the composition of households this century and on employment patterns among women.

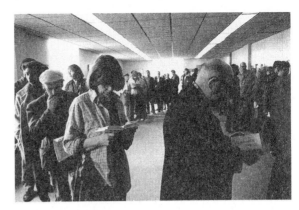

After the full employment years of the 1950s and 1960s, the dole queue has again become a commonplace feature of life in late twentieth-century Britain.
(Photo: Crispin Hughes/Photo Co-op)

■ The British population, like that of all Western nations, has aged dramatically; the extent of employment amongst women has greatly increased; and new social groups have emerged, notably single-parent households.

These changes had two effects. First, they led to an increase in the numbers of people in need, placing demands on the welfare state that were not anticipated, and which could only have been met by substantial increases in taxation. Second, they required a large number of *ad hoc* alterations and additions to the regulations governing entitlement to different benefts, creating a system of such complexity that few but the very expert could understand it.

If post-war policies to reduce poverty and economic inequality have failed, what are the options for the future?

Looking to the future

In the United Kingdom, a number of sharply contrasting approaches to reducing poverty can be distinguished among policy-makers and political strategists, not all of which would redress economic inequality. The Conservative governments of the 1980s and early 1990s argued that a **market approach to reducing poverty** is the only one that will succeed. The central concern for those who wish to reduce poverty by this means must be to control inflation, develop a rigorous and growing market economy, and so generate incentives for people to create wealth. This in turn will, it is argued, gradually 'trickle down' to increase the standard of living for society as a whole.

□ How do you think the market approach would affect economic inequalities?

■ Economic competition would lead (at least in the short-term) to an *increase* in economic inequalities—this is the main incentive for generating more economic growth and hence more wealth.

In other industrialised countries the debate about the reduction of poverty and economic inequalities has taken a somewhat different form to that apparent in the United Kingdom. In the 1960s, for example, the American 'War on Poverty' was based on the premise that poverty would only be reduced by enhancing educational standards amongst poor people, and by developing stronger local resources and networks in poor areas through **community development initiatives**.

A similar approach was adopted for a brief period in the United Kingdom in the 1970s by the Home Office, which sponsored the Comprehensive Community Programme involving a number of projects in inner city areas around the country. (An account of the experiences of these projects is provided in a book by a group of academics and former officials involved in the programme, see Higgins *et al.*, 1983 in the Reference list.) Though short-lived, the Comprehensive Community Programme was followed by a large number of smaller-scale community development initiatives around the country. Additionally, the community development approach has been adopted by many agencies, including Health Promotion Departments within some health authorities, as a way of working with people living in economically disadvantaged areas.

Such initiatives do not, however, form a significant part of the policies being proposed by those outside government in the early 1990s to combat poverty and reduce economic inequality nationally. There is a vigorous debate between those who favour intervening through the tax and benefit systems and those who favour wider structural changes in the way that society and the economy are organised. We shall look at each of these approaches in turn.

Despite the failure of post-war tax and benefit policies in the United Kingdom, many people still believe that a **tax and benefit approach** to dealing with poverty and inequality will be the most fruitful. For this reason, a large number of complex proposals to ensure a *minimum income*—regardless of employment status—have been developed. Several widely differing types of reform have been proposed—each with its particular advantages and drawbacks.

Basic income schemes

At one extreme there are those who believe in a **basic income** for all, provided in the form of a cash payment and financed through general taxation. This is sometimes described as a 'social dividend' or 'citizen's income'. This idea is once again fashionable, but it has a respectable pedigree, running back to the work of Lady Juliette Rhys Williams who campaigned for such a scheme in the 1950s.

At present, most of us receive some income from the state in the form of *transfer payments*. These include: universal cash benefits paid regardless of income, such as Child Benefit; means-tested benefits, such as Family Credit or Housing Benefit, payable at a rate which falls as income rises; or tax allowances and exemptions (for a mortgage for instance). A basic income scheme would sweep away this paraphernalia of different transfer payments, and replace them with a single cash payment, set at the level of subsistence and varying only according to the number of dependants.

There would be no tax allowances, so tax would be payable from the first pound earned, at a rate sufficient to provide the basic income for all. However, in order to achieve a basic income for all, the tax rate would have to be very high, probably around 55–65 pence in the pound.

Negative income tax schemes

The high tax rate associated with the basic income strategy has led to alternative proposals, including various **negative income tax schemes**. These schemes also involve setting an income threshold. Tax would be payable on earnings above this level, as happens with the present income tax system. But anyone with an income *below* the threshold would receive a payment or *negative tax* which would raise their income nearer to the threshold level.

Advocates of negative income tax schemes argue that they would be much simpler than the present system and—as long as the negative tax payments were set at an appropriate level—would eliminate absolute poverty at much less cost than a full-blown basic income scheme.

Social dividends

A third alternative falling somewhere between the two extremes of basic income and negative income tax schemes was considered by the Meade Committee on tax reform in the 1970s (Meade, 1978). This involved providing two forms of **social dividend**. An 'unconditional' payment would be made to everyone, regardless of their situation—a sort of child benefit for grown-ups too. However, this would be set *below* the level of subsistence (which, of course, would need to be agreed at a politically acceptable level), and would therefore require much lower tax rates to finance than a basic income scheme.

For those still left below the level of subsistence, a second social dividend would be provided—conditional on *circumstances* (e.g. payable because of unemployment or disability), rather than being means-tested. This would simply replace the existing national insurance benefits.

The three schemes described above, despite their striking differences, all depend on changes in the tax and benefit systems *per se*. In that respect, they are all developments of Beveridge's approach which, as the earlier discussion suggests, has been far from successful in reducing poverty and economic inequality. The supporters of the schemes just described would argue that if the major demographic and social changes that have occurred since World War II had been better monitored, and the effects of post-war policies had been properly evaluated, then the tax and benefit approach could have been adapted and made more effective.

However, this strategy has some critics among those who are also committed to achieving less poverty and greater equality. They argue that this approach would again result in a bewildering array of *ad hoc* changes to the tax and benefit systems, and it would continue to depend on redistributing resources 'after the event', i.e. after they had been distributed unequally through the labour market. These critics claim that governments must interfere in the market *before* inequalities are created, if they are ever to reduce either poverty or economic inequality.

Tackling inequalities at their source

The arguments for tackling economic inequalities at their source are most articulately and loudly put by pressure groups such as the Child Poverty Action Group (CPAG) and the Low Pay Unit. However, a diverse mixture of academic, voluntary and church groups (such as the Anglican Church Action on Poverty) also support this approach. There is not the scope in this chapter to provide a detailed account of the many different policy dimensions that advocates argue would be needed, but we can describe the broad contours of the proposed strategy and leave it to the interested reader to pursue the details elsewhere.

The strategy includes policies to make the tax system more equitable and more redistributive, for example by introducing a wealth tax or a more effective inheritance tax. Changes in the principles upon which the social security system is based are also proposed. These include the provision of adequate benefits to meet people's social, physical and cultural needs—not a basic *minimum* as at present. Benefits would be provided universally and not through means-testing. Payment of benefits would be on an individual basis, so that women and men could claim in their own right. Finally, advocates argue for equal access without discrimination and for clearly stated rights combined with simplicity and flexibility.

Parallel changes in the labour market, in employment policies and in public services are also included in this version of a 'strategy for equality'.

□ On the basis of what you have read so far, can you suggest the three main aspects of employment policy that the advocates of this approach are likely to propose?

■ First, a return to full employment is set as the primary objective of economic policy; second, there are proposals aimed at dealing with low pay, through a statutory minimum and maximum wage and improved equal pay laws; and third there are proposals aimed at improving access to employment for groups who are disadvantaged in the labour market, such as people from minority ethnic groups, people with disabilities and women.

Advocates of these policies argue that they would need to be supported by, and in some cases would be dependent on, changes in the provision of public services. Women's access to paid employment, for example, is linked to the expanded provision of good quality child-care facilities. Similarly, young people's employment opportunities are seen to be dependent on the quality of the education and training they receive. Good quality and accessible housing and health care are also important.[8]

It is often argued that such a strategy—involving full employment, improved services and increases in income for the poor—would be too expensive. However, its proponents believe that such an approach would result—in the long term—in *smaller* burdens on the state and the taxpayer.

□ Can you suggest how this might come about?

■ Reducing unemployment also cuts the cost of unemployment benefit, and generates extra income for government through the taxes that those now in work can contribute. Raising income above the poverty line reduces the need for individuals and families to claim benefits such as Family Credit, Income Support and Housing Benefit.

---

[8]The association between education, housing quality and health is discussed in *World Health and Disease*, Chapter 10.

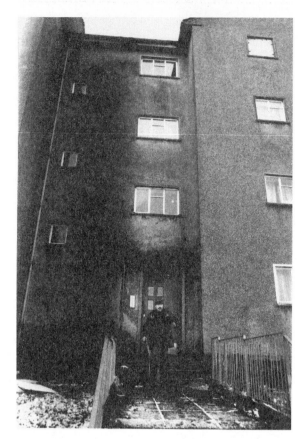

Addressing the health and social problems associated with poor quality housing in many British towns and cities presents a formidable challenge to policy-makers. (Photo: Glaswegians Photo Archive/Cranhill)

In addition, improved child-care facilities would provide employment and allow parents to contribute to economic activity if they wish to do so, using their skills and energy to increase overall prosperity as well as that of their family. And if the strategy succeeded not only in reducing poverty but in reducing ill-health as well, it would further reduce the financial burden on the state. Arguments against the implementation of such a strategy centre on the perceived damage it would do to economic growth—a subject to which we now turn.

Implementing anti-poverty strategies: dilemmas and difficulties

The suggestion that we should pursue strategies for economic equality for the good of our 'communal health' poses a number of dilemmas and difficulties. Three of these are particularly important. First, there is an apparent dilemma between the pursuit of greater economic equality and the overall standard of living of the country as a whole. Second, there is the question of how effective such policies can be expected to be in improving the nation's health. Finally, assuming a strategy focused on reducing economic inequalities can be shown to be effective on both economic and health grounds, how likely is it that the policies involved would gain widespread public support?

Health or wealth?

Any policies involving significant redistribution of resources from the rich to the poor would seem to pose a considerable dilemma for would-be reformers. In the past half-century in Britain, policies to improve living standards have to a large extent been based on an acceptance of what has been termed the *ideology of inequality*. As already discussed, these policies have attempted to redistribute resources 'after the event' to those in need without interfering to any great extent in the operation of the economic system. To do so, it was and is still widely believed, would have grave consequences for the economy.

According to this argument, inequalities in income and wealth rightly reflect differences in individual abilities and are the driving force for the economic system. Any attempt to reduce inequalities at their source would reduce the incentive people have to work and to create wealth, interfere with market forces of supply and demand and therefore lead to economic decline. This would mean that the lot of the poor would worsen as overall living standards declined.

But just how real is this dilemma? One contemporary social policy analyst, Julian Le Grand, has argued (1982) that many of the elements of this 'ideology of inequality' are actually empirical questions open to testing, and that they are not supported by the available evidence. For example, looking at the determination of wages amongst top managers, Dorothy Wedderburn—a member of the Royal Commission on the Distribution of Income and Wealth, dismantled in 1979—noted that:

> If economic determinants were all important, we would expect to find some correlation between the level of salary of top managers and the profitability of their company, its rate of growth or its size, for these factors might help to determine what the senior executive is 'worth' in market terms. But the correlation is, in fact, very weak. (Wedderburn, 1980, p. 13)

Similarly, evidence suggests that the accumulation of wealth is more closely related to inheritance than to individual merit and effort (Pond, 1983).

What then of the argument that inequalities are the driving force of the economic system—that, whether we approve of them or not, they are functional and necessary if overall living standards are to continue to rise and the plight of the poor is to be improved?

There is very little empirical evidence to support or refute this position. There are countries, such as Japan, Sweden, and New Zealand, which have a more equal distribution of income and wealth than the United Kingdom. Until at least the late 1970s this was achieved with stronger economies, but even though these countries are experiencing considerable economic difficulties in the 1990s and have made radical changes in their welfare systems, they still retain a more equal income distribution than the United Kingdom. Similarly, every other member of the European Community, except Ireland, already has a national minimum wage. Yet, although British wages are relatively low by European standards, so too is our productivity, making us less competitive.

The case that a major redistribution of resources in society would damage economic growth is far from proven. However, it is a measure of the extent to which ideas about the functional importance and justice of economic inequalities are built into dominant beliefs and values in our society that they are sustained with such little empirical support one way or another.

What then of the evidence that a strategy to reduce economic inequalities at their source would be effective in improving health?

Which strategy for health?

Measures to reduce the most extreme aspects of poverty, even without a change in the overall distribution of income and wealth, would undoubtedly have some effect on the health of the poorest members of our society. However, recent research by Allison Quick and Richard Wilkinson, building on work conducted by Wilkinson over a number of years, suggests that this would not be the most effective way of improving health. They argue that:

> Overall health standards in developed countries are highly dependent on how equal or unequal people's incomes are. The most effective way of improving health is to make incomes more equal. (Quick and Wilkinson, 1991, p. 5)

Some of the evidence they use to support this argument is shown in Figures 11.1 and 11.2.

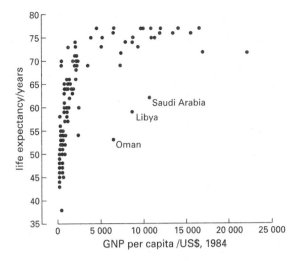

Figure 11.1 *The relationship between Gross National Product (GNP) per capita and average life expectancy in rich and poor countries. The rich Middle Eastern oil-producing countries with low life expectancy are named. (Source: Marsh, C., 1988,* Exploring Data, *Polity Press, Cambridge, p. 213)*

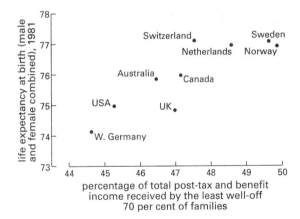

Figure 11.2 *The relationship between life expectancy and the distribution of income in different societies, measured by the percentage of total post-tax and benefit income received by the least well-off 70 per cent of families. (Source: World Bank, 1990, Luxembourg Income Study,* Working Paper 26, World Tables, *Harvester-Wheatsheaf, New York and London)*

☐ Describe and contrast the relationships shown in Figures 11.1 and 11.2.

■ Figure 11.1 suggests that life expectancy is strongly related to national wealth (measured in terms of GNP per capita) in countries below $5 000

GNP per capita. Above this level of GNP the curve levels out, indicating that there is no relationship between further increases in GNP and life expectancy. This suggests that with increasingnational wealth, improvements in health show what economists would call 'diminishing returns'. In Figure 11.2, by contrast, the curve suggests a very strong positive relationship—the more equal the income distribution in a country, the longer the life expectancy of the population.

□ Can you suggest any problems with interpreting the data in Figures 11.1 and 11.2 to conclude that there is a causal relationship between income, economic inequality and health?

■ There are a number of aspects of the data that must be kept in mind. First, the data are cross-sectional and countries have been selected for consideration; it cannot be assumed that the same relationships would be found if different years and/or different countries had been examined. Second, you cannot conclude that the relationship between income and health is causal: they may be independently related through a third factor (e.g. more egalitarian societies may have better public services, including health care). Third, life expectancy is being used as a proxy for health, which is a complex and contested phenomenon. Finally, life expectancy will reflect *past* experience whilst current income distribution is likely to influence *future* life expectancy.

However, Quick and Wilkinson have considered other evidence to support their argument. For example, in countries surveyed by the Organisation for Economic Development (OECD) for which comparable data are available, they found a strong relationship between the annual rate of change in life expectancy and the annual rate of change in income distribution, over different time periods. As income distribution became more equal, life expectancy increased more rapidly. They also cite the rapid increase in life expectancy which took place in Britain during the two World Wars as further evidence for the relationship between income distribution and health. Although they acknowledge the improvements in diet that are frequently credited with the health improvement noted during World War II, they argue that:

> What both periods have in common…is that both wars were periods of dramatic income redistribution. As well as seeing the virtual elimination of unemployment and very favourable trends in earnings differential, both wars saw

attempts to ensure at least minimum standards of provisions for all. (Quick and Wilkinson, 1991, p. 15)

By the early 1950s, Britain was a more equal society than it had been before World War II but, most importantly, the differences in the mortality rates between social classes were then at their smallest on record.

A comparison between Britain and Japan published in 1989 by two epidemiologists and public health experts, Michael Marmot and George Davey Smith, also supports the argument that reducing economic inequalities is a more effective strategy for improving the nation's health than could be achieved by simply reducing poverty. At the beginning of the 1970s, both countries had roughly similar income distributions and life expectancies. In the years that followed, Japan became a much more equal society, a process which was accompanied by improvements in life expectancy. The Japanese now have the greatest longevity, and the most equal distribution of income, in the developed world.

But how could a more equal income distribution increase life expectancy? The data in Figure 11.3 are taken from the *Health and Lifestyle* survey of over 9 000 British adults, published in 1990.[9] The graphs show the effect of £50-a-week increments in household income on age-standardised health ratios for women and men, i.e. the ratio of women and men reporting and not reporting symptoms within different weekly income groups.

□ Look carefully at Figure 11.3(b) and describe what happens to the illness ratio for women and men in the lowest weekly income groups and in the highest weekly income groups as income increases by £50 a week.

■ The graph suggests that as income *increases* in the lower income groups the ratio of those reporting illness compared to those not reporting illness declines rapidly—that is, there appears to be a very substantial improvement in health. As income increases still further, the illness ratio levels off and then begins to rise slightly amongst the highest income groups—suggesting that a *reduction* in income might be related to better health in this richer section of society.

[9]The *Health and Lifestyle* survey and in particular the work of Mildred Blaxter on lay health beliefs was featured in a television programme for Open University students called 'Why me? Why now?', associated with the first book in this series, *Medical Knowledge: Doubt and Certainty* (Open University, revised edition, 1994).

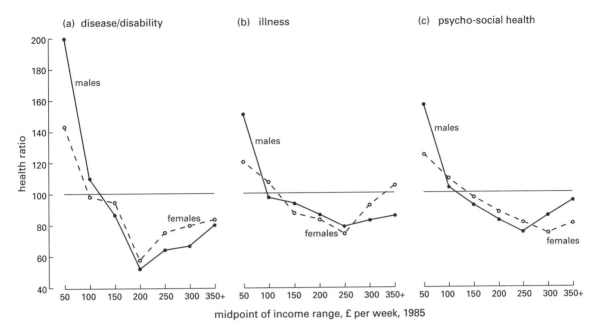

Figure 11.3   *Age-standardised health ratios in men and women aged 40–59 years in Britain in 1985, in relation to weekly income. (a) Disease/disability ratio, based on reported medically-defined conditions and the degree of disability which accompany them, (b) illness ratio, based on reports of symptoms suffered, and (c) psycho-social health ratio, based on reports of psycho-social symptoms. (All in the age group expressed as 100). (Source: Blaxter, M., 1990,* Health and Lifestyle, *Tavistock, London, p. 73)*

Again, the data in Figure 11.3 relate to a single year, so they must be interpreted cautiously, but the fact that three separate measures of health give similar results is noteworthy. Data such as these indicate that the greater longevity of a population that occurs as income rises is at least partly due to better health among the poorest members of society, resulting from an improvement in their living standards.

However, Quick and Wilkinson argue that the health of 'less poor' sectors of the population will also benefit from a more equal income redistribution. In fact, the greatest gains in *national* life expectancy occur when income is more equally distributed across the bottom 50–60 per cent of the population, rather than targetting benefits only at the poorest sector. They acknowledge that the precise mechanisms responsible for the beneficial effects of widespread income redistribution on health (beyond simply making the poor less poor) have still to be identified, but they point to some of the possible pathways.

> Much the largest part of the problem is not the material concomitant or consequences of relative deprivation, but the fact of relative deprivation itself. This means that we have to address ourselves to the psychological and social implications of income differences, of relative poverty and of having to live in conditions which are recognisably substandard—regardless of what affluence may have done to the standard.... The key element in understanding the health effects not only of poverty but also of income differentials more generally is likely to be the combination of stress, insecurity, and poor social relationships. (Quick and Wilkinson, 1991, pp. 29 and 31)

Whatever the mechanisms involved, the evidence—if it is as good as it seems—suggests that a strategy to reduce socio-economic inequalities would be an effective method of reducing health inequalities. But proof of effectiveness may not be sufficient to ensure that such a strategy is developed and implemented. This would depend in part on public attitudes towards the policies suggested.

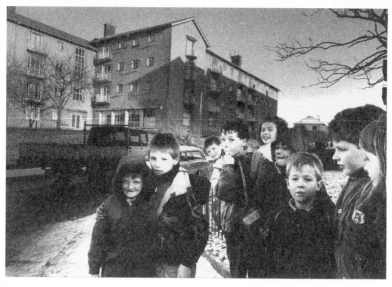

If a more equal distribution of income is pursued in the years ahead, it could affect the life expectancy of today's children in more affluent as well as in poorer areas of the country. (Photo: Glaswegians Photo Archive/Cranhill)

Public attitudes to poverty and economic inequality

The available evidence suggests that public attitudes towards the causes of poverty are contradictory. For example, a survey by the European Commission on perceptions of poverty in 1989 (published the following year), found that a fifth of the United Kingdom sample of adults attributed poverty to *laziness*—a higher proportion than in all other countries in the European Community except Greece and Luxembourg. In contrast, however, a third of Britons attributed poverty to welfare cuts, 60 per cent to long-term unemployment, and 30 per cent to injustice in society (European Commission, 1990, p. 41). (The percentages add up to more than 100 because people were allowed to give more than one answer to the question.)

These data suggest that a considerable number of people may accept that the poor are not to blame for their plight. But there is evidence that despite this, there would be little public support for policies aimed at reducing economic inequality. A recent British survey, for example, found that the majority of people who recognised the existence of poverty defined it in absolute terms:

The most prevalent definition remains the most austere, insisting on inadequacy of food and basic living needs before the term becomes relevant. The British do like their poor to look the part. (Golding, 1991, p. 41)

We began this book with an exploration of Aneurin Bevan's vision of the NHS as an opportunity to *universalise the best* in health care. Earlier chapters have highlighted the considerable difficulties and dilemmas that lie in the path of achieving his vision. In this final chapter, we end the book by reflecting on the *limitations* of health care as a vehicle for improving health status at the national level. As we have shown, there is evidence that major improvements in the health of populations come predominantly through large-scale social and economic changes. However, the difficulties and dilemmas that lie in wait along this path are no less profound than those involved in changing health-care systems. It remains to be seen how much progress is made along either course into the twenty-first century.

OBJECTIVES FOR CHAPTER 11

When you have studied this chapter you should be able to:

11.1 Explain the differences between absolute poverty, relative poverty and economic inequality, commenting on problems in defining these terms.

11.2 Give a rough estimate of the numbers of people living in poverty in Britain in the late 1980s, and identify the main demographic and social factors associated with an increased risk of poverty.

11.3 Contrast strategies for reducing poverty and economic inequality based on the 'tax and benefit systems' with those aimed at tackling inequality 'at source'. Summarise the main criticisms of, and constraints on implementing, these approaches.

11.4 Discuss the extent to which evidence supports a causal relationship between national wealth, the distribution of income and the distribution of health and illness in a society.

QUESTIONS FOR CHAPTER 11

Question 1 (*Objective 11.1*)

In 1989, John Moore, the then Conservative Secretary of State for Social Security, argued in a speech that:

...by almost every material measure it is possible to contrive: health, longevity, real income, ownership of consumer durables, number and length of holidays, money spent on entertainment, number in further education...not only are those on lower incomes not getting poorer, they are substantially better off than they ever were before. (Moore, 1989, p. 13)

Discuss the approach to defining poverty that is implicit in this quote and state on what grounds it might be criticised.

Question 2 (*Objective 11.2*)

Describe the main risk factors associated with the experience of poverty in contemporary Britain.

Question 3 (*Objective 11.3*)

What was the underlying rationale for British post-war anti-poverty policies and what factors obstructed the aims of these policies being achieved?

Question 4 (*Objective 11.4*)

On what basis could the following claim be made?

'To at least half our fellow citizens we can say inequality damages your health.'

Appendix

Table of abbreviations used in this book

Abbreviation	What it stands for
AIDS	acquired immune deficiency syndrome
ASH	Action for Smoking and Health
BMA	British Medical Association
BSE	bovine spongiform encephalopathy
CABG	coronary artery bypass graft (or grafting)
CASS	Coronary Artery Surgery Study
CEPOD	confidential enquiry into peri-operative deaths
CHC	Community Health Council
CHD	coronary heart disease
CPAG	Child Poverty Action Group
CSM	Committee on Safety of Medicines
CT	computed tomography
DH	Department of Health
DHA	District Health Authority
DHSS	Department of Health & Social Security
DSS	Department of Social Security
EN	Enrolled Nurse
EOC	Equal Opportunities Commission
FHSA	Family Health Services Authority
FPC	Family Practitioner Committee
GHS	General Household Survey
GNP	Gross National Product
GP	General Practitioner
HDL	high-density lipoprotein
HIV	human immunodeficiency virus
HRT	hormone replacement therapy
HSA	Health System Agency

Abbreviation	What it stands for
IQ	intelligence quotient
ITU	Intensive Therapy Unit
LDL	low-density lipoprotein
MRC	Medical Research Council
MRI	magnetic resonance imaging
NACNE	(Health Education Council's) National Advisory Committee on Nutritional Education
NHS	National Health Service
NMR	nuclear magnetic resonance
NTD	neural tube defects
PAMs	professions allied to medicine
PSSRU	Personal Social Services Research Unit
QALY	Quality-Adjusted Life Year
R&D	research and development
RAWP	Resource Allocation Working Party
RCT	randomised controlled trial
RGN	Registered General Nurse
RHA	Regional Health Authority
RMI	Resource Management Initiative
RN	Registered Nurse
RPI	Retail Price Index
SEN	State Enrolled Nurse
SHO	Senior House Officer
SMR	standardised mortality ratio
SRN	State Registered Nurse
UGM	Unit General Manager
UKCC	United Kingdom Central Council for Nursing, Midwifery and Health Visiting

References and further reading

References

Aaron, H. and Schwarz, W. (1984) *The Painful Prescription: Rationing Health Care*, Brookings Institution, Washington.

Acheson, Sir D. (1991) quoted in Brindle, D., Chief urges anti-poverty fight? *Guardian*, 13 September, p. 4.

Acquire (Alcohol Concern's Quarterly Information and Research Bulletin)(1992) **1**(1), Summer, p.1.

Adler, M. W. (1978) Changes in local clinical practice following an experiment in medical care: evaluation of evaluation, *Journal of Epidemiology and Community Health*, **32**, pp. 143–6.

Adler, M. W., Waller, J. J., Creese, A. and Thorne, S. C. (1978) Randomised controlled trial of early discharge for inguinal hernia and varicose veins, *Journal of Epidemiology and Community Health*, **32**, pp. 136–42.

Alford, R. R. (1975) *Health Care Politics: Ideological and Interest Group Barriers to Reform*, University of Chicago Press, Chicago.

Allen, D. (1981) An analysis of the factors affecting the development of the 1962 Hospital Plan for England and Wales, *Social Policy and Administration*, **15**(1), pp. 3–18.

Annual Abstract of Statistics (various years), HMSO, London.

Atkinson, A. B. (1991) *Poverty, Statistics and Progress in Europe*, The Welfare State Programme, discussion paper, April, London School of Economics.

Audit Commission (1986) *Making a Reality of Community Care*, HMSO, London.

Audit Commission (1990) *A Short Cut to Better Services: Day Surgery in England and Wales*, HMSO, London.

Audit Commission (1992) *Community Care: Managing the Cascade of Change*, HMSO, London.

Bailit, H., Newhouse, J., Brook, R. *et al.* (1985) Does more generous dental insurance coverage improve oral health? *Journal of the American Dental Association*, **110**(5), pp. 701–7.

Ball, K. P. (1979) *The Heart Patient I, Epidemiology*, Update Publications, Guildford.

Baly, M. E. (1987) *A History of the Queen's Institute: 100 Years 1887–1987*, Croom Helm, London.

Banyard, R. (1988) Watching the revolution, *Health Service Journal*, 11 August, pp. 916–7.

Barker, D. J. P. and Martyn, C. N. (1992) Maternal and fetal origins of cardiovascular disease, *Journal of Epidemiology and Community Health*, **46**(1), pp. 8–11.

Barking and Havering Family Health Services Authority (1991) *Addressing Inequalities: Short Term Plan 1991/92*, Barking and Havering Family Health Services Authority, London.

Baxter, C. (1987) *The Black Nurse: An Endangered Species*, Training in Health and Race, National Extension College, Cambridge.

Beresford, P. (1991) *The Sunday Times Book of the Rich*, Penguin, Harmondsworth.

Berry, D. (1992) A system in need of change, *Guardian*, 4 March.

Beveridge, W. (1942) *Report on Social Insurance and Allied Services*, Cmd. 6404, HMSO, London, (the 'Beveridge Report').

Blane, D., Davey Smith, G. and Bartley, M. (1990) Social class differences in years of potential life lost: size, trends and principal causes, *British Medical Journal*, **301**, pp. 429–32.

Blaxter, M. (1990) *Health and Lifestyles*, Tavistock, London.

Bosanquet, N. and Gray, A. (1989) *Will You Still Love Me?* National Association of Health Authorities, Birmingham.

Boulton, M., Tuckett, D., Olson, C. and Williams, A. (1986) Social class and the general practice consultation, *Sociology of Health and Illness*, **8**, pp. 325–50.

Breslow, L. (1990) A health promotion primer for the 1990s, *Health Affairs*, Summer, pp. 6–21.

Brisson, G. (1982) *Lipids in Human Nutrition*, MTP Press, Toronto.

British Medical Association (1990) *The BMA Guide to Living with Risk*, Penguin, London.

British Medical Association (1992) *Stress and the Medical Profession*, BMA, London.

Brook, R., Ware, J. E., Rogers, W. H. *et al.* (1983) Does free care improve adults' health?, *New England Journal of Medicine*, **309**(23), pp. 1 426–34 .

Brophy, M. and McQuillan, J. (1989) *Charity Trends*, 12th edn, Charities Aid Foundation, Tonbridge.

Brotchie, J. (1990) *Help at Hand*, Bedford Square Press, London.

Bryan, B., Dadzie, S. and Scafe, S. (1985) *The Heart of the Race: Black Women's Lives in Britain*, Virago Press, London.

Buchan, J. and Seccombe, I. (1991) *Nurses' Work and Worth: Pay, Careers and Working Patterns of Qualified Nurses*, IMS Report No. 213, Institute of Manpower Studies, Brighton.

Buck, N., Devlin, B. and Lunn, J. N. (1987) *Report of a confidential enquiry into peri-operative deaths*, Nuffield Provincial Hospitals Trust, London.

Buckingham, R. W., Lack, S. A., Mount, B. M., MacLean, L. D. and Collins, J. T. (1976) Living with the dying: use of the technique of participant observation, *Canadian Medical Association Journal*, **115**, pp. 1 211–15.

Bunting, M. (1991) Crippled by the system, *Guardian*, 13 November.

Burstall, M. L. (1990) *1992 and the Regulation of the Pharmaceutical Industry*, IEA Health Series, No. 9, Institute of Economic Affairs, London.

Butler, K., Carr, S. and Sullivan, F. (1988) *Citizen Advocacy: A Powerful Partnership*, National Citizen Advocacy, London.

Butler, P. (1992) Academics urge trust managers to take on doctors over performance, *Health Service Journal*, 26 June, p. 6.

Buxton, M., Packwood, T. and Keen, J. (1991) *Final Report of the Brunel University Evaluation of Resource Management*, Brunel University, London.

Bynner, J. and Stribley, K. M. (eds) (1978) *Social Research: Principles and Procedures*, Open University Press, Milton Keynes.

Campbell, D. T. (1969) Reforms as experiments, *American Psychologist*, **24**, pp. 409–29.

Cancer Research Campaign (1991) *Breast Cancer*, Factsheet 6.2, CRC, London.

Cancer Research Campaign (1992) *Lung Cancer and Smoking*, Factsheet 11.1, CRC, London.

Carr-Hill, R., Dixon, P., Gibbs, I. *et al.* (1992) *Skill Mix and the Effectiveness of Nursing Care*, Centre for Health Economics, University of York.

CASPE (Clinical Accountability, Service Planning and Evaluation) (1988) Patient Satisfaction Questionnaire, King's Fund, London.

CASS (1983) Coronary Artery Surgery Study (CASS): a randomized controlled trial of CABG survival data, *Circulation*, **68**(5), pp. 939–50.

Centre for Health Economics (1992) *How Much is a Doctor Worth?*, York University, York.

Chaitman, B. R. *et al.* (1981) Effect of coronary bypass surgery on survival patterns, *American Journal of Cardiology*, **48**, pp. 765–77.

Challis, D. and Davies, B. (1986) *Case Management in Community Care*, Gower, Aldershot.

Clay, T. (1986) Where have all the women gone?, *Lampada*, Spring, **7**, pp. 20–2.

Cochrane, A. L. (1971) *Effectiveness and Efficiency: Random Reflections on Health Services*, Nuffield Provincial Hospitals Trust, London.

Cohen, D. and Henderson, J. (1983) *A Minister for Prevention: An Initiative in Health Policy*, HERU Discussion Paper 2/83, University of Aberdeen.

Cox, D. (1991) Health service management—a sociological view: Griffiths and the non-negotiated order of the hospital, in Gabe, J., Calnan, M. and Bury, M. (eds) *The Sociology of the Health Service*, Routledge, London and New York.

Culyer, A. J. (1992) The morality of efficiency in health care: some uncomfortable implications, *Health Economics*, **1**(1), pp. 7–18.

Daly, E., Vessey, M. P., Barlow, D., Gray, A., McPherson, K. and Roche, M. (1993) Hormone replacement therapy in a risk-benefit perspective, paper delivered at the 7th International Congress on the Menopause, Stockholm, June.

Davey Smith, G. and Marmot, M. (1991) Trends in mortality in Britain, *Annals of Nutrition and Metabolism* (Suppl.), pp. 61–2.

Davey Smith, G. and Pekkannen, J. (1992) Should there be a moratorium on the use of cholesterol lowering drugs?, *British Medical Journal*, **304**, pp. 431–4.

Davey Smith, G. and Shipley, M. J. (1991) Compounding of occupation and smoking; its magnitude and consequences, *Social Science and Medicine*, **32**(11), pp. 1 297–300.

Davies, C. and Rosser, J. (1986) *Processes of Discrimination: A Study of Women Working in the NHS*, DHSS/HMSO, London.

Davison, C., Davey Smith, G. and Frankel, S. (1991) Lay epidemiology and the prevention paradox: the implications of coronary candidacy for health education, *Sociology of Health and Illness*, **13**, pp. 1–19.

Day, P. and Klein, R. (1991) Britain's Health Care Experiment, *Health Affairs*, Fall, pp. 39–59.

Delamothe, A. (1991) Social inequalities in health, *British Medical Journal*, **303**, pp. 1 046–50.

Dennis, G. (ed.) (1993) *Annual Abstract of Statistics 1993: no. 129*, HMSO, London.

Department of Health (1989a) *Working for Patients*, Cmnd. 555, HMSO, London.

Department of Health (1989b) *Medical Audit*, Working Paper No. 6, HMSO, London.

Department of Health (1989c) *Caring for People*, Cmnd. 849, HMSO, London.

Department of Health (1990) *NHS Workforce in England*, Department of Health Leaflets Unit, Stanmore.

Department of Health (1991a) *The Patient's Charter*, HMSO, London.

Department of Health (1991b) *Return of Written Complaints by or on Behalf of Patients: England 1990/91*, Government statistics service and management information division, Branch SM12.

Department of Health (1991c) *Women Doctors and their Careers*, Report of the Joint Working Party, HMSO, London.

Department of Health (1991d) *Review Body on Doctors' and Dentists' Remuneration*, 21st Report, Cmnd. 1412, HMSO, London.

Department of Health (1991e) *Review Body on Nursing Staff, Midwives and Health Visitors*, 8th Report, Cmnd. 1410, HMSO, London.

Department of Health (1991f) *Research for Health: a Research and Development Strategy for the NHS*, HMSO, London.

Department of Health (1991g) *The Health of the Nation: A consultation document*, Cmnd. 1523, HMSO, London.

Department of Health (1992) *The Health of the Nation: A Strategy for Health in England*, Cmnd. 1986, HMSO, London.

Department of Health (various years) *Health and Personal Social Services Statistics for England*, HMSO, London.

Department of Health and Social Security (1976) *Priorities for Health and Personal Social Services in England: A Consultative Document*, HMSO, London.

Department of Health and Social Security (1981a) *Care in the Community: A Consultative Document on Moving Resources for Care in England*, HC(81) 9/LAC, (81)5, HMSO, London.

Department of Health and Social Security (1981b) *Care in Action: A Handbook of Policies and Priorities for the Health and Personal Social Services in England*, HMSO, London.

Department of Health and Social Security (1981c) *Report of Study on Community Care*, DHSS, London.

Department of Health and Social Security, Scottish Office, Welsh Office and Northern Ireland Office (1981) *Growing Older*, Cmnd. 8173, HMSO, London.

Department of Health and Social Security (1985) *Government Response to the Second Report from the Social Services Committee, 1984–85 Session: Community Care*, Cmnd. 9674, HMSO, London.

Department of Health and Social Security (1987) *Promoting Better Health*, HMSO, London.

Department of Health and Social Security (1988) *Review of the Resource Allocation Working Party Formula: Final Report by the NHS Management Board*, DHSS, London

Department of Social Security (1992) *Households Below Average Income—A Statistical Analysis, 1979–1988/89*, HMSO, London.

Dingwall, R., Fenn, P. and Quam, L. (1991) *Medical Negligence: A Review and Bibliography*, Centre for Socio-legal Studies, Oxford.

Doll, R. and Peto, R. (1976) Mortality in relation to smoking: 20 years' observation on male British doctors, *British Medical Journal*, **2**, pp. 1 525–36.

Dowling, S. and Barrett, S. (1991) *Doctors in the Making: The Experience of the Pre-registration Year*, SAUS Publications, Bristol.

Doyal, L., Hunt, G. and Mellor, J. (1981) Your life in their hands: migrant workers in the National Health Service, *Critical Social Policy*, **1**(2), pp. 54–71.

Drucker, P. F. (1979) *Management*, Heinemann, London.

Elston, M. A. (1991) The politics of professional power: medicine in a changing health service, in Gabe, J., Calnan, M. and Bury, M. (eds), *The Sociology of the Health Service*, Routledge, London and New York.

Equal Opportunities Commission (1990) *Equality Management: Women's Employment in the NHS*, EOC, Manchester.

Equal Opportunities Task Force (1990) *Racial Equality: the Nursing Profession*, Occasional Paper No. 6, King's Fund, London.

European Commission (1990) *Eurobarometer: The Perception of Poverty in Europe*, EC, Brussels.

European Commission (1991) *Final Report on the Second European Poverty Programme, 1985–1989*, EC, Brussels.

Fall, C. H. D., Barker, D. J. P. and Osmond, C. (1992) Relation of infant feeding to adult serum cholesterol concentration and death from ischaemic heart disease, *British Medical Journal*, **304**, pp. 801–5.

Flynn, R. (1991) Coping with cutbacks and managing retrenchment in health, *Journal of Social Policy*, **20**(2), pp. 215–36.

Foot, M. (1975) *Aneurin Bevan, 1945–60,* Paladin, London.

Frayman, H. (1991) *Breadline Britain 1990s*, Domino Films/London Weekend Television, London.

Freidson, E. (1975) *Profession of Medicine: A Study of the Sociology of Applied Knowledge*, Dodd Mead, New York.

Fuchs, V. (1972) The basic forces influencing costs of medical care, in Fuchs, V. (ed.), *Essays in the Economics of Health and Medical Care*, Columbia University Press, New York.

Gehlen, A. (1980) *Man in the Age of Technology*, Columbia University Press, New York.

Golding, P. (1991) Poor attitudes, in Becker, S. (ed.) *Windows of Opportunity*, Child Poverty Action Group, London.

Goodin R. E. and Wilenski, P. (1984) Beyond efficiency: the logical underpinnings of administrative principles, *Public Administration Review*, **6**, pp. 512–7.

Gray, M. (1979) *Man against Disease,* Oxford University Press, Oxford.

Green, H. (1988) *Informal Carers*, Office of Population Censuses and Surveys (OPCS), Social Survey Division, HMSO, London.

Green, J. (1988) On the receiving end, *Health Service Journal*, 4 August, pp. 880–1.

Griffiths, R. (1983) *NHS Management Inquiry*, DHSS, London. [The 'Griffiths report' was in the form of a 24-page letter from Roy Griffiths to the then Secretary of State for Health and Social Services, Norman Fowler.]

Griffiths, R. (1988a) *Community Care: Agenda for Action*, HMSO, London.

Griffiths, R. (1988b) Does the public service serve? The consumer dimension, *Public Administration*, **66**, pp. 195–204.

Griffiths, R. (1992) speech to the Audit Commission in 1991 published in full under the title 'Seven years of progress: general management in the NHS', *Health Economics*, **1**(1), pp. 61–70.

Haffenden, S. (1991) *Getting it Right for Carers*, Department of Health, Social Services Inspectorate, HMSO, London.

Hall, C. (1992) Clot-busting drugs 'cut heart deaths', Report on 14th Congress of the European Society of Cardiology in Barcelona, *Independent*, 3 September, p. 5.

Ham, C. (1985) *The Governance of Health Services,* Topic Paper No. 18, University of Birmingham, Department of Social Administration, Birmingham.

Harrison, S., Hunter, D. J., Johnston, I. H., Nicholson, N., Thunhurst, C. and Wistow, G. (1991) *Health Before Health Care*, Institute for Public Policy Research, London.

Harrison, S. and Wistow, G. (1992), The purchaser/provider split in English health care, *Policy and Politics*, **20**(2), pp. 123–36.

Haywood, S. (1979) Team management in the NHS: what is it all about?, *Health and Social Service Journal*, 5 October (special insert).

Health Education Authority (1992) *Tobacco and the BBC*, HEA, London.

Hersen, M. A. and Bellack, A. S. (1988) *Dictionary of Behavioural Assessment Techniques*, Pergamon Press, New York.

Higgins, J., Deakins, N., Edwards, J. and Wicks, M. (1983) *Government and Urban Poverty: Inside the Policy-making Process*, Basil Blackwell, London.

Himmelstein, D. and Woolhandler, S. (1984) Pitfalls of private medicine: health care in the USA, *Lancet*, **2**, pp. 391–3.

House of Commons Health Committee (1991–2) *Second Report on Maternity Services*, HMSO, London (the 'Winterton Report').

House of Commons Social Services Committee (1988) *Public Expenditure on the NHS: A Memorandum Received from the DHSS*, Session 1987–88, HMSO, London.

House of Commons Social Services Committee (1990) *Community Care: Carers*, Fifth Report, Session 1989–90, HMSO, London.

House of Lords Select Committee on Science and Technology (1988) *Priorities in Medical Research*, Third Report, HMSO, London.

Hunt, S. M., McEwen, J. and McKenna, S. P. (1986) *Measuring Health Status*, Croom Helm, London.

Hunter, D. J., Judge, K. and Price, S. (1988) *Community Care: Reacting to Griffiths*, King's Fund Institute Briefing No. 1, King's Fund Centre, London.

Hunter, D. J. and Wistow, G. (1987) *Community Care in Britain: Variations on a Theme*, King's Fund, London.

Illsley, R. (1980) *Professional or Public Health?* Nuffield Provincial Hospitals Trust, London.

Institute for Fiscal Studies (1990) *Poverty in Official Statistics*, IFS Commentary No. 24, London.

Institute of Medicine (1985) *Assessing Medical Technologies*, National Academy Press, Washington D.C.

ISIS-3 (Third International Study of Infarct Survival) Collaborative Group (1992) A randomised comparison of streptokinase *vs* tissue plasminogen activator *vs* anistreplase, and of heparin *vs* aspirin alone, among 41 299 cases of suspected acute myocardial infarction, *Lancet*, **339**, pp. 753–70.

Isles, C. G., Hole, D. J., Hawthorne, V. M., Lever, A. F., *et al.* (1992) Relation between coronary risk and coronary mortality in women of the Renfrew and Paisley Survey, compared with men, *Lancet*, **339**, pp. 702–6.

Jacobson, B., Smith, A. and Whitehead, M. (eds) (1991) *The Nation's Health: A Strategy for the 1990s*, King's Fund, London.

Jarman, B. and Bosanquet, N. (1992) Primary health care in London—changes since the Acheson report, *British Medical Journal*, **305**, pp. 1 130–6.

Johns, C. (1992) Developing clinical standards, in Vaughan, B. and Robinson K. (eds), *Knowledge for Nursing Practice*, Butterworth Heinemann, Oxford, pp. 156–71.

Joseph, K. and Sumption, J. (1979) *Equality*, John Murray, London.

Kalache, A. and Vessey, M. P. (1982) Risk factors for breast cancer, *Clinics in Oncology*, **1**(3), pp. 661–78.

Kane, R. L., Wales, J., Bernstein, L., Leibowitz, A. and Kaplan, S. (1984) A randomised controlled trial of hospice care, *Lancet*, **(i)**, pp. 890–4.

Khaw, K-T. and Barrett-Connor, E. (1986) Family history of heart attack: a modifiable risk factor?, *Pathophysiology and Natural History—Coronary Heart Disease*, **74**, pp. 239–43.

Kirchberger, S. (ed.) (1991) *The Diffusion of Two Technologies for Renal Stone Treatment across Europe*, King's Fund Centre, London.

Kitson, A. (1986) Quality assurance: rest assured, *Nursing Times*, 27 August, pp. 29–31.

Klein, R. (1989) *The Politics of the NHS*, Longman, London and New York.

Knapp, M., Beecham, J., Anderson, J., Dayson D., Leff, J., Margolius, O., O'Driscoll, C. and Wills, W. (1990b) *Predicting the Community Costs of Closing Psychiatric Hospitals: The TAPS Project*, Discussion Paper 640, Personal Social Services Research Unit, Canterbury.

Knapp, M., Cambridge, P., Thomason, C., Beecham, J., Allen, C. and Darton, R. (1990a) *Care in the Community: Lessons from a Demonstration Programme*, Personal Social Services Research Unit, Canterbury.

La Vecchia, C., Levi, F., Franceschi, S. and Boyle, P. (1991) Assessment of screening for cancer, *International Journal of Technology Assessment in Health Care*, **7**(3), pp. 275–85.

Le Grand, J. (1982) *The Strategy of Equality*, George Allen and Unwin, London.

Leathard, A. (1990) *Health Care Provision: Past, Present and Future*, Chapman and Hall, London.

Lichtenstein, S. *et al.* (1978) Judged frequency of lethal events, *Journal of Experimental Psychology: Human Learning and Memory*, **4**, p. 551.

Lindblom, C. E. (1959) The science of 'muddling through', *Public Administration Review*, **19**(3), pp. 79–88.

Lomas, J., Enkin, M., Anderson, G. M., Hannah, W. J., Vayda, E. and Singer, J. (1991) Opinion leaders *vs* audit and feedback to implement practice guidelines, *Journal of the American Medical Association*, **265**, pp. 2 202–7.

London Health Planning Consortium (The Acheson Committee) (1981) *Primary Health Care in Inner London*, London Health Planning Consortium, London.

Loomes, G. and Sugden, R. (1982) Regret theory: an alternative theory of rational choice under uncertainty, *The Economic Journal*, **92**, pp. 805–24.

Mack, J. and Lansley, S. (1991) *Poor Britain*, HarperCollins, London.

Mackay, L. (1989) *Nursing a Problem*, Open University Press, Milton Keynes.

Mahoney, F. I. and Barthel, D. W. (1965) Functional evaluation: the Barthel Index, *Maryland State Medical Journal: Annual Meeting*, pp. 61–5.

Mallett, J. (1991) Shifting the focus of audit, *Health Services Journal*, 28 February, pp. 24–5.

Marmot, M. G. and Davey Smith, G. (1989) Why are the Japanese living longer?, *British Medical Journal*, **299**, pp. 1 547–51.

Marsh, C. (1988) *Exploring Data*, Polity Press, Cambridge.

McKee, M. and Lessof, L. (1992) Nurse and Doctor: Whose task is it anyway?, in Robinson, J., Gray, A. and Elkan, R. (eds) *Policy Issues in Nursing*, Open University Press, Buckingham, pp. 60–7.

McKinlay, J. B. (1981) From 'promising report' to 'standard procedure': seven stages in the career of a medical innovation, *Milbank Memorial Fund Quarterly/Health and Society*, **59**, pp. 374–411.

Meade, J. E. (1978) *The Structure and Reform of Direct Taxation*, George Allen and Unwin, London.

Medical Research Council Working Party (1992) Medical Research Council trial of treatment of hypertension in older adults: principal results, *British Medical Journal*, **304**, pp. 405–12.

Mihill, C. (1991) GPs who refuse second opinions, *Guardian*, 12 February.

Mihill, C. (1991) Patients 'being left in ignorance', *Guardian*, 7 February.

Millar, B. (1991) Wrong drug, wrong leg, wrong compensation, *Health Service Journal*, 17 January, p. 16.

Ministry of Health (1944) *A National Health Service*, Cmd. 6502, HMSO, London.

Ministry of Health, Scottish Home and Health Department (1966) *Report of the Committee on Senior Nursing Staff Structure*, HMSO, London (the 'Salmon Report').

Mitchell, J. R. A. (1984) What constitutes evidence on the dietary prevention of coronary heart disease? Cosy beliefs or harsh facts?, *International Journal of Cardiology*, **5**, pp. 287–97.

Moore, J. (1989) The end of the line for poverty, speech delivered by the Secretary of State for Social Security, 11 May, Department of Social Security, London.

Moores, B. (1987) The changing composition of the British hospital nursing workforce 1962–84, *Journal of Advanced Nursing*, **12**, pp. 499–504.

National Advisory Committee on Nutritional Education (NACNE) (1983) *Discussion Paper on Proposals for Nutritional Guidelines for Health Education in Britain*, Health Education Council, London.

Neilson, D. D. and Sorenson, D. D. (1979) Alcohol policy: alcohol consumption, alcohol prices, delirium tremens and alcoholism as cause of death in Denmark, *Social Psychiatry*, **14**, begins p. 133.

Oakley, A. (1980) *Women Confined: Towards a Sociology of Childbirth*, Martin Robertson, Oxford.

Oakley, A. (1984) *The Captured Womb: A History of Medical Care of Pregnant Women*, Blackwells, Oxford.

OECD (Organisation for Economic Cooperation and Development) (1990) *Health Care Systems in Transition: the Search for Efficiency*, OECD Social Policy Studies, No. 7, OECD, Paris.

Office of Technology Assessment, US Congress (1976) *Development of Medical Technology: Opportunities for Assessment*, US Government Printing Office, Washington D.C.

Office of Technology Assessment, US Congress (1982) *Strategies for Medical Technical Assessment*, US Government Printing Office, Washington D.C.

Oliver, M. (1992) Letter, *British Medical Journal*, **304**, pp. 393–4.

OPCS (1992) *Social Trends 22*, HMSO, London.

OPCS (1993) *Social Trends 23*, HMSO, London.

Oppenheim, C. (1990) *Poverty: The Facts*, Child Poverty Action Group, London.

Owens, P. and Glennerster, H. (1990) *Nursing in Conflict*, Macmillan, Basingstoke.

Paffenbarger, R. S. *et al.* (1986) Physical activity, all cause mortality and longevity of College Alumni, *New England Journal of Medicine*, **314**, pp. 605–13.

Paterson, E. (1981) Food-work: maids in a hospital kitchen, in Atkinson, P. and Heath, C. (eds) *Medical Work: Realities and Routines*, Gower, Farnborough.

Payer, L. (1988) *Medicine and Culture: Varieties of Treatment in the United States, England, West Germany and France*, Henry Holt & Co, New York.

Pearson, M. (1987) Racism: the great divide, *Nursing Times*, 17 June, **83**(24), pp. 24–6.

Pendleton, D. and Bochner, S. (1980) The communication of medical information in GP consultations as a function of social class, *Social Science and Medicine*, **14a**, pp. 669–73.

PEP (Political and Economic Planning) (1944) Medical care for citizens, *Planning*, **222**.

Phillips, A. N., Shaper, A. G., Pocock, S. J. and Walker, M. (1988) Parental death from heart disease and the risk of heart attack, *European Heart Journal*, The European Society of Cardiology, **9**, pp. 243–51.

Plamping, D. (1991) The new NHS: better to go forwards than backwards, *British Medical Journal*, **302**, pp. 737–8.

Pollitt, C. (1987a) Performance measurement and the consumer: hijacking the bandwagon?, in *Performance Measurement and the Consumer*, National Consumer Council, London.

Pollitt, C. (1987b) Capturing quality? The quality issue in British and American health policies, *Journal of Public Policy*, **7**(1), pp. 71–92.

Pond, C. (1983) Wealth and the two nations, in Field, F. (ed.) *The Wealth Report 2*, Routledge and Kegan Paul, London.

Pond, C. and Popay, J. (1983) Tackling inequalities at their source, in Glennerster, H. (ed.) *The Future of the Welfare State: Remaking Social Policy*, Heinemann Educational, London.

Popham, R. E., Schmidt, W. and de Lint, L. (1975) The prevention of alcoholism: epidemiological studies of the effect of government control measures, *British Journal of Addiction*, **70**, begins p. 125.

Quick, A. and Wilkinson, R. (1991) *Income and Health*, Socialist Health Association, London.

Ravnskov, U. (1992) Cholesterol lowering trials in coronary heart disease, frequency of citation and outcome, *British Medical Journal*, **305**, pp. 15–19.

Regan, D. E. and Stewart, J. (1982) Essay in the government of health, *Social Policy and Administration*, **16** (1), pp. 19–43.

Relman, A. S. (1980) The new medical–industrial complex, *New England Journal of Medicine*, **303**, pp. 963–70.

Robb, B. (ed.) (1967) *Sans Everything—A Case to Answer,* Nelson, London.

Rose, G. and Marmot, M. (1981) Social class and CHD, *British Heart Journal,* **45**, pp. 13–9.

Royal College of Nursing (1992) *Cost Effective Care,* RCN Briefing, September, Royal College of Nursing, London.

Royal College of Physicians of London (1991) *Preventive Medicine: A Report of a Working Party of the Royal College of Physicians,* Royal College of Physicians of London, London.

Royal Commission on the National Health Service (1978) *Patients' Attitudes to the Hospital Service,* Research paper No. 5, HMSO, London.

Royal Commission on the National Health Service (1979) *Report,* HMSO, London.

Rue, R. (1991) Evaluation of resource management, *British Medical Journal,* **302**, pp.1 291–2.

Seale, C. (1990) Caring for people who die: the experience of family and friends, *Ageing and Society,* **10**, pp. 413–28.

Sheldon, T. (1991), The good, the bad, and the relatives, *Health Service Journal,* 14 November, p. 13.

Small, N. (1989) *Politics and Planning in the National Health Service,* Open University Press, Buckingham.

Smith, A. (1812) *The Wealth of Nations,* Ward Lock, London (first published 1776).

Stacey, M. (1976) The health service consumer: a sociological misconception, in Stacey, M. (ed.) *The Sociology of the National Health Service,* Sociological Review Monograph No. 22, University of Keele, Keele.

Stacey, M. (1991) *The Sociology of Health and Healing,* Routledge, London and New York.

Stamler, J. and Epstein, F. (1972) CHD risk factors as guides to preventive action, *Preventive Medicine,* **1**, p. 27.

Stocking, B. (1984) *Initiative and Inertia: Case Studies in the NHS,* Nuffield Provincial Hospitals Trust, London.

Stocking, B. (1991) *Factors Affecting the Diffusion of Three Kinds of Innovative Medical Technology in European Community Countries and Sweden,* King's Fund, London.

Strong, P. and Robinson, J. (1990) *The NHS: Under New Management,* Open University Press, Buckingham.

Sykes, W., Collins, M., Hunter, D. J., Popay, J. and Williams, G. (1992) *Listening to Local Voices in the NHS,* Nuffield Institute for Health and PHRRC, Leeds and Salford.

Szczepura, A. K., Fletcher, J. and Fitz-Patrick, J. D. (1991) Cost effectiveness of magnetic resonance imaging in the neurosciences, *British Medical Journal,* **303**, pp. 1 435–9.

Tawney, R. H. (1964) *Equality,* George Allen and Unwin, London (first published 1931).

Titmuss, R. (1961) Community care: fact or fiction?, in Titmuss, R. (1968) *Commitment to Welfare,* Allen and Unwin, London.

Torrance, G. W. (1986) Measurement of health state utilities for economic appraisal: a review, *Journal of Health Economics,* **5**, pp. 1–30.

Townsend, P. (1979) *Poverty in the United Kingdom,* Allen Lane, Harmondsworth.

Townsend, P. (1991) *The Poor are Poorer: A Statistical Report on Changes in the Living Standards of Rich and Poor in the United Kingdom, 1979–1989,* University of Bristol.

U205 Course Team (1985) *Caring for Health: Dilemmas and Prospects,* The Open University Press, Milton Keynes.

Uttley, S. (1991) *Technology and the Welfare State: The Development of Health Care in Britain and America,* Unwin Hyman, London.

Veitch, A. (1985) Lack of cash 'killing' transplant patients, *Guardian,* 28 January.

Waitzkin, H. (1979) A Marxian interpretation of the growth and development of coronary care technology, *American Journal of Public Health,* **69**, pp. 1 260–8.

Walker, C. and Cannon, G. (1984) *The Food Scandal,* Century Publishing, London.

Wedderburn, D. (1980) Inequalities in pay, in Routh, G., Wedderburn, D., and Wootton, B. (eds) *The Roots of Pay Inequalities,* Low Pay Unit, London.

Wertheimer, A. (ed.) (1991) *A Chance to Speak Out,* King's Fund Centre, London.

West, C. (1992) A general manager's view of contemporary nursing issues, in Robinson, J. Gray, A. and Elkan, R. (eds) *Policy Issues in Nursing,* Open University Press, Buckingham, pp. 52–9.

Wildavsky, A. (1979) *The Art and Craft of Policy Analysis,* Macmillan, London.

Williams, A. (in press for 1994 publication) Priority setting in the NHS, in Davey, B., Gray, A. and Seale, C. (eds) *Health and Disease: A Reader* (2nd edn), Open University Press, Buckingham.

Winkler, F. (1987) Consumerism in health care: beyond the supermarket model, *Policy and Politics,* **15**(1), pp. 1–8.

Winkler, F. (in press for 1994 publication) Transferring power in health care, in Davey, B., Gray, A. and Seale, C. (eds) *Health and Disease: A Reader* (2nd edn), Open University Press, Buckingham.

Wistow, G. and Hardy, B. (1991) Joint management in community care, *Journal of Management in Medicine,* **5**(4), pp. 40–8.

Wood, J. (1984) Patient participation in general practice, in Maxwell, R. and Weaver, N. (eds), *Public Participation in Health,* King's Fund, London.

World Bank (1990) *Poverty, Inequality and Income Distribution in Comparative Perspective: the Luxembourg Income Study,* Working Paper 26, World Tables, Harvester-Wheatsheaf, New York and London.

World Health Organisation (1984 to 1991, annual publication) *World Health Statistics,* WHO, Geneva.

Wright, K. (1987) *Cost-Effectiveness in Community Care,* Discussion Paper 33, Centre for Health Economics, University of York, York.

Further reading

A very wide range of topics and issues is covered in *Dilemmas in Health Care*. The Reference list above is comprehensive and can usefully be consulted as a source of additional reading. However, we have chosen a short selection of recommended titles (listed under *General* below), which are relevant to many areas of contemporary health care in the United Kingdom in the 1990s, and which are easily obtainable, inexpensive and accessibly written for the general reader. As elsewhere in this book, we are using the widest possible definition of health care to include health-service activity, social and community services, disease prevention and health promotion, and fiscal and social policies that may have an impact on health. Recommended further reading relating to specific areas of interest contained largely within one chapter is listed below under the relevant chapter number. Note that there are no specific titles for Chapters 1, 3 or 10.

General

Blaxter, M. (1990) *Health and Lifestyles,* Tavistock/Routledge, London and New York. Discusses the results of a large-scale British survey of many aspects of health, including lay health beliefs, and their relationship to 'lifestyle'.

Bulmer, M. (1986) *Social Science and Social Policy,* Allen and Unwin, London. An account of the extent to which people who make public policy are influenced by the findings of social science.

Department of Health (1992) *The Health of the Nation: A Strategy for Health in England,* HMSO, London. Official government policy for reducing the mortality from common diseases, specifying targets to be achieved by the end of this century.

Gabe, J., Calnan, M. and Bury, M. (1991) *The Sociology of the Health Service,* Routledge, London and New York. A collection of essays about policy issues, including professional power and health care evaluation.

Johnson, T. J. (1972) *Professions and Power,* Macmillan, London. A general discussion of professional autonomy, considered to be a classic text.

Klein, R. (1989) *The Politics of the NHS,* Longman, London and New York. One of the best books available on this subject, with an extensive analysis of the community interest in the NHS, among many other topics.

Chapter 2

Culyer, A. J. (1992) The morality of efficiency in health care: some uncomfortable implications, *Health Economics,* **1**(1), pp. 7–18. A careful exposition of the argument that only *effective* health care should be provided by the NHS.

Harrison, S. (1988) *Managing the National Health Service: Shifting the Frontier?,* Chapman and Hall, London. Summarises some twenty-five pre-Griffiths research studies of NHS management.

Harrison, S., Hunter, D. J., Johnston, I. H., Nicholson, N., Thunhurst, C. and Wistow, G. (1991) *Health Before Health Care,* Institute for Public Policy Research, London. The argument that the NHS should be transferred to local government control to assist the integration of health services with other relevant services is evaluated in the new context of the 'purchaser–provider split' in health care.

Harrison, S., Hunter, D. J., Marnoch, G. and Pollitt, C. (1992) *Just Managing: Power and Culture in the National Health Service,* Macmillan, London. Summarises some twenty-five post-Griffiths research studies of NHS management.

Schulz, R. and Harrison, S. (1986) Physician autonomy in the Federal Republic of Germany, Great Britain, and the United States, *International Journal of Health Planning and Management,* **1**(5), pp. 335–55. A discussion of professional autonomy as it applies specifically to medicine.

Chapter 4

Black, N. (1990) Quality assurance of medical care, *Journal of Public Health Medicine,* **12**(2), pp. 97–104. Summarises major developments in practitioner-based self-evaluation in Great Britain.

Bowling, A. (1991) *Measuring Health: A Review of Quality of Life Measuring Scales,* Open University Press, Buckingham. A discussion of a selection of health measures which together measure quality of life.

Campbell, D. T. and Stanley, J. C. (1966) *Experimental and Quasi-experimental Design for Research,* Rand McNally, Chicago. A classic statement of the logic of quasi-experimental evaluation design.

Coulter, A. (1991) Evaluating the outcomes of health care, in Gabe, J., Calnan, M. and Bury, M. (eds) *The Sociology of the Health Service,* Routledge, London and New York, Chapter 5. Summarises many considerations in the evaluation of health care, with a case study of the evaluation of hysterectomy.

Chapter 5

Age Concern (1989) *Guidelines for setting up Advocacy Schemes,* Age Concern, London. Contains practical advice for those contemplating setting up such schemes.

Alford, R. R. (1975) *Health Care Politics,* University of Chicago Press, Chicago. An American analysis of the three key interest groups with a say in health services, with an explanation for the weakness of the community interest.

Fitzpatrick, R. (1984) Satisfaction with health care, in Fitzpatrick, R., Hinton, J., Newman, S., Scambler, G. and Thompson, J. (eds), *The Experience of Illness,* Tavistock Publications, London. A discussion of methods and results of assessing patient satisfaction.

Klein, R. (1984) The politics of participation, in Maxwell, R. (ed.), *Public Participation in Health: Towards a Clearer View,* King's Fund, London. An account of community participation in the British NHS.

Marmor, T. R. and Morone, J. A. (1980) Representing consumer interests: imbalanced markets, health planning and the Health Systems Agencies, *Milbank Memorial Fund Quarterly,* **58**(1), pp. 125–65. An account of an experiment in participation in America, written with reference to the framework proposed by Robert Alford (see second reference above).

Chapter 6

Beardshaw, V. and Robinson, R. (1990) *New for Old? Prospects for Nursing in the 1990s,* Research Report 8, King's Fund, London. A report on the key issues in British nursing, aimed at a non-nursing audience, principally health-care policymakers.

Elston, M. (1991) The politics of professional power: medicine in a changing society, in Gabe, J., Calnan, M. and Bury, M. (eds) *The Sociology of the Health Service, London and New York*, Routledge, London and New York. The chapter title fully reflects the content.

Mackay, L. (1989) *Nursing a Problem*, Open University Press, Buckingham. An ethnographic study of the experience of nursing work.

Miles, A. (1991) *Women, Health and Medicine*, Open University Press, Buckingham. Chapter 5 gives an account of theories about the division of health labour and reviews the position of women in health professions. Chapter 6 looks at some of the consequences of gender divisions for the control of health care and encounters between carers and cared for.

Robinson, J., Gray, A. and Elkan, R. (eds) (1992) *Policy Issues in Nursing*, Open University Press, Buckingham. This collection of essays represents a wide range of viewpoints on nursing and the nursing workforce, with articles from nurses, sociologists and general managers.

Stacey, M. (1991) *The Sociology of Health and Healing*, Routledge, London and New York. Chapters 6 and 13 give a historical and sociological account of the division of paid health work; they are rich in detail and especially alive to class and gender issues.

Chapter 7

McKinlay, J. B. (1981) From 'promising report' to 'standard procedure': seven stages in the career of a medical innovation, *Milbank Memorial Fund Quarterly/Health and Society*, **59**, pp. 374–411. This paper outlines the typical career of a medical innovation, explains why so few innovations are subjected to adequate clinical trials, and sets out an alternative approach based on evidence from randomised controlled trials (RCTs).

Chapter 8

Audit Commission (1992) *The Community Revolution: Personal Social Services and Community Care*, HMSO, London. Provides a good summary of the move to community care and assesses the problems confronting local authorities as they implement the reforms.

House of Commons Social Services Committee (1990) *Community Care: Planning and Cooperation*, Eighth Report, Session 1989–90, HMSO, London. Provides a succinct review and critique of the government's community care reforms in the key area of planning across agency boundaries.

Tomlinson, D. (1991) *Utopia, Community Care and the Retreat from the Asylums*, Open University Press, Buckingham. Analyses the process of closure of two large mental hospitals and the development of community services for discharged hospital residents.

Twigg, J., Atkin, K. and Perring, C. (1991) *Carers and Services: A Review of Research*, HMSO, London. Examines the issues affecting carers resulting from the move to community care.

Chapter 9

Forrest, Sir P. (1987) *Breast Cancer Screening: Report to the Health Ministers of England, Wales, Scotland and Northern Ireland*, HMSO, London. The basis of current policy on breast cancer screening in the United Kingdom, with a thorough discussion of its justification.

Rose, G. (1992) *The Strategy of Preventive Medicine*, Oxford University Press, Oxford. A good basic introduction to the policy of disease prevention, discussing why and how, and emphasising the distinction between concentrating on high risk individuals as opposed to mass intervention in populations.

Sikora, K. and Thomas, H. (1989) *Fight Cancer: How to Prevent it and How to Fight it*, BBC Books, London. An introduction to all aspects of reducing the burden of cancer.

Chapter 11

Frayman, H. (1991) *Breadline Britain 1990s*, Domino Films/LWT, London. This booklet was produced to accompany the television series, Breadline Britain 1990s, broadcast by London Weekend Television. It gives the summary results of the national survey commissioned for the series, and provides a picture of the overall level of poverty, public attitudes towards the poor, and case studies of individuals and families.

Le Grand, J. (1982) *The Strategy of Equality*, George Allen and Unwin, London. Julian Le Grand is an economist with an interest in health and social policy issues. In this book, he examines who benefits from different forms of public spending, including spending on health. He concludes that the welfare state actually delivers more help to higher socio-economic groups than to poorer sections of society, and argues that a more direct approach to tackling inequalities is necessary.

Le Grand, J. (1991) *The Distribution of Public Expenditure on Health Care Revisited*, Discussion Paper WSP/64, June, London School of Economics, London. His conclusions from the 1982 analysis are updated to the 1990s.

Mack, J. and Lansley, S. (1991) *Poor Britain*, HarperCollins, London. A more detailed account of relative poverty in the 1990s, written by the programme makers responsible for the Breadline Britain television series.

Oppenheim, C. (1993) *Poverty: The Facts*, 2nd edn, Child Poverty Action Group, London. A revised and updated edition, which provides a succinct and readable analysis of the scale and causes as well as the experience of poverty in Britain in the 1990s.

Quick, A. and Wilkinson, R. (1991) *Income and Health*, Socialist Health Association, London. This small book by researchers at the University of Sussex provides a comprehensive and readable summary of the arguments and evidence of the link between inequality and health, using comparisons over time and between countries.

Answers to self-assessment questions

Chapter 1

1 The authors consider that surgical procedures that are appropriate for day-case admission would be carried out more *effectively* in a unit dedicated to those procedures than in a general surgical ward dealing with a wide range of surgical treatments. Day surgery is thought to be more *humane* because it reduces the time patients are separated from their homes and support networks, and decreases the likelihood of distressing last-minute cancellations. This last point should also improve *equity* because patients are more likely to be prioritised according to need for surgery, rather than face the cancellation lottery. Greater equity would also result from the predicted reduction in waiting lists. Day surgery is expected to offer a more *efficient* use of resources, especially those arising from the 'hotel' costs of an in-patient stay (nursing, catering, cleaning, etc.)

2 The effectiveness of the rapid use of clot-busting drugs in reducing mortality after a heart attack could lead to a decision at the *strategic* level of management in the health service to recommend that all GPs carry the drugs with them at all times. This has consequences for *operational* management, for example in hospitals that admitted patients who would otherwise have died. Doctors who carry these drugs would, by using them, be changing their *clinical* management of a recent heart attack.

3 An increase in day surgery creates dilemmas for *managers* who must find the resources to set up, or improve, appropriate facilities and staffing before any efficiency savings can be made. They may also find themselves in uncomfortable negotiations with surgeons who are uncertain about the benefits of day surgery to themselves and their patients. Some *consultants* will be anxious that pressure to admit patients for day surgery will undermine their clinical freedom to prescribe treatment, or see it as an erosion of their allocation of beds. Others may be concerned that reduction in waiting lists will also reduce their income from private patients, who could in future get minor surgery performed quickly as an NHS 'day case' rather than pay for a private in-patient bed. *Patients* who prefer to stay in hospital overnight after minor surgery may find this option closed. Patients who have no one to care for them when discharged so soon after an operation face the dilemma of whether to accept earlier treatment as a day patient under these circumstances. Early discharge of patients may create a new demand for community care and hence have unforeseen resource implications, or place greater burdens on informal carers.

Chapter 2

1 For most of the history of the NHS, doctors have been its most influential group, having utilised their 'clinical freedom' not only to determine the overall pattern of services to patients, but, on occasions, to obstruct changes of which they disapproved. In this climate, citizen representatives were weak, and the role of managers bore little resemblance to textbook prescriptions (such as Drucker's principles). In the 1980s, the Griffiths (general management) changes, combined with financial stringency, began to tilt this balance somewhat in the direction of managers, particularly through information systems which rendered doctors' work more visible. The NHS reforms of the 1990s may have accelerated this process.

2 The *Working for Patients* changes will continue the trend towards greater information for managers about the work of doctors (referred to in the answer to Question 1). In addition, managers are now much more involved in decisions about the appointment and working arrangements of doctors, particularly in the new NHS Trusts. Finally, the purchaser–provider split, which makes hospitals dependent for finance on the numbers of patients treated, seems to have provided additional managerial leverage over doctors.

3 (a) An increase in the influence of doctors can be justified on the grounds that clinical autonomy is essential to safeguard the best treatment for patients, against increasing pressure from managers to contain costs.

   (b) By the same token, an increase in managerial influence may be pursued to ensure that variations in performance are made more visible and subjected to more rigorous scrutiny. Such activities on the part of management may be seen to represent an extension of the public interest over the self-serving behaviour of doctors.

(c) Similarly, citizen representatives may more directly express the preferences of health-service users about the quality of services and the range of treatments which should be offered.

4 The basic responsibility of managers in a *purchasing* organisation is to consider questions, from the perspective of the local population as a whole, about who gets care, how and with what results. More particularly, managers in a purchasing organisation must be involved in identifying the needs for health care of that population and allocating resources to meet those needs in accordance with defined priorities and standards. In short, therefore, purchasers 'buy' health services to meet the needs of the local population for which they are responsible. In turn, it is *provider* organisations that supply those services as specified in contracts with purchasers. Thus they are responsible for the 'hands-on' management and delivery of health services to individual patients within the terms of contracts won from purchasers and the budgets accompanying those contracts.

Chapter 3

1 The *need* for treatment is clear from the fact that people died while waiting for it. The *demand* for treatment came into being because of the availability of the operation: before the 1980s the operation was not available in the United Kingdom and consequently there was no demand. The existence of a waiting list could be interpreted as evidence that the demand exceeded the *supply* of the treatment.

2 Rationing is inevitable because the demand for health care is very great while the supply of care is limited. Moreover, because health care is permeated by the agency relationship, in which doctors act as the agent of the patient in deciding what treatment to demand, increases in supply usually bring forth an increase in demand.

In the NHS, health care is rationed by restrictions on the total amount of care available, which are imposed when the government decides an annual resource allocation to the NHS. This results in patients having to queue (on waiting lists), and doctors having to set treatment criteria in the light of a realistic assessment of the availability of care. Direct charges, for instance for prescriptions or dental care, are another form of rationing.

3 Until the 1970s, English RHAs were allocated health resources largely on the basis of their existing level of hospital services: the more they had, the more they received. This perpetuated geographical inequalities in provision that had been a feature of health care before the NHS. The RAWP formula was designed to reduce these. Since its introduction there has undoubtedly been some narrowing of geographical inequalities (Figure 3.4), but more rapid progress has been prevented by tight restrictions on total NHS spending since the late 1970s: in these circumstances, greater equality would require some levelling down of resources—a much more painful procedure than levelling up.

4 You may have suggested the following:
(a) Measuring cost-effectiveness requires accurate information not only on effectiveness (life expectancy and quality of life), but on costs, which can also be difficult to obtain.
(b) The cost-effectiveness of any single treatment means almost nothing in itself: what is relevant is how this compares with other treatments. Cost-effectiveness is a relative measure.
(c) Few people would accept that cost-effectiveness was a *sufficient* criterion on which to decide if something is worth doing. As discussed in the chapter, many other moral and political issues are likely to enter such decisions.

Chapter 4

1 A number of patients suffering from depression would be randomly assigned to two groups, a treatment group receiving ECT and a control group not receiving it. To control for the placebo effect, which might occur if the subjects of the experiment knew whether or not they were getting ECT, a 'sham' or 'dummy' treatment would have to be given to the control group. As patients are anaesthetised before ECT, this would present no practical problems (although ethical ones are not ruled out) since patients could all be anaesthetised, with only those in the treatment group being given ECT.

A threat to *internal* validity that remains is the effect of experimenter bias: those giving the treatments might convey in subtle ways that they had different expectations for the recovery of those receiving treatment. A threat to *external* validity would occur if the people in the experiment were not representative of all patients suffering from depression, for whom the results might be believed relevant.

2 The first task would be to define the *hoped-for* outcomes, so that the processes believed to lead to these can be identified. In this case, change in health status or quality of life could be taken to be the desired outcome.

Process and outcome give varying amounts of information about the four elements of good health care.

(a) A study of the *process* of care might help assess the *humanity* of the care, perhaps by qualitative description of the experience of participants. The degree to which resources within the programme were being used economically could also be illuminated by such study, helping us to assess efficiency. A study of the process by which people gain entry to the programme would shed light on *equity* issues, but to establish whether there was equal access to the programme would require a study of the population potentially served by the programme.

(b) A study of the *outcomes* of care would help in the evaluation of its *effectiveness*, as this would provide evidence about changes in health status or quality of life resulting from the programme. Relating the cost of care to outcomes would give a measure of cost-effectiveness, an aspect of *efficiency*.

3 The consultants would be particularly concerned to record outcome in terms of morbidity and mortality in the mothers and babies. If high levels of these were found for deliveries outside the hospital (controlling for the fact that one place of delivery might attract disproportionate numbers of high-risk mothers) they would feel that their case was supported. The Community Health Council might be more interested in women's satisfaction with care as an outcome measure. They might also want to measure the incidence of post-natal depression. If low levels of satisfaction and high levels of depression were found for hospital care, they would feel that their case was supported.

4 The basic objective of medical audit is to encourage discussion between doctors, so that they become aware of the extent to which their clinical practice meets, or falls below, the best standards. If this awareness leads to constructive change, a better quality service to patients will have been provided. However, medical audit by doctors is an activity in which the areas investigated and the criteria for success are decided by the doctors themselves. There is a potential conflict of interest in providers evaluating their own practice.

5 The age-structure of the female population in the two areas could influence the need for hysterectomy (it would be more prevalent in an older population). The manager would also need some indication of the relative incidence of symptoms amenable to treatment by hysterectomy. Without this there is no indication of whether the variation in rates of surgery are the result of variability in clinical judgements, or whether they are the result of

differences in need. Ideally, the manager would possess information about improvements in health status that occurred as a result of operations in the two areas in order to assess the optimum level of surgery. Information of this last sort, however, would require a costly exercise in data collection.

Chapter 5

1 Unlike the consumer of most goods and services in the private sector, the consumer of health services (whether public or private) may not have sufficient information, expertise or opportunity to make an informed choice between one provider and another. It may be inappropriate to regard the *current user* of the service as the consumer when others—carers, potential users, taxpayers—may be as important. The key private-sector principle of improving quality by consumer choice may be difficult to apply to health and social services when quasi-political rationing decisions are being taken. In the case of health care, completely free choice by consumers could lead to unbalanced resource allocation at the expense of those with weak 'purchasing' power.

2 The health service shows all the signs of having become more consumer conscious in the 1980s with, for example, increased use of surveys of patient satisfaction and efforts to improve the ease with which patients can make complaints. However, Winkler suggests that such 'supermarket consumerism' is superficial, reflecting managers' desire to gain the upper hand over doctors rather than a real concern for patients. For Winkler, the consumer voice in decision-making can only be effective if managers and doctors are willing to concede power.

3 (a) At the individual level, consumers can vary in the extent to which they can represent themselves. It may be easier to be heard in private health-care settings than in public health care. Certain individuals who are less articulate may need help in expressing their needs and wants, by advocacy for example. Getting access to information on the quality of clinical aspects of care may be difficult for an individual.

(b) At the group level, citizen representatives may also vary in their power to influence decisions. This can be because they are overwhelmed by concentrated professional or managerial expertise in committees, or because they are not elected by a particular constituency, so cannot draw on that source of legitimacy. Even more fundamental is the extent to which representatives of local community interests are allowed to participate in decision-making through health-authority member-ship—a right that was lost in the reforms of the 1990s.

4 Although earlier legislation made it easier for patients to change their GP, the setting up of the internal market does not in itself enhance the power of individual con-sumers to choose services. Purchasers (GPs and health authorities) act as *proxy* consumers, a situation that may be appropriate in a market where specialist expertise is required to judge quality and so make good choices. The information systems that are generated by the needs of the internal market may, in theory, be used to give individual consumers better information about the quality of clinical care, thus enhancing their ability to make informed choices. Access to this information, though, is likely to be fiercely contested.

Chapter 6

1 You may have suggested the following:

(a) Attempts to contain NHS costs are likely to be felt directly by health workers, as they are the major cost to the health budget.

(b) A large and complex workforce poses dilemmas about its organisation and control; boundary disputes over work roles and occupational stress are likely to increase as the labour process is made more cost-effective and jobs are shed.

2 In 1990, the most recent year for which figures are available, about three-quarters of GPs were male; but the proportion of female GPs increased steadily and substan-tially from 15.3 per cent in 1979 to 23.8 per cent in 1990. The proportion of GPs born in Great Britain (i.e. England, Scotland and Wales) was close to 73 per cent during the whole period. By 1990 there were, however, fewer GPs born in other parts of the United Kingdom or the Irish Republic, and more who were born elsewhere. Almost a quarter of GPs were born outside the United Kingdom and Ireland. These data tell us nothing about the *ethnic status* of GPs; some of those born in the United Kingdom will belong to ethnic minorities, and some GPs born elsewhere will belong to the ethnic majority.

3 (a) The proportion of men in senior nursing posts is likely to increase for two reasons: women will take most of the part-time jobs, which involve lower status, and men may benefit from active discrimination in promotion competitions (recall that male nurses reach senior grades much more quickly than women).

(b) Increased part-time work will tend to decrease the proportion of young nurses because part-time work predominates among older women with children.

4 The extension of clinical skills is a reference to the pressure to adopt an extended clinical role in the 'hands-on' treatment of patients, for example, by taking over some tasks previously performed by junior doctors. Although managers are in favour (they save money and gain a more flexible workforce), many nurses and doctors oppose them. Nurses are concerned that the focus of nursing will be shifted towards medical (rather than nurs-ing) skills and, by implication, a return to the 'hand-maiden role'. Doctors are concerned about being underpriced and losing jobs. The reference to increased managerial skills relates to the increasing need for all staff to be involved in resource management. While managers and many nurses are enthusiastic about this, some nurses are concerned that it will erode their focus on clinical nursing skills and divert them from patient care.

5 The key elements identified in this chapter are: con-trol of access to the nursing profession via a specified training and registration, and continuing standards of conduct, overseen by the UKCC; enhanced academic levels of nurse training in the 1990s, following the Project 2000 review; the development of nursing practices (such as primary nursing) and a clinical nursing hierarchy to consultant level, which develop nursing roles with prime responsibility for patient care.

6 Managerial strategies include: increasing flexibility of work roles and responsibilities (for example, allowing nurses to discharge day-surgery patients, as in the Audit Commission's recommendations); employing a higher proportion of less-skilled workers (following a 'skill-mix review' in the current jargon); employing more part-time workers; exerting tighter control over working practices and the volume of work, based on evaluation exercises (as described in Chapter 4).

Chapter 7

1 Until recently, new drugs tended to be developed almost exclusively by the large multi-national pharamaceutical companies in their own R&D facilities. More recently, there has been an increasing number of products that originated in universities and independent research institutes, especially in the field of biotech-nology, and that have been rapidly capitalised upon by a range of companies, frequently involving the researchers

directly (see, for example, the case of Tracy, the genetically engineered sheep). This is part of a general trend towards the commercialisation of scientific research and a breaking down of the barriers between 'pure' and 'applied' research.

Change in organisational systems in the NHS can occur at the level of the entire service, as in the 1989 *Working for Patients* legislation, in which case it tends to be driven by government and political conviction. Organisational innovation at other levels is constantly taking place on a more modest scale. It is generally the result of the interplay between managers, health-care workers and consumer groups.

2   First came the product innovation of modern anaesthetics which then enabled the process or organisational innovation of the day-case surgical ward to be implemented successfully. Once this technology had spread within the health system, surgeons began to experiment with new instruments (products) to expand the scope of day surgery (a process).

3   Mainly science-push. The basic technique, nuclear magnetic resonance, was developed by physicists motivated by a desire to understand atomic processes. It was used in basic science laboratories by physicists and chemists for many years before its medical potential became apparent and new types of machine were designed. (Note: this example demonstrates the difficulty of separating science-push and market-pull. The first MRI instruments were produced in basic science laboratories but the scientists, although not directly commissioned, were certainly orienting their work towards an area where long-term commercial relevance might be expected to encourage funding.)

4   Although day surgery has been made possible by product innovations such as quick-recovery anaesthetics, its implementation requires a process innovation. Hospitals have to reorganise their internal activities which can have knock-on effects beyond the day-surgery area. Such changes are typically difficult to introduce, especially on the basis of recommendations by outsiders, unless staff are convinced of their worth or have strong incentives to cooperate. Day surgery may benefit the hospital's finances and patient satisfaction without directly benefitting the staff (although the Report argues that nurses prefer the regular working hours of day units). By contrast, MRI is a product innovation which a high-status segment of the medical profession (e.g. neurosurgeons) believes extends the range and quality of their diagnoses. It does not interfere with current working practices and is perceived to enhance them. It enables clinicians to become associated with the prestige of high-technology medicine.

Chapter 8

1   You may have suggested the following dilemmas (there are others):

(a)   Confusion over the definition of 'community care' has (among other consequences) led to financial incentives that favoured an expansion of private residential care rather than care in the community; the dilemma is whether community care should be developed in accordance with a normalisation strategy, or whether the prime objective should be to keep priority groups out of hospitals.

(b)   Care *in* the community has quite different implications for the provision and source of support than care *by* the community; should care come from formal services, or from informal sources (e.g. families), or voluntary bodies, or is a 'mixed market' approach the best solution?

(c)   Informal carers do most of the caring, but demographic and social trends are likely to result in increased pressures on them and in a decline in their numbers; should new types of integrated care worker be trained to make up the shortfall? (Chapter 6 should have alerted you to the possibility that this could raise boundary disputes with other professionals, or be seen as substituting a less-trained and cheaper worker for existing grades.)

(d)   The cost of community care must inevitably rise (the evidence about whether it is cheaper or more expensive than institutional care is unclear, although it may be more cost-effective); will governments of the future commit the necessary resources to it, or should social care insurance schemes bear the brunt of the increase?

2   (a)   The main ideological factor that has led to support for community care is the belief that it is both humane and cheaper to maintain people in their own homes rather than care for them in isolated institutions.

(b)   Policy over community care has shifted over the years from a belief that it is *cheaper* than hospital care, to a belief that it is a more *appropriate* form of care in meeting people's needs which, even if it is not cheaper, is more *cost-effective* (i.e. better value for money). Community care policy has also displayed confusion about its purpose, namely, about whether it is concerned with relocating people from long-stay hospitals or with providing support to keep people in the community.

(c)   The main factors creating additional pressures on community-care resources are: an ageing population coupled with an increase in the inability to cope independently; a decline in the available pool of informal carers (mainly women) for demographic reasons and changes in family structure and employment practice; and changes in hospital acute care leading to faster throughput and earlier discharge.

3   The indicators concerning informal carers show that they shoulder a considerable responsibility for providing care and support. The implications are that unless carers are encouraged to remain carers through improved financial support and direct practical support, then they will be unable to cope, will simply not be available (see the answer to Question 2c) or both. It cannot be assumed in future that carers will continue to behave in the way they have done in the past. An ageing population which will comprise a larger number of those requiring intensive levels of support will add to the pressures on carers.

4   The community care reforms are mainly a result of the criticisms of successive governments' policy in this area. Governments of both political persuasions have been accused of neglecting community care in favour of acute health services. An inability among service professionals and agencies to work together has resulted in fresh attempts to secure more coherent community-care provision and overcome concern about the slow progress in meeting targets in community-based services.

5   Scotland stands out as having places available for a considerably greater proportion of its elderly people in residential homes than is the case in England and Wales; this emphasis on institutional care is also consistent with the far greater proportion of elderly people in hospital in Scotland, and with the low expenditure on day-care and domiciliary services. The comparatively low provision of places in residential homes for people with mental illness or mental handicap (as health-service statistics still refer to them) is offset by the substantially higher provision of hospital beds for these groups. Community care policy has developed more slowly in Scotland in part because of a political commitment there to hospital services, the power of the medical lobby, and more favourable resource allocation which has provided less incentive for change.

By contrast, Wales has the highest proportion of mentally ill or mentally handicapped people in residential homes, but this is supplemented not by hospital services but by greater expenditure on day-care and domiciliary support. This reflects policy initiatives backed by leading local politicians, such as the All Wales Mental Handicap Strategy, to support people in the community rather than in hospitals. The relatively lower provision of residential care in England can be traced to the more stringent resource constraints that have been imposed there, and is not offset by more hospital beds or community services.

Chapter 9

1   (a) is tertiary prevention aimed at preventing the worst effects of kidney failure.

(b) to (d) are all primary prevention strategies, aimed at preventing the onset of possible disease, respectively: asbestos-related diseases such as lung cancer; vitamin-deficiency diseases in newborn babies, possibly including spina bifida (see Chapter 4); and deformities such as blindness in newborns infected with rubella early in embryonic development.

(e) is secondary prevention, aimed at early detection of eye diseases common in elderly people, such as cataract and glaucoma (damage from high pressure in the eyeball).

2   The emphasis is clearly on individual responsibility for nutritional health, supported by relevant health education targeted at 'consumers'. Government responsibility consists of funding research, seeking expert advice and seeking ways to disseminate information. Legislation to enforce labelling of foods or nutritional standards in catering outlets is not considered. You may have noted some other areas of potential government intervention that the strategy did not address, such as setting nutritional standards in the public sector (e.g. for school and hospital meals), or pricing policies to make healthier foods more affordable and to deter purchase of less healthy foods (much as pricing deterrents now operate to some extent against tobacco, alcohol and leaded petrol).

3   In theory, a randomised controlled trial (RCT) is the most reliable method, but in practice it would never be chosen. In an RCT, the IQ scores of children randomly allocated to live in an environment where lead pollution had fallen following the petrol-price intervention would be compared with the IQs of similar children whose exposure to lead had not changed. The practical difficulties of such an evaluation are enormous. First, consider the impossibility of allocating children at random to live in environments which differ only in their levels of lead pollution. Second, the effect on IQ is unlikely to be seen in all the children in the intervention group, so a large number is required in each group to make a valid comparison. Third, they must be followed up over a long

period of time before any effect of the intervention on IQ will be detected. These three problems create a fourth: the prohibitive cost of such an evaluation.

4   The most basic criterion that a screening programme must meet is that it *increases the quantity and/or quality of life*. This can only be argued convincingly for breast cancer screening of women between the ages of 50 and 64. For younger women, mammography is not sensitive enough to distinguish tumours from dense breast tissue. Screening must also be *acceptable* and, although the test is effective among women over the age of 65, the uptake rate is too low to justify the expense. A screening programme must also be *affordable*: the cost per QALY gained by breast cancer screening is relatively high (£5 550 at 1993 prices) and, since both the sensitivity and the specificity of mammography is around 95 per cent at first-time screening, it is hard to justify the expense of testing more frequently than every three years.

5   The dilemma arises from tension between individual freedom and the 'public good'. Smoking is clearly harmful to the health of a high proportion of smokers, though not every smoker is harmed by it. You might agree with Mill that society should not exercise power over individuals for their own good, especially where some are not in fact at risk from their behaviour. Conversely, cigarette smoke can harm non-smokers who inhale it over a prolonged period (so-called *passive* smoking), so Mill might accept that banning in public places was justified 'to prevent harm to others'.

Chapter 10

1   One example of a process innovation would be a reorganisation or expansion of the ambulance service and an increase in 'paramedics' as a means of getting people who suffered a heart attack into hospital faster and getting resuscitation equipment or drugs more quickly to the patient. The establishment of coronary care units and 'fast-track' admission routes in many hospitals are two other process innovations.

The difficulties that might block the adoption and diffusion of these innovations are principally the *financial costs* of more (and more highly-trained) staff, extra ambulances, etc. and the *coordination* of a range of services and personnel (GPs, emergency services, casualty departments, etc.)

2   You should look for reliable evidence that:
   (a)   the method of intervention would achieve a reduction in cholesterol;

   (b)   that achieving that reduction would reduce the incidence of CHD;
   (c)   that the intervention was not harmful to health in other respects;
   (d)   that it would be readily acceptable to the subjects; and
   (e)   that the intervention would be cost-effective.

3   You might justify such a campaign on the grounds that:
   (a)   there is an association between the number of cigarettes smoked and the incidence of CHD mortality (Figure 10.8);
   (b)   the association appears to be causal, given that stopping smoking reduces the risk of CHD;
   (c)   there are important benefits in reducing the incidence of other diseases (e.g. lung cancer);
   (d)   such a campaign may be relatively inexpensive, in that no medical screening is required to identify the individuals who have that risk factor.

Arguments against a *mass* intervention campaign are that the risk of CHD associated with smoking may have been overestimated because of a confusion between smoking rates and other aspects of social class (though this is not the case with the lung cancer risk), and because the risk principally affects those smokers with a family history of CHD.

4   Money for primary prevention is limited and therefore rationed (Chapters 3 and 9). Campaigns to reduce CHD risk factors such as elevated blood pressure or blood cholesterol have to compete for resources with programmes such as routine cervical smear testing or mammography—which may have a greater chance of benefitting the population (Chapter 9). Rationing of treatment might take several forms (Chapter 3): e.g. limiting the number of specialist coronary care units; establishing waiting lists for surgical intervention in patients requiring CABG or angioplasty; and preferentially prescribing expensive treatments for younger patients.

The lack of certainty about the value of, or best strategy for, intervening to reduce CHD mortality and morbidity, is not for want of evaluation. CHD has been one of the most studied of all diseases, and interventions (both treatment and prevention) have been subjected to numerous RCTs (Chapter 4). This illustrates the difficulty of generating reliable information about a disease which has multiple interacting causes.

The adoption, diffusion and (in some cases) eventual decline in popularity of innovations in medical treatment (Chapter 7) are well represented by anti-coagulant therapy, CABG, angioplasty and clot-busting drugs. The fervent promotion of dietary cholesterol as a major cause of CHD, despite evidence to the contrary, illustrates the power of influential professional figures and organisations, backed by media pressure, to preserve the 'orthodox view' from challenge.

Chapter 11

1   In this quote John Moore is focusing on people who receive what he refers to as 'lower incomes'. He does not define this term, so it could apply to any point on the income distribution in society, but usually official statements on 'lower incomes' refer to people living on incomes below half the national average. He is implicitly defining poverty in *absolute* terms when he argues that the material living standards, health, longevity, etc. of lower income groups in Britain in 1989 are 'substantially better' than they were in the past. The absolute approach to poverty identifies a subsistence level of income and other resources sufficient to supply the *minimum* necessities of nutrition, clothing, etc. People who have an income above this subsistence level are not considered to be living in poverty.

There are two main criticisms of defining poverty in absolute terms. The first is that it takes no account of the living standards of the rest of society. If, over the same period of time, those on 'higher incomes' had increased their material living standards at a faster rate than those on 'lower incomes', then the lower income group will have become poorer *relative* to the better-off in society. Second, it does not acknowledge that people's needs, even for food, are shaped by the society in which they live; thus the subsistence level varies between societies and changes over time. Moore's statement that lower income groups are better off than ever before could be translated to mean that more people are now living above a level of subsistence that would have been considered just sufficient at some point in the *past*, but which is no longer sufficient *today*.

2   The four most widely recognised risk factors associated with the experience of poverty are unemployment, long-term illness or disability, lone parenthood, and old age, but several other less-visible factors are also important. The presence of children in households increases the risk of poverty, as shown by the high risk associated with lone parenthood—but note that couples with children are twice as likely to be on incomes below half national average as those without (see Table 11.2). Women are at greater risk of poverty than men because they are less likely to have paid work, and more likely to have low-paid or part-time work, than men. Even within households with overall incomes above the national average, women may have very limited access to money

and experience relative poverty in the private sphere of the family. People from minority ethnic groups are also at greater risk of poverty than white Britons, at least in part due to discrimination in the labour market.

3   The main strategy for reducing poverty and inequality during the post-war years was to use taxation and public expenditure. It was assumed that taxes (to which the richest contribute the most) would finance public expenditure (from which the poor would benefit the most). The advocates of the tax and benefit strategy argued that this was preferable to direct intervention in the processes that generate poverty and inequality, since it would involve less distortion to the operation of market forces.

Opponents argue that this approach was bound to fail, since it tried to cure the symptoms of inequality without addressing the causes (principally unemployment and low wages). In an already unequal society, the better-off gained more than the poor from the welfare state and the tax and benefit system. Beveridge argued that post-war policies could only reduce poverty if full employment and adequate child benefit levels were maintained—neither of which has occurred. Finally, the welfare state was unable to meet rising and changing demands resulting from unforeseen social and demographic changes (e.g. an ageing population).

4   There is growing evidence that the experience of health and illness in society is at least as closely linked to the way that income and personal wealth is distributed across the population as it is to the level of average income. The evidence takes two forms. First, there is a strong correlation between the extent to which national income is evenly distributed across all sections of a society, and the *current* life expectancy of its citizens. This correlation is strongest when income is redistributed across the bottom 50–60 per cent of the population, i.e. the improvement in national life expectancy is greater than when benefits are targeted only at the poorest sector. However, it cannot be assumed that equality in income distribution *causes* longer lifespan from epidemiological data alone. Second, a number of 'natural experiments' support the argument that a move towards more equal income distribution leads to improvements in life expectancy (e.g. the United Kingdom during two World Wars, and Japan since the 1940s).

If this analysis is further substantiated, then it is likely that economic inequality damages the health of at least 50 per cent of the population of the United Kingdom in the 1990s, and possibly more. The gap between the richest and poorest in our society has widened in recent years, and is now back at the levels of economic inequality experienced in the early 1950s.

Index

Entries and page numbers in **bold type** refer to key words which are printed in **bold** in the text. Indexed information on pages indicated by *italics* is carried mainly or wholly in a figure or table.

α₁-antitrypsin, 104
Aaron, Henry, 34, 39, 170
Abortion Act (1967), 50
absenteeism, alcohol-related, 149
absolute poverty, **186**
accidents, medical, 73, 74
Acheson Committee, 36
Acheson, Sir Donald, 184
activity data, **28**
activity-related budgets, 17
acute services, *38*
Adler, Michael, 45
administrative and clerical workers, *84*, 85
adoption and diffusion of innovations, **113**–18
advertising
    alcohol, 148–50
    cigarette, 149–50, *161*
    HRT, 147
    medical, 78
age, and health care expenditure, 29
Alcohol Concern, 149
alcohol consumption, 148–50
Alford, Robert, 15, 18
All Wales Mental Health Strategy, 138, *139*
Allen, David, 46
ancillary health workers, *84*, 85
    of overseas origin, 90
Ancoats Hospital, Manchester, *75*
angina, 168, 169
angioplasty, **171**
Association for Victims of Medical Accidents, 74
atherosclerosis, 167
Atkinson, A. B., 188
Audit Commission, 8
    report on day surgery, 8–9, 33, 69, 118, 129
    reports on community care, *123*, 125, 132–4, *136*, 137–9

Ball, K. P., *173*
Baly, Monica, 99
Banyard, Richard, 17
Barker, David, 179
Barking and Havering Family Health Services Authority, 78
Barrett-Connor, Elizabeth, 179
Barthel Index, 54
basic disciplines of management, 14
basic income schemes, **192**
before–after studies, 50
benefits system, 190–2
Bevan, Aneurin, 5, 27, 28
Beveridge Report, 28
Beveridge, William, 188, 191, 193
biotechnology, 120
    see also genetic engineering

birthweight, and blood pressure, 179
Black, Andy, 23
Blane, D., *180*
Blaxter, Mildred, 160, 162n., 196n., *197*
'blind' trials, 49
blood pressure
    and birthweight, 179
    see also hypertension; hypotension
Bochner, Stephen, 55, 56
Bosanquet, N., *29*, 36
Bottomley, Virginia, 136
Boulton, Mary, 56–8
breast cancer, 152–8
    and HRT, 147
    screening for, 155, 156–8, 160
    treatment, 47
breastfeeding, and CHD, 179
breathalyser, evaluation of introduction, 50
Breslow, Lester, 145, 146–7, 148
Brisson, G., *175*
British Council of Organisations of Disabled People, 129
British Medical Association
    campaign against 1991 reforms, 47
    objections to general management, 17
British Medical Journal, reports of medical audit initiatives, 60
Brophy, M., *112*
Bryan, B., 90
Buck, N., *59*, 60
Buckingham, Robert, 51, 53
Burstall, M. L., 111
Butler, K., 76–7
Butler, P., 23

CABG, **169**
    see also coronary artery by-pass grafts
Campbell, Donald, 44
cancer
    endometrial, 147
    lung, 152–5
    research, 111
    screening, 155–8
    skin, 162
    see also breast cancer
Cancer Research Campaign, 111
Cannon, Geoffrey, 175
Care in the Community Initiative (Department of Health), 131
Care in the Community Project (Darlington), 131–2
care standards, 51
carers, 121–2, 127–8
    health, 127–8
    stress on, 127
    see also formal carers; informal carers
Caring for People, 123, 125, 126–7, 132, 135
case (care) management, 131
case-note review, **59**, 60
cash limits on health care, **32**
CASPE, patient satisfaction questionnaire, *70*, 71

CASS trial of coronary artery surgery, 170
Centre for Health Economics, report on doctors' pay, 23
CEPOD *see under* peri-operative death
Chaitman, B. R., *170*
charities and trusts
    funding of R&D, 111–12
    health promotion, 146
    see also pressure groups; support groups
Chawner, John, 23
CHCs *see* Community Health Councils
CHD *see* coronary heart disease
child care, 193
childbirth, control of, 93, 95
children, affected by poverty, 187
cholesterol, blood levels, 166, 174–7, 181–2
    combined with lipoproteins, 175, 177
    screening, 155
cigarette advertising, 149–50, *161*
Cinderella services, **38**, 39
cirrhosis of the liver, 148, 149
citizen representatives, 74
    interest group in NHS, 14–15, 18, 19–20, 24–5
    see also user participation
Citizen's Charter, 64
civil servants, risks of CHD, 180, *181*
Clay, Trevor, 89
clinical autonomy (or freedom), **16**, 21–2
clinical iceberg, **28**
clinical level of health care management, 7–**8**, 9, 14
clinical psychologists, gender divisions, 87–8
'clot-buster' drugs, 6, **171**–2
Cochrane, Archie, 47, 48, 58
Cohen, D., *151*
Committee on Safety of Medicines (CSM), 110–11
communication, doctor–patient, 53, 57–8, 119
community care, 8, 39, 121–41, **122**
    agencies involved, *123*, 124
    Audit Commission reports, *123*, 125, 132–4, *136*, 137–9
    coordination of health and social services, 124, 136–7
    cost, 121, 130–32
    defined, 122–5
    funding, 121, 135–6, 139
    future scenarios, 139–41
    initiatives and projects, 131–2
    progress towards, 132–8
community development initiatives, **192**
Community Health Councils (CHCs), 13, 24, 74, 75–6
    reduction in influence, 19, 76
community participation
    health promotion, 146–7, 148
    policy formulation, 74–6
competitive tendering, **84**, 91, 100
complaint and redress, **72**–4
    see also negligence; medical malpractice claims
Comprehensive Community Programme, 192
computer-aided tomography (CT), 34, 116–17, 118
computers, use in health-care system, 109
Consolidated Fund, 32
consultants
    gender divisions, 87
    information given to patients, 66
    pay, 91
    relationship with managers, 19
consumer choice, 68, 77–9
consumerism in health care, 65–9, 79–80
    management-led, 69–72, 80
    representation and participation approach, 74–7, 80

Consumers' Association, 66
contamination effects in RCTs, **49**
coronary artery by-pass grafts (CABG), 166, **169**–72
Coronary Artery Disease Research Association, *111*
coronary artery surgery, in UK and USA, 34
coronary care units, USA, 113
coronary heart disease, 165–82, **167**
    and blood cholesterol, 155, 174–7
    and diet, 166–7, 174–6, 181–2
    and early environment, 179–80
    epidemiological distribution, 168
    and health education, *159*
    heritable risks, 178–9
    prevention, 172–9, 181–2
    risk factors for, 172–81
    screening, 155, 166
    and smoking, *159*, 172–3, 179, 180–81, 182
    and social class, 179, 180–81
    treatment, 6, 166, 168–72
    use of 'clot-buster' drugs, 6, 171–2
    in women, 147, 174, 177–8
cost–benefit ratio, 45
cost-effective treatment, **40**
cost-effectiveness analysis, 38, 39–**40**, 55
    disease prevention, 159
cost-utility studies, **40**
Cox, David, 91–2
CSM *see* Committee on Safety of Medicines
CT *see* computer-aided tomography

Daly, E., *158*
Davey, Basiro, 5
Davey Smith, George, *168*, 172, 176, *180*, 196
Davies, Celia, 89
Day, Patricia, 16, 20
day surgery, 8, 104
    Audit Commission report, 8–9, 33, 69, 118, 129
decision-making in health care, 7–8, 16, 17, 26, 43–7
demographic changes, 29
    impact on community care, 126–7, 129, 139–40
    impact on welfare system, 191
Denmark, beer prices and consumption, 149
Dennis, G., *126*, *140*
dental service, charges, 32
dentures, demand for, 28
DHAs *see* District Health Authorities
diagnostic imaging *see* computerised tomography; magnetic resonance imaging
dicoumarol (Warfarin), 166
diet
    fat, *159*, 166, 174–6, 182
    salt, 166
diffusion of innovations, **113**–18
dilemmas in health care, **6**–11, 13
    in anti-poverty strategies, 194–8
    in CHD prevention, 166–7, 172, 180
    in CHD treatment, 171–2
    in community care, 121–2
    in decision-making processes, 25
    in decisions on rationing, 27, 39
    definition of good care, 44
    democracy *v.* efficiency, 46
    ethical, in evaluation, 47–8
    in health promotion and disease prevention, 143–4, 147, 155, 158, 163, 166–7, 172, 180
    in health research, 110
    in health work, 81–2, 98–100

in hospital management, 20–21, 71–2, 97, 116
in HRT, 147
individual need *v.* general need, 66, 68, 80
in limitations of health care, 184
need *v.* cash limits, 26
in professionalisation of nurses, 99–100
in redress and complaint, 73
Dingwall, Robert, 73
disabled people, independence, 128–9
disease prevention, 143–63
    costs and benefits, 150–55
    defined, 144–5
    evaluation of effectiveness, 150
    screening strategies, 155–8
    strategies, 146–50
district general hospitals, 20–21, 46
District Health Authorities (DHAs)
    consultations with public, 24–5
    medical audit advisory committees, 60
    membership, 19
doctors
    boundaries of responsibility, 93–5
    clinical autonomy, 16, 21–2
    experience of stress, 82
    hospital
        gender divisions, 87
        pay, 91
        see also junior doctors
    incentive systems, 22, 23
    interest group in NHS, 14, 18
    management role, 95, 96
    of overseas origin, 90
    pre-Griffiths influence, 16
    relationship with managers, 19
    role in innovation diffusion, 114
    and smoking, 154, *161*
    see also consultants; general practitioners; medical audit
Doll, Sir Richard, *173*
'double blind' trials, 49
Doyal, Lesley, 90
Drucker, Peter, 14
drugs
    anti-coagulant, 166
    anti-hypertensive, 173, *174*, 182
    β-blockers, 173, *174*
    cholesterol-lowering, *176*, 177, 182
    'clot-buster', 6, 171–2, 182
    consumption in European countries, *106*
    diuretic, 173, *174*
    evaluation, 48, 49, 144
    marketing costs, 114
    'me-too', 110
    patented, 110
    pricing structure, 111
    see also pharmaceutical industry

economic inequality and health, 184–98, **189**
effectiveness of health care, **5**, 44–5, 46, 55, 71
    see also evaluation
efficiency of health care, **6**–7, 21, 39–41, 44–5, 46
elderly people
    care for, *38*, 124–6, 135, 140
    as carers, 126
    cost of community care, 130–1
    demand for health care, 29, *30*, 39
    and poverty, 141
    projected numbers, 126, 140

residential care, *see* nursing homes; residential homes
elective surgery, **9**
    waiting lists, 33
Elston, Mary Ann, 95
employment and poverty, 191, 192, 193
empowerment, **76**, 148
endometrial cancer, 147
endoscopy, 118–19
Enrolled Nurses, 90n., 99
environmental health hazards, 162
equity of health care, **6**–7, 21, 25, 44
    in GP consultations, 55–8
    search for, 35–9
ethical difficulties
    in CHD treatment/prevention, 172, 182
    in disease prevention/health promotion, 144, 155
    in genetic screening, 182
    in medical innovation, 119
    in RCTs, 47–8
ethnic divisions
    in experience of poverty, 189
    in NHS workforce, 90
ethnic monitoring, 90
European Commission, report on poverty, 186, *187*, 189, 198
evaluation
    of coronary artery by-pass grafts, 170
    of disease prevention/health promotion strategies, 143–4, 150
    of health care, 5–6, 40, 43–62
    illuminative approach, 51–3
    see also health status measurement; randomised controlled trials
exercise
    and age of menarche, 154–5
    and CHD, 174
expenditure on health care, 29, 30–32
    capital costs in NHS, 118
    cash limits, 32
    impact of innovations, 119
    in priority and non-priority services, 38–9
    in UK and USA, 34
external validity of quasi-experiments, **50**

Fall, C. H. D., 179
false negatives (screening tests), **157**
false positives (screening tests), **157**
families
    as carers, 121
    changes in structure, 126, *127*
    history of CHD, 178–9
Family Health Services Authorities, medical audit advisory committees, 60
Family Planning Association, 112
family practitioner services, workers, *84*
fat
    dietary, *159*, 166, 174–6, 182
    saturated and unsaturated, defined, 174n.
felt need (for health care), **28**
Fitz-Patrick, J. D., 118
Fletcher, J., 118
Flynn, Rob, 18
formal carers, 129
Fowler, Norman, 125
Frayman, H., 186, *187*
Freidson, Eliot, 95

Gehlen, Arnold, 104
gender
    divisions in NHS workforce, 86–9, 90, 93
    significance in hierarchies, 95
General Household Survey, informal carers, 127
general management, 13, **16**
    future prospects, 18–20
    introduction, 16–18
    nurses' role in, 95–6
    see also Griffiths report
general practitioners
    access to technology, 12
    changing, 78
    cognitive outcomes of consultations, 57–8
    defining patients' needs, 28–9
    disease prevention, 150
    distribution, 36
    equity in consultations, 55–8
    formation of patient groups, 77
    fund-holding, 8, 42
        increasing influence, 19
    impact of complaints, 73
    non-fund-holding, limits on choice, 79
    pay, 78
    'practice leaflets', 78
    refusal of second opinion, 66
    resource rationing, 34
    role in community care, 139
genetic engineering
    animals, 103–4
    drugs, 110
genetic screening, 155, 182
geriatric services, *38*
Germany, hypotension treatment, 106
Glennerster, Howard, 92, 97
Goodin, R. E., 24
government
    action on alcohol consumption, 148–50
    community care policy, 125, 129
    decision-making responsibility, 7
    decisions, 20, 26, 30
    funding of R&D, 108–9
    legislation on environmental hazards, 162
Gray, Alastair, 27, *29*
Green, H., 128
Griffiths, Sir Roy, 24, 69
    report on NHS management ('Griffiths Report'), 12, 13,
        46, 100
        general managers, 16, 18
        nurses as managers, 96
    review of community care, 132, 133–5
        care workers, 129
        funding, 139–41
        hospital closures, 136–7
Gross National Product (GNP), defined, 31n.
Growing Older, 129
Guillebaud Committee, 130
gynaecology, performance indicators, 61–2

Haffenden, S., 128
Ham, Chris, 25
Harrison, Stephen, 12, 19, 24, 25
Haywood, Stuart, 17
HDL-cholesterol, 175, 177
health care
    availability of, 36–9
    cash limits on, 32

    demand for, 27–30
    need for, 28–9
    see also dilemmas in; effectiveness; efficiency; equity;
        humanity
Health for All by the Year 2000, 143
health education, **146**, 159
Health Education Authority, *159*
Health Education Council, 175
health insurance, in USA, 35
health promotion, 143–63, **145**
    costs and benefits, 150–52
    defined, 145–6
    evaluation of effectiveness, 150
    strategies, 146–50
health status, measurement, 44, **53–5**
Health Systems Agencies (HSAs), 74–5
health visitors, professionalisation, 98
health workers, 81–100
    boundary disputes, 81, 93–5
    controlling, 95–6
    defining and counting, 82–5
    ethnic divisions, 90
    gender divisions, 86–9, 90, 93
    occupational divisions, 85–6
    professionalisation, 92, 96
    resources for, 96–8
    variations in income, working conditions and status, 91–2
health-care assistants, 99
heart, anatomy, *167*
heart attacks, **168**, 169
heart disease *see* coronary heart disease
hernia, hospital stay after repair, 45–6
Higgins, J., 192
high-risk screening, **155**
HIV *see* human immunodeficiency virus
Holmes, Richard, 165
home helps, *124*, 125
hormone replacement therapy (HRT), **147**–8, *158*, 178
hospice care
    evaluation using secret participation, 51, 53
    RCT, 48–9, 51
Hospital Plan (1962), 46
hospitals
    'bed blocking', 136
    closing of long-stay, 121–2, 136–7
    coronary care units, USA, 113
    district general, 20–21, 46
    'hotel' aspects, 71
    kitchen maids, 92
    'league tables', 78
    length of patient stay, 139
    nursing staff numbers, 98
    patient satisfaction questionnaire, *70*
    patient waking times, 115–16
    psychiatric, 38
    re-admission rates, 60
    respite care in, 51, 52
    ward design, 116
household income, distribution, 189–90
housing, *194*
    and community care, 130
HRT, **147**
    see also hormone replacement therapy
HSAs *see* Health Systems Agencies
human immunodeficiency virus (HIV), 108
    screening for, 155
humanity of health care, **6**, 41, 44

Hunt, S. M., 54
Hunter, David, 121, 134
Huntington's disease, screening for, 155
hypercholesterolaemia, 177
hypertension and CHD, 173–4, 182
hypotension, treatment, 106

ideology of inequality, 194
Illsley, Raymond, 51
illuminative approach to evaluation, **51**–3
immunisation, 143
Imperial Cancer Research Fund, 111
income distribution and life expectancy, *195*, 196
income redistribution, **190**–4, 196
income support, 124, 133, 188
individual, as responsible for own health, 158–60
industry
    funding of R&D, 109–11
    see also pharmaceutical industry
inequality *see* economic inequality; social inequality
inflation, 31
informal carers, 121, 125–7, 128, 132
information systems, 23, 79, 120
innovations, 7, 97, 103–20, **107**, 120
    adoption and diffusion, 113–18
Institute of Fiscal Studies, report on poverty, *187*, 190
insurance
    health, 35, 73, 74
    medical malpractice claims, 73
    social care, 141
intensive care beds, in UK and USA, 34
interest groups in NHS, 13, 14–16, 18, 26
internal market in health care, 37, 47
    limits on GPs choice, 79
    evaluation by RCT, 49
internal validity (of quasi-experiments), 50
invention, **107**
ischaemic heart disease (IHD), 167
    see also coronary heart disease
Isles, C. G., *177*

Japan, life expectancy and income distribution, 196
Jarman, B., 36
Jenkin, Patrick, 76
Johns, C., 52
Joseph, Sir Keith, 186
junior doctors, *82*
    gender divisions, 87
    supervised/trained by nurses, 94–5
    tasks delegated to nurses, 94

Kalache, A., *154*
Kane, Robert, 48–9, 53
Kent Community Care Project, 131
Kent University, Personal Social Services Research Unit *see* PSSRU
Khaw, Kay-Tee, 179
kidney failure
    rationing of treatment, 34, 68
    treatment in Europe, 105
    treatment in UK and USA, 34
kidney stones, treatment *see* lithotripters
King's Fund Centre, 60
    Equal Opportunities Task Force, 90
Kirchberger, S., *105*
Kirke, Peader, 47
kitchen maids, 92

Klein, Rudolf, 16, 20, 68
Knapp, M., 131–2

La Vecchia, Carlo, 155–6, 157
Lambert, Helen, 143
Lansley, Stewart, 186
lay health care, 82–3
LDL-cholesterol, 175
Le Grand, Julian, 194
lead-time bias in screening, **156**–7
Leathard, A., *15*
Lessof, Leila, 94
Lichtenstein, S., *160*
life expectancy
    and income distribution, *195*, 196
    and national wealth, 195–6
'lifestyle', as a determinant of
    CHD, 172–7
    disease, 158–61
Lindblom, C. E., 46
lipoproteins, combined with cholesterol
    high-density (HDLs), 175, 177
    low-density (LDLs), 175
lithotripters, distribution in Europe, 105
local authorities, and community care, 134–6, 139
Local Government Finance Act 1982, 8
London, primary health care in, 36
London Health Planning Consortium, 36
Loomes, G., 112
Lorber, John, 48, 49–50
lung cancer, 152–5

McEwen, James, 54
Mack, Joanna, 186
Mackay, Lesley, 89, 97
McKee, Martin, 94
McKinlay, John, 106
McPherson, Klim, 143
Macmillan nurses, 112
magnetic resonance imaging (MRI), 116–18
Mahoney, F. I., 54
Mallett, Jane, 60–61
mammography, **156**–7
management, **13**–14
    by consensus, 46
    of NHS, 7–8, 12–25, 100
        see also general management
    of nursing, 95–6, 97
management-led consumerism, 69–72, 80
managers
    and performance indicators, 61–2
    interest group in NHS, 14, 26
    relationship with doctors, 19
    strategies to contain costs, 17–19, 94, 100
market approach to reducing poverty, **191**–2
market-pull model of innovation **107**, 115
Marmot, Michael, *168*, *181*, 196
Marsh, C., *195*
Martyn, C. N., 179
mass screening, **155**
matching in RCTs, **50**
Mays, Nicholas, 103
Medicaid, Oregon experiment, 41–2
medical audit, 18, **58**–61
    access to results, 78
medical–industrial complex, 113
medical malpractice claims, 73

Medical Practices Committees, 36
Medical Research Council (MRC), 108
medical technology, 103, **104**–6
    'career', 106–7
    consequences, 118–19
    evaluation, 144
    funding of R&D, 107–12
    impact on community care, 129
    impact of innovations on nurses, 97
    technological imperative, 112–13
    see also innovations; magnetic resonance imaging
Medicines Act 1968, 110
menarche, age of, and breast cancer, 153–4
menopause, 147–8
mental-health nursing, gender divisions, *88*, 89
mentally handicapped people *see* people with learning
    difficulties
mentally ill people, 38, 122
    cost of community care, 131
    residential homes, 142
midwives, 81
    boundaries of responsibility, 93, 95
    gender divisions, 88–9
    medical control, 95
    professionalisation, 92, 98
Mitchell, J. R. A., 181
mortality rates, tables, 78
MRC *see* Medical Research Council
MRI *see* magnetic resonance imaging
myocardial infarction, 168

National Advisory Committee on Nutritional Education
    (NACNE), 175
National Health Service Management Executive, 7, 71, 109
National Health Service Trusts, 8
    hospital doctors' pay, 23
    management teams, 20
National Insurance contributions, 32
national minimum wage, 195
National Society for Cancer Relief, 112
negative income tax schemes, **192**
negligence, medical, 73, 74
Neilson, D. D., *149*
neural tube defects, prevention, 47–8, 49–50
'New Right', 67
NHS and Community Care Act 1990, 8, 132, 134
Nichol, Duncan, 64
no-fault compensation, **74**
normalisation philosophy, **130**
Northern Ireland, health and social services boards, 138
Nottingham Health Profile, 54
nuclear magnetic resonance (NMR), 117
    see also magnetic resonance imaging
nurse education, *88*, 89, 98
nurses, 81, *84*, 85, 86
    boundaries of responsibility, 93–5
    gender divisions, 87, 88–9
    and management, 95, 97
    of overseas origin, 90
    part-time work, *88*, 89
    primary, 99n.
    professionalisation, 92, 98, 99
    reduction of workforce, 100
    shortage in 'Cinderella services', 39
    staff grades, 90n.
    stress on, 97–8
    talking to patients, 97

nursing, standard setting in, 51, 52
nursing homes, private, 33, 121, 125
Nursing, Midwifery and Health Visiting Act 1979, 98

Oakley, Ann, 95
obstetric services, *38*
    caesarian deliveries in USA, 73
obstetricians, boundaries of responsibility, 93, 95
oestrogen, 147, *158*, 177–8
Oliver, Michael, 182
operational level of health care management, 7–**8**, 9, 14
Oppenheim, C., *188*, 189
optimal health, **145**–6
Oregon experiment, 41–2
osteoporosis, 147
Ottawa Charter for Health Promotion, 143
outcome and **process** evaluations of health care, **51**, 58
Owens, Patricia, 92, 97
ozone layer, 162

Paffenbarger, R. S., 174
PAMs *see* professions allied to medicine
Panting, Gerard, 73
Pascall, Gillian, 81
patented drugs, **110**
paternalism, 72
Paterson, Elizabeth, 92
patient advocacy, **76**–7
patient participation, 76–7
patient satisfaction surveys, **69**–71
patients
    as consumers, 67–8
    direct charges, 28, 32–3
    needs, 22
    talking to, 97, 119
    unwilling to engage in decision-making, 72
    waking times, 115–16
Patients' Charter, 22, 23, 26, 64–5, 66, 68–9, 71–2, 78
Payer, Lynn, 106
peer review, **59**
    medical audit, 59
    MRC priorities, 108
Pekkannen, J., 176
Pendleton, David, 55, 56
penicillin, 107n.
people with learning difficulties, 38, 123–4, 124n., 130
    care policy in Wales, 138
    cost of community care, 131
    residential homes, 142
performance indicators, 17, 19, **61**–2
peri-operative death, assessment of causes (CEPOD), 59–60,
    78
pharmaceutical industry, 109–11, 114
Pharmaceutical Proteins, *104*, 107
Phillips, A. N., *178*
placebo, 47
placebo effect, 49, 173
Plamping, Diane, 79
Pollitt, Christopher, 67, 78
Pond, Chris, 184, 195
Popay, Jennie, 184
Popham, R. E., *148*
population screening, **155**
population structure, 29
poverty, 141, 162
    absolute, 186
    causes, 188–9

defining and measuring, 185–8
and health, 184–98
relative, 186
prescribing restrictions, 17
pressure groups
   health promotion, 146
   health service users, 66, *67*
   reduction of economic inequality, 193
primary health care, 120, 139
primary nurses, 99n.
primary prevention of disease, **144**–5, 155
   CHD, 176
   lung cancer, 152–5
Priorities in Medical Research, 108
priority groups, 38–9, 71
   health care provision in Scotland, 138
   Oregon experiment, 41–2
private health care, 33
privatisation of services *see* competitive tendering
process and **outcome** evaluations of health care, **51**, 58
process innovations, **104**, 109, 119
product innovations, **104**, 107, 109, 119
professional and technical health workers, 84, 85
professionalisation of health workers, 92, 96, 98, 99–100
professionally defined need (for health care), **28**
professions allied to medicine (PAMs), 85
progesterone, 147
Project 2000, 98–9
Promoting Better Health, 78
PSSRU, community care costs study, 131–2
psychiatric hospitals, 38
public attitudes
   health-care priorities, 39, 41
   health education, 159–60
   poverty and economic inequality, 184, 197–8
purchaser–provider split, 7, 19, 20, 25, 134
purchasing authority managers, 21, 42
   consultations, 24
   increasing influence, 19, 79

quality-adjusted life years (QALYs), **40**–41, 42, 55
   gain from breast cancer screening, 158
quality assurance, **61**
quasi-experimental designs, 49–**50**
   threats to validity, 50
Quick, Allison, 195–7

racism, 90
radiologists, interventional, 119
Rand health insurance experiment, 33
randomised controlled trials (RCTs), **47**–51, 106
   contamination effects in, 49
   coronary artery by-pass grafts, 170
   disease prevention strategies, 150
   ethical objections, 47–8
   screening strategies, 157
rationing of health care, 27–42, 68, 71, 114, 118, 152
Ravnskov, Uffe, 181
RAWP formula, **36**–8
RCTs, **47**
   see also randomised controlled trials
re-admission rates to hospital, 60
Regan, D. E., 25
Registered General Nurses (RGN), 90n.
Registered Nurses (RN), 90n., 92, 99
relative poverty, **186**
   consensus on basic necessities, 186

relative poverty line, **186**
relative risks, breast cancer, **153**–4
Relman, Arnold, 113
reminiscence therapy, 95
representation and participation, **74**–7, 80
reprovision studies (cost of community care), 131
research and development (R&D)
   funding, 107–12
      charitable, 111–12
      industrial, 109–11
      state, 108–9
residential homes, 142
   private, 33, 121, 125
Resource Allocation Working Party, 36
   see also RAWP formula
resource constraints, 20, 21
resource management, 19, 46, 104
Resource Management Initiative (RMI), 46
respite care, standard of care statement on access, 51, 52
resuscitation teams, 172
Retail Price Index (RPI), **31**
RHAs *see* Regional Health Authorities
Rhys Williams, Lady Juliette, 192
risk factors, **153**
   breast cancer, 153–4
   and health education, 159–60
risk factors for heart disease, **172**
RMI *see* Resource Management Initiative
road deaths, drink-related, 149
Robb, Barbara, 38
Robinson, Jane, 18
Robinson, Kate, 81
Rose, G., *181*
Rosser, Jane, 89
Rowntree, Seebohm, 188
Royal College of Nursing, 89
   support for professionalisation, 99
   survey of working hours, 98
Royal College of Physicians, report on preventive medicine, *145*, *148*, 149
Royal Commission on the NHS, 69
RPI, **31**

Salmon Report, 96
salt, dietary, 166
Schwarz, William, 34, 39, 170
science-push model of innovation, **107**, 115
Scotland
   hospital and community care, 138
   residential homes, 142
screening, bias
   lead-time, 156–7
   length-time, 156
   selection, 156
screening strategies, **155**–8
   for cancer, 155–8, 160
   for CHD, 155, 166
   high-risk (or individual), 155
   population (or mass), 155
screening tests
   sensitivity and false negatives, 157
   specificity and false positives, 157
scurvy, treatment, 46
Seale, Chris, 43, 64, *127*
Second Report on Maternity Services *see* Winterton Report
secondary prevention of disease, **144**–5, 155
secret participant observation, 51, 53

self-governing trusts *see* National Health Service Trusts
sensitivity of screening tests, **157**
Sheldon, Tony, 20
Shipley, M. J., 172, 180–81
Simanowitz, Arnold, 74
skin cancer, 162
Smith, Adam, 185–6
smoking
    and heart disease, *159*, 172–3, 179, 180–81
    and lung cancer, 152, 154, 155, 165
    see also cigarette advertising
SMRs *see* Standardised Mortality Ratios
social class, 160–2
    and CHD, 172, 179, 180–81
    and GP consultations, 55–8, 77
social dividend, **192**–3
social inequality and health, 185
social work, suggested RCTs, 48
socio-economic factors in health behaviour, 160–62
Spastics Society, *67*, 112
specificity of screening tests, **157**
spectacles, demand for, 28
speech therapists, gender divisions, 87–8
Stacey, Margaret, 67–8, 85, 86
Stamler, J., *174*
standard of care statements, 51, 52
standard setting, **51**
Standardised Mortality Ratios (SMRs), and performance
    indicators, 61–2
Stewart, John, 25
Stocking, Barbara, 113–14, 115–16, 118, 119
strategic level of health care management, **7–8**, 14
streptokinase, 171
stress
    on carers, 127
    and CHD, 181
    on health workers, 82
    in nursing, 97–8
stroke, prevention, 174
Strong, Philip, 18
structural interests (in health care), 15, 18
subsistence level, 188
Sugden, R., 112
supplier-induced demand for health care, 29, 35
supply of health care, 30–33
support groups, health service users, 66
surgery
    assessment of causes of death, 59–60
    inguinal hernia repair, 45–6
    see also coronary artery by-pass grafts; day surgery
Sutherland, Holly, 188
Szczepura, A. K., 118

Tawney, Richard, 190
tax and benefit approach to poverty/inequality, **192**–3
tax system, 190–92
technological imperative, **112**–13
technology, **104**
tertiary prevention of disease, **144**–5
thalidomide, 110
Thatcher, Margaret, 12
therapies, evaluation, 43–4, 47
Thorne, S. C., *45*
threats to internal (and external) validity (of quasi-
    experiments), **50**
Titmuss, Richard, 122
Torrance, G. W., 40

Townsend, Peter, 186
treatment protocols, **59**
Tuckett, D., 56, *57*, *58*

unit general managers, 17
United Kingdom Central Council for Nursing, Midwifery and
    Health Visiting (UKCC), 90, 92n., 98–100
universities, research at, 110
USA
    coronary artery by-pass grafts, 170–71
    coronary care units, 113
    CT scanners, 116
    defensive medical practice, 73
    health care, compared with UK, 34–5
    Health Systems Agencies (HSAs), 74–5
    information available to service-users, 79
    mass screening for CHD, 155
    mortality rates, tables, 78
    MRI scanners, 117
    Oregon experiment, 41–2
    Rand health insurance experiment, 33
    'War on Poverty', 192
user participation, 74–6, 129
    Listening to Local Voices in the NHS, 71
Uttley, Stephen, 103

volume planning of health care, **32**

waiting lists, 33–4
Waitzkin, Howard, 113
Waldegrave, William, 64
Wales
    All Wales Mental Health Strategy, 138, *139*
    residential homes, 142
Walker, Caroline, 175
Warfarin (dicoumarol), 166
wealth, **190**
    inequality in, 190
    inheritance of, 195
    national, and life expectancy, 195–6
Wedderburn, Dorothy, 194
West, Chris, 100
Which? Way to Health, 66
White Paper
    on care of the elderly (1981) *see Growing Older*
    on community care (1989) *see Caring for People*
    on *Health of the Nation* (1992), 143, 185
    on the NHS (1944), 35
    on the NHS (1989) *see Working for Patients*
    on primary care (1987) *see Promoting Better Health*
Wildavsky, Aaron, 136
Wilenski, P., 24
Wilkinson, Richard, 195–7
Williams, Alan, 40, 45
Winkler, Fedelma, 71–2, 75–6, 79, 80
Winterton Report, 93
Wistow, Gerald, 12, 19, 24, 137
women
    and CHD, 147, 174, 177–8
    employment, 193, 194
    in poverty, 188–9
    see also breast cancer; gender; menopause
Working for Patients, 15, 19–20, 26, 37, 60, 76, 100
World Health Organisation, 143

X-ray examinations, in UK and USA, 34